# MULTIPLE SYSTEM ATROPHY

*ALSO FROM THE SAME AUTHOR:*

Lectures on the Physics of Radiology

The Odyssey of Humanity’s Diseases – Volumes 1, 2, 3

From the Heart to the Brain

The Human Brain

Cancer

Glioblastoma - Management and Treatment

Nanomedicine

Lyme Disease

Pandemics

COVID-19

(Co-authored and co-edited with N.R.A. Romm and J. Kapalanga)

Alzhei...Who?

Parkin...ss...oo...nn

Dementia

Epilepsy

Multiple Sclerosis

... and other books

# MULTIPLE SYSTEM ATROPHY

## The chronic, progressive, neurodegenerative synucleinopathic disease

ALAIN L FYMAT

Multiple System Atrophy


The information in this book has been compiled by way of general guidance concerning the specific subjects addressed. It is not a substitute, and should not be relied on, for medical, healthcare, pharmaceutical or other professional advice on specific circumstances, and in specific locations. Please consult your General Practitioner or Physician Specialist before starting, changing, or stopping any medical treatment. So far as the author is aware, the information given is correct and current as of April 2023. Practice, laws, and regulations all change and the reader should obtain up-to-date professional advice on any such issue. As far as the laws allow, the author disclaims any liability arising directly or indirectly from the use or misuse of the information contained in this book.



tellwell

Tellwell Talent
www.tellwell.ca

ISBN
978-0-2288-9443-8 (Hardcover)
978-0-2288-9442-1 (Paperback)

*To:*

Claudius Galenus (Κλαύδιος Γαληνός) or Galen of Pergamon (129 – c AD–216)
Greek physician, surgeon, and philosopher
"Father of Medicine"
who influenced the development of Neurology
among many other medical and philosophical fields,
and recognized the specialized autonomic nervous system

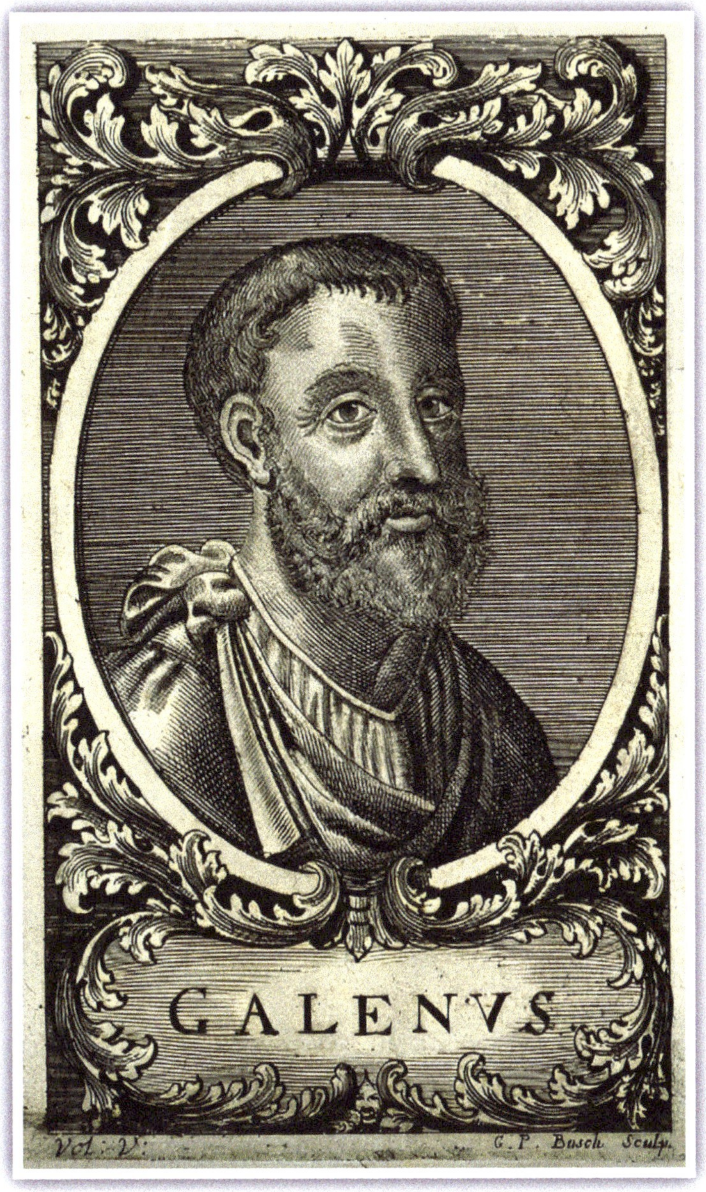

# Table of Contents

# Preface

Alpha-synucleinopathies refer to age-related neurodegenerative and dementing disorders characterized by the accumulation of the alpha-synuclein protein in neurons and/or glia. The process of protein accumulation and aggregation within oligodendrocytes is accepted by many as one of the main pathological events underlying the diseases. Recent research suggests that abnormal alpha-synuclein accumulation in nerve cells and their supporting cells leads to cellular dysfunction and progressive loss of nerve cell function (neurodegeneration).

The anatomical location of alpha-synuclein inclusions and the pattern of progressive neuronal death give rise to distinct neurological phenotypes that include Parkinson's disease, dementia with Lewy bodies, and multiple system atrophy. Common to these disorders is the involvement of the central and peripheral autonomic nervous system where pure autonomic failure is thought to be an ideal model to assess biomarkers that may predict its phenoconversion to these other diseases. Such biomarkers would aid in clinical trials in the development of disease-modifying drugs/therapies.

Of paramount importance here is multiple system atrophy - a neurodegenerative disease caused by the progressive loss of brain cells over time and by the abnormal folding and accumulation of the alpha-synuclein protein inside of brain cells. It is accompanied by diverse clinical manifestations that may include parkinsonism, cerebellar syndrome, and autonomic failure. This disease and other debilitating movement disorders are often hard to distinguish from one another. Pathologically, it is characterized by glial cytoplasmic inclusions in oligodendrocytes that contain fibrillary forms of α-synuclein. Unfortunately, studies on its pathogenesis are scarce relative to studies of the pathogenesis of the other synucleinopathies.

Multiple system atrophy remains a challenging neurodegenerative disorder with a difficult and often inaccurate early diagnosis and a still lacking effective treatment. It is characterized by a highly variable clinical presentation with a rapid progression and an aggressive clinical course. The definite diagnosis is only possible *post-mortem* when the presence of distinctive oligodendroglial cytoplasmic inclusions, mainly composed of misfolded and aggregated alpha-synuclein protein, is demonstrated. It is considered a multifactorial disorder with multiple pathogenic events acting together including neuroinflammation, oxidative stress, and disrupted neurotrophic support, among others.

With the increase in life expectancy due to advancement of medical diagnosis and treatments, the incidence of age-dependent neurodegenerative diseases increased, including Alzheimer's disease, parkinsonian syndromes, small vessel disease, and motor neuron disease. In spite of the progress of knowing the pathogenesis of various neurodegenerative diseases at molecular and genetic levels, they are still very incompletely understood and often cause diagnostic and therapeutic challenges to physicians. Due to the overlapping presentations and similar brain pathologies, especially in the early stage of the diseases, it is difficult to differentiate idiopathic Parkinson's disease from atypical parkinsonian syndromes, such as multiple system atrophy and progressive supranuclear palsy. Similarly, distinguishing Alzheimer's disease bodies, corticobasal degeneration, and vascular dementia can be difficult. In addition, co-morbidities are common in the elderly, further complicating the diagnosis. It is, therefore, necessary to develop accurate and comprehensive diagnostic tests to properly prognosticate the diseases, start treatments in the early stages of the diseases, and maximize the accuracy of drug trials for more effective preventive and therapeutic measures.

Cognitive neurodegenerative diseases are a major public health issue. At present, the diagnosis of certainty is still based on anatomopathological analyses. Even if the diagnostic tools available to clinicians have made it possible to improve probabilistic diagnosis during the patient's lifetime, there are still too many diagnostic errors and sub-diagnoses in this field. The arrival of biomarkers has made it possible to reduce these diagnostic errors, which were of the order of 25% to 30%, the high error rate being due to different parameters. At present, the only cerebrospinal fluid biomarkers that are routinely used for the biological diagnosis of neurodegenerative cognitive pathologies are those specific to Alzheimer's disease (Aβ42, Aβ40, tau-total, and phosphor-tau). These biomarkers represent an almost indispensable tool in the diagnosis of dementia. It is, therefore, important to determine whether Alzheimer's biomarkers can be disrupted in other neurodegenerative cognitive pathologies, but also to find biomarkers specific to these different pathologies. This could be facilitated by the implementation of clinical studies, which will thus make it possible to improve their diagnosis.

In the U.S., multiple system atrophy affects roughly 13,000 people. Symptoms, which may include stiffness, slowness, imbalance and tremor, and autonomic dysfunction can be complex and require special considerations for care. It is not yet known why people develop this disease and arriving at the correct diagnosis can be a lengthy and confusing process. While treatment cannot slow the progression of the disease at this time, there are options to manage symptoms and support the needs of patients and families. Healthcare professionals and researchers are working diligently to understand, prevent, and treat multiple system atrophy and other neurodegenerative diseases.

Having deeply immersed myself in the subject of multiple system atrophy and other rare and neglected disorders, I hope this book will also interest those other individuals and organizations who could do their part, however small, in helping get rid of this scourge that has terribly afflicted humanity almost since its beginnings and continues unabated. Otherwise, it would be a tragic dereliction of our collective duties and responsibilities to humanity as a whole. It is also hoped that patients (and other interested readers) will be empowered to get hold of, and contribute to, the better understanding and treatment options for their disease.

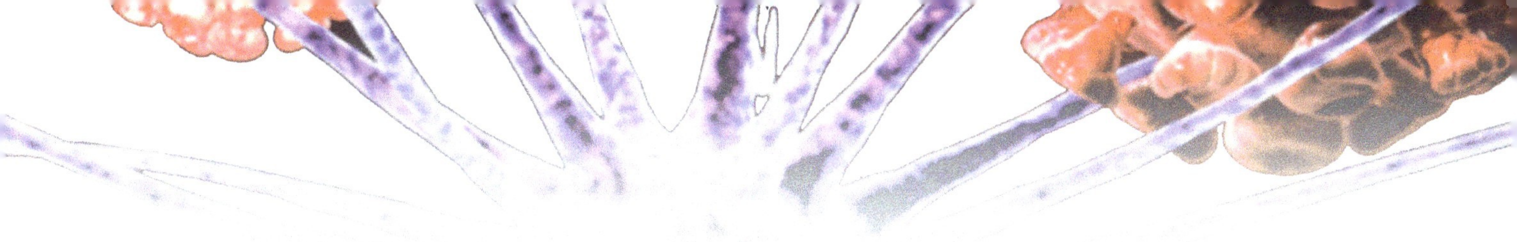

# Introduction

This book is divided into five sequentially arranged parts (Parts A through E). **Part A** ('Once upon a time') includes two chapters (Chapters 1 and 2). **Chapter 1** provides a brief chronicle of multiple system atrophy (MSA) since its beginnings. To personify such a history, who else but Willis? **Chapter 2**, therefore, briefly retraces the life, works, and accomplishments of Thomas Willis, a pre-eminent English doctor considered to be the father of clinical neuroscience. He also played an important part in the history of anatomy, neurology, psychiatry, and was one of the founding members of the Royal Society. It recounts his illustrious scientific career, contributions to neurological science, and neurological and other activities.

**Part B** ('The disease and its particulars') encompasses seven chapters (Chapters 3-9). Multiple system atrophy affecting both the autonomic nervous system and the motor system, two brief primers on these topics are provided in the following two chapters. Thus, **Chapter 3** discusses what is the nervous system and its parts, particularly the autonomic nervous system structure, internal and external regulation, innervation, and function. It discusses the sympathetic, parasympathetic and enteric nervous systems, and the interaction of the autonomic nervous system with the immune system. It also describes the various neuron types (structural, functional, directional), their morphology (white and gray matter), neurotransmitters, and how do neurons function. Lastly, it presents the various glial cells (oligodendrocytes, astrocytes/astroglia, ependymal cells, and microglia). A sidebar lists some of the conditions and disorders affecting the nervous system. As indicated in **Chapter 4**, the motor system is a biological system with close ties to the muscular and circulatory systems. Here, the pyramidal and extrapyramidal systems are reviewed along their motor and descending (efferent) pathways and, likewise, for the sensory and ascending (afferent) pathways with emphasis on their clinical significance. **Chapter 5** defines MSA as a sporadic, progressive, and fatal neurodegenerative synucleinopathic disease that is characterized by autonomic failure (cardiovascular and/or urinary), parkinsonism, cerebellar impairment, and corticospinal signs. Its varied symptoms reflect the death of different types of nerve cells in the brain and spinal cord and the progressive loss of associated functions. Its clinical presentation, symptoms, and progression as well as the several affected brain regions are elaborated upon. MSA is one of several neurodegenerative diseases known as synucleinopathies, having in common an abnormal accumulation of the alpha-synuclein protein in various parts of the brain. Although historically many terms were used to refer to MSA, including striatonigral degeneration, olivopontocerebellar atrophy, and Shy–Drager syndrome, these terms were discontinued by consensus in 1996 and replaced with MSA and its subtypes (MSA-Parkinsonism, MSA-cerebellar, and MSA-mixed), as described in **Chapter 6.** Other variants may also exist such as MSA with combined features of dementia with Lewy bodies or frontotemporal lobar degeneration. The signs and symptoms of MSA are presented in **Chapter 7. Chapter 8** sets forth the hallmarks of the disease as widespread glial cytoplasmic inclusions whose main components are Papp-Lantos inclusion bodies that are mainly constituted of misfolded, hyperphosphorylated fibrillary α(alpha)-synuclein – the same protein that is involved in Parkinson's disease. Multiple system atrophy can be explained as cell loss and gliosis (a proliferation of astrocytes in damaged areas of the central nervous system forming a scar called a glial scar). The causes of the disease are unknown, although genetics, environmental processes (toxins), and lifestyle factors (trauma) may contribute to the underlying pathological processes. However, conflicting results indicate the possibility of heterogeneity of the disease in different genetic backgrounds. Lastly, **Chapter 9** reviews the current (very sketchy) epidemiology of MSA. While MSA-P predominates in the Western Hemisphere, MSA-C predominates in the Eastern Hemisphere although the subtypes of MSA vary among Asian countries. Genders are apparently equally distributed.

**Part C** ('Diagnosis, treatment, and prognosis') covers eight chapters (Chapters 10-17). As stated in **Chapter 10,** diagnosis of MSA is clinically based on the combination of signs and symptoms, medical history, physical examination, laboratory test results, various autonomic insufficiency tests, neuroradiological imaging studies, and response to certain treatments. The tests can help determine whether the diagnosis is 'probable MSA' or 'possible MSA'. Unfortunately, no laboratory or imaging studies are able to definitively confirm the diagnosis. Reaching a diagnosis can be challenging and difficult, particularly in the early stages, in part because many of its features are similar to those observed in Parkinson's disease, parkinsonism, and a number of other confounding diseases. Because of this difficulty, some people are actually never properly diagnosed. The main differential diagnoses seek to rule-out any one or more of the following confounding diseases: Alzheimer's, corticobasal degeneration, Creutzfeldt-Jakob, dementias (Lewy bodies, multi-infarct), frontotemporal degeneration, Lytico-Bodig (Guam) syndrome, Huntington's disease, Parkinson's disease, parkinsonism (including atypical syndromes), progressive supranuclear palsy (Steele-Richardson-Olszewski), tremors (benign essential, cerebellar, drug- or toxin-induced, psychogenic), and Wilson's disease. Here, brief primers are provided only on Parkinson's disease and parkinsonism. The complete panoply of MSA diagnostic tests is reviewed, including: Autonomic function testing (blood pressure, thermoregulatory sweat, bladder function, bowel function, electrocardiogram, sleep, diminished respiratory sinus arrhythmia, olfactory testing, skin biopsy, abnormal response to the Valsalva maneuver, diminished response to isometric exercise, diminished response to cold pressor stimuli); neuropathological testing; radiopharmaceutical imaging (DaTscanTM, Iodine-123 scintigraphy); neuroradiological imaging (CT or MRI brain scans), positron emission tomography (scanning with fluorodopa, Iodine-123—FP-CIT), single photon emission computerized tomography; transcranial sonography; and genetic testing.

**Chapter 11** deals with the various approaches for symptom management. Whilst no specific treatment can reverse or halt the progression of the disease, symptoms can be managed for orthostatic hypotension, postural hypotension management, constipation, and urinary incontinence and falls. For movement disorders, treating with drugs but their effectiveness may be limited. For functional capacity, recombinant erythropoietin has been shown to correct anemia and improve standing blood pressure. Pharmacological therapy is required because the disorder is progressive and fatal. Most of the available drugs have been indicated, including detailed Facts Sheets. The next four chapters (Chapters 12-15) dwell on the treatment portfolio. **Chapter 12** elaborates on pharmacological treatments although there are currently no treatments available to delay or arrest the progressive neurodegeneration of the disease, and there is no cure. The condition varies in its gradual progression, does not go into remission, and eventually leads to death. There is no neuroprotective treatment available. However, potential drug candidates have been considered, including: Minocycline, Rasagiline, and Rifampicin. A sidebar is provided on pharmacovigilance, that is the science and activities relating to the detection and reporting of side effects of a medicine, together with measures to minimize those risks. Compassionate use is also discussed including, in particular, what is and what is not a compassionate use program, the underling regulations, the conditions required for the use of medicines on a compassionate basis, and the availability of such medicines. In **Chapter 13,** the use of orphan, repurposed, off-label, and compassionate use medicines is taken up. Orphan medicines are intended for the diagnosis, prevention or treatment of rare diseases. The process of developing them is regulated from the application stage to the development stage to the follow-up as to their efficacy and safety. An off-label use is the use of a drug prescribed for a different disease or when the dosage differs from the one stated on its label. A compassionate use is the use of a medicinal product available for compassionate reasons to patients with a chronically, seriously debilitating, or life-threatening disease and who cannot be treated satisfactorily by an authorized medicinal product. **Chapter 14** deals with clinical trials. These are prospective biomedical or biobehavioral research studies on human participants, designed to answer specific questions about biomedical or biobehavioral interventions, including new treatments and known interventions that warrant further study. Treatments might be new drugs or new combinations of drugs, new surgical procedures or devices, or new ways to use existing treatments. They can also look at other aspects of care, such as improving the quality of life for people with chronic illnesses. The overriding goal of clinical trials is to determine if a new test or treatment is safe and effective. **Chapter 15** reviews the status of experimental disease-modifying drugs. Current approaches point to putative targets for disease modification: α-synuclein pathology, neuroinflammation modulation, and neuroprotection enhancement. The majority of the developed therapeutic approaches has been focused on enhancing α-syn degradation and preventing or disrupting its aggregation. Despite the existence of prominent therapeutic strategies, major obstacles and open questions remain, including the absence of useful biomarkers (whether early in the disease or as the disease progresses), the challenge in making an early diagnosis, the discrepancies in the design of preclinical and clinical studies, the failure of treatment outcome measurements in clinical trials, the limited knowledge about the root cause of the disease, and the failure in defining the best therapeutic target(s) for disease modification. **Chapter 16** reviews the new therapeutic options of growth hormone therapy, immunotherapy, gene therapy, and mesenchymal stem cell therapy as potential components of the treatment portfolio. Growth hormone therapy uses the drugs Mynocycline, Rasagiline, and Rifampicin. It appears to slow the progression of the disease but not significantly. The principle of immunotherapy (passive or active) is based on the specific binding of the antigen α-syn and its respective antibody, followed by clearance of the complexes. Active immunotherapy employs certain antibodies (Affitope® PD01 and PD03, Anle138b). Gene therapy is the insertion of genes into an individual's cells and tissues to treat hereditary diseases where deleterious mutant alleles can be replaced with functional ones. It can also be used to correct non-genetic deficiencies such as the loss of dopamine in MSA, to modify the function of a group of cells, or to provide a source of growth factors. Stem cell therapies have been of interest in MSA for a long time. Thus, mesenchymal stem cells applied intravenously were found to suppress the exacerbated neuroinflammatory cellular environment by producing anti-inflammatory cytokines and neurotrophic factors and exerting neuroprotection. Unfortunately, no reliable approach has yet been identified, despite the extensive preclinical evidence. The prognosis and future outlook for MSA are explored in **Chapter 17.** Older people with parkinsonian features, (MSA-P) and those with severe autonomic dysfunction have a poorer prognosis. By contrast, those with predominantly cerebellar features (MSA-C) and those who display autonomic dysfunction later have a better prognosis. As the disease worsens, many people need additional procedures or interventions to maintain or modify body processes and avoid dangerous complications. The outlook for MSA is poor. The disease progresses without remission at a variable rate. Symptoms get progressively worse and always disrupt body function, leading to deadly complications. The mean life expectancy following the onset of symptoms is about 6 – 10 years and approximately seven years after diagnosis. In less severe cases, people can survive up to 15 years. In very severe cases, survival time may be much lower. The most common causes of death are: Sudden death and death caused by infections, which include urinary catheterization infections, feeding tube infections, bronchopneumonia, pulmonary embolus, and cachexia.

**Part D** ('Living with the disease') includes four chapters. (Chapters 18-21). **Chapter 18** deals with the issues of living with MSA and the help available. As with common diseases, the personal and economic burdens of rare diseases are immense. Most rare diseases have no cure, so living with a rare disease is an ongoing learning experience for patients and families. Thankfully, valuable assistance is available with access care aid, caregiver aid, emergency relief, educational support, and end-of-life issues. In **Chapter 19,** patient advocacy and support organizations are listed whether **wor**ldwide, international, national, or private. They offer many valued services and often drive the research and development of treatments for their disease(s) of interest. Because these organizations include the life experiences of many different people who have a specific disease, they may best understand the resources needed by those in their community. They usually have information and services focused more on specific medical condition(s), but may also have information about associated diseases. **Chapter 20** attempts to answer most frequently asked questions about the disease. For this purpose, the questions have been categorized as about: the disease; learning from others; seeking a health provider; normal living; the disease course; symptoms management; treatments; prognosis and life expectancy; fatality and terminal illness; and the Research Registry. **Chapter 21** deals with the impact of the COVID-19 pandemic during the medical establishment faced (and continues to face) major hurdles that required extraordinary measures to confront its challenges. It became necessary to adjust how clinical trials are managed, including changes and protocol deviations needed in their conduct such as, for example, self-isolation or quarantine of participants, access to public places (including hospitals), and reallocation of healthcare professionals. The pandemic also negatively affected rare disease patients in terms of access to regular health care, treatment, hospitalization, and special diet even among those who reported acquiring the infection.

**Part E** ('Hope for the future') includes two chapters (Chapters 22 and 23). **Chapter 22** reports on past, current, and future research in Europe and across the USA, including he latest updates on multiple system atrophy. Although researchers have not yet been able to identify the root cause of MSA with any certainty, there has been excellent progress in other areas of MSA research, especially in the development of new treatments to prevent exacerbations of the disease. New discoveries are constantly changing MSA treatment options and helping to reduce MSA-related disability. From the concluding chapter, **Chapter 25**, it is very clear that, as with most other neurodegenerative disorders, the proximal trigger is unknown. Regardless, what is evident is that understanding the mechanisms of chronic progression in MSA is currently the major challenge because this is the phase that contributes most to irreversible disability. The lack of insight into mechanisms of progression is largely responsible for the extremely limited treatment options currently available. A shift in thinking about the disease, with greater consideration given to a potential underlying degenerative etiology, will spur new and original research directions that will eventually unravel the mystery and provide more effective therapeutics to mitigate the disabling progressive phase of MSA.

For the reader's convenience, each Chapter ends with a take-away points section to summarize what we have learned from it. Sidebars are provided at the end of Chapters 3, 5, 11, 12, 14, and 22 for those readers interested in the more specialized aspects they describe.

# A. ONCE UPON A TIME

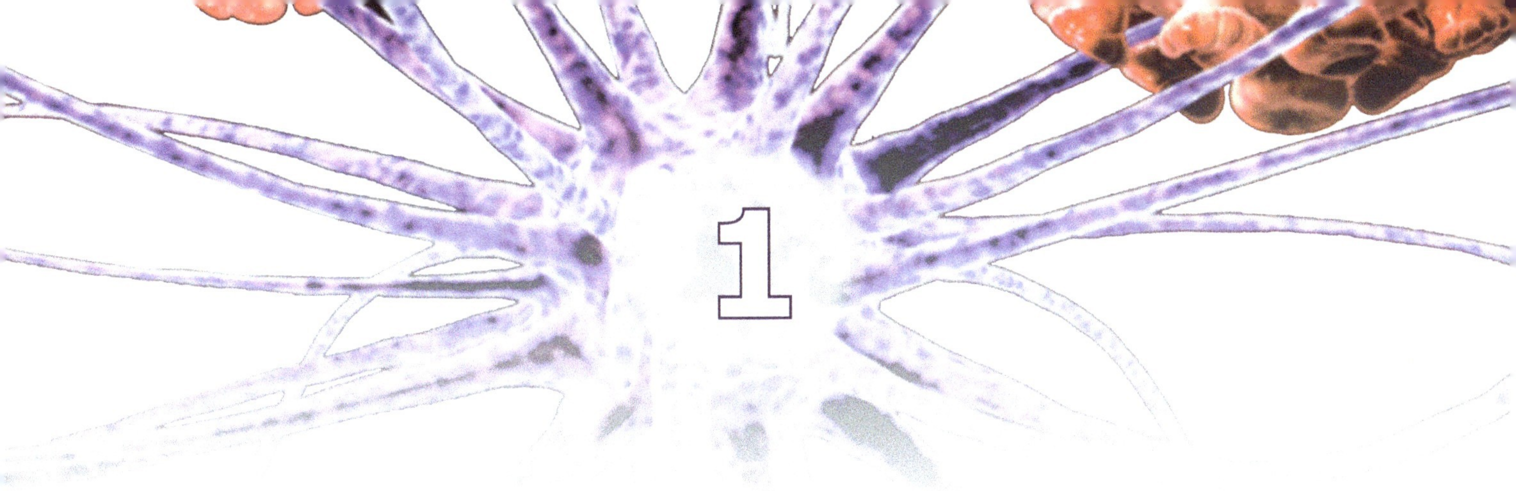

# 1

# A brief chronicle of MSA

The history of multiple system atrophy (MSA) appears to have begun during the second century of the current era when Aelius Galenus or Claudius Galenus (Κλαύδιος Γαληνός; 129 – c. AD 216), often Anglicized as Galen or Galen of Pergamon, a Greek physician, surgeon, and philosopher with Roman citizenship, recognized the autonomous nervous system. Considered to be one of the most accomplished of all medical researchers of Antiquity and the father of medicine, Galen influenced the development of various scientific disciplines, including anatomy, physiology, pathology, pharmacology, and neurology as well as philosophy and logic. However, it was not until nearly fifteen centuries later that the field of clinical neuroscience, including MSA, came to light under Thomas Willis FRS (1621 – 1675), an English doctor, founding member and Fellow of the Royal Society and considered the father of clinical neuroscience, played an important part in the history of anatomy, neurology, and psychiatry, and used the terminology of the disease.

Skipping over much of the intervening centuries, the following chronicle retraces the modern developments in the study of the nervous system and, particularly, MSA.

**1656:** Willis published a significant medical work: *De Fermentatione.*

**1659:** Willis published another significant medical work: *De Febribus.*

**1663:** Willis published his *Diatribae duae medico-philosophicae – quarum prior agit de fermentatione.*

**1664:** Willis published his *Cerebri anatome: Ccui accessit nervorum descriptio et usus,* (*Anatomy of the brain, with a description of the nerves and their function),* an important work on the anatomy of the brain and nerves.

**1667:** Willis published *Pathologicae cerebri, et nervosi generis specimenet*, another important work on the pathology and neurophysiology of the brain.

**1672:** Willis published his *De Anima Brutorum*.

**1672:** Publication by Willis of the earliest English work on medical psychology. He was also the first to identify achalasia cardia.

**1675:** Willis published his *Pharmaceutice rationalis. Sive Diatriba de medicamentorum operationibus in humano corpore* [A plain and easy method for preserving (by God's blessing) those that are well from the infection of the plague, or any contagious distemper in city, camp, fleet, &c., and for curing such as are infected with it.]"

**1670s:** Willis numbered the cranial nerves in the order in which they are now usually enumerated by anatomists, noting the parallel lines of the mesolobe (corpus callosum). These were later minutely described by Félix Vicq-d'Azyr.

**1681:** Publication by Willis of his *Clarissimi Viri Thomae Willis, Medicinae Doctoris, Naturalis Philosophiae Professoris Oxoniensis ... Opera Omnia : Cum Elenchis Rerum Et Indicibus necessariis, ut & multis Figuris aeneis.*

**1900:** Dejerinne and Thomas at the Hopital Salpetriere, Paris, France, published their landmark paper on olivopontocerebellar atrophy (OPCA) in which they reported on patients presenting with ataxia, dysarthria, akinesia, rigidity, brisk reflexes, and urine incontinence.

**1900:** John Newport Langley used the term defining the two divisions as the sympathetic and parasympathetic nervous systems.

**1925:** Bradbury and Eggleston reported on patients who presented with postural hypotension, anhydrosis, hyperactive or asymmetric reflexes, and extensor plantar responses pointing to an association between autonomic failure and neurological dysfunction.

**1960:** Milton Shy, National Institute of Health, and Glen Drager, Baylor College of Medicine in Houston, Texas described in the *Archives of Neurology* two individual patients who shared common clinical symptoms, including parkinsonian symptoms. The postmortem examination of one of them provided evidence that he had a distinct and unique disease. To acknowledge their contribution, this disorder was named "Shy-Drager Syndrome" (SDS). Among the many names for this disorder, multiple system atrophy (MSA) is the most commonly used today, but many physicians still use such other terms as striatonigral degeneration (SND) or sporadic olivopontocerebellar atrophy (sOPCA).

**1961:** Adams *et al.* described striatonigral degeneration (SND).

**1961:** Birkmayer and Hornykiewicz in Europe and Barbeau in Canada first described the benefits of low doses of L-dopa in Parkinson's disease.

**1964:** Steele, Richardson and Olszewski described progressive supranuclear palsy (PSP).

**1967:** Hoehn and Yahr described the progression of parkinsonism.

**1967:** Cotzias confirmed that large doses of L-dopa were dramatically effective in Parkinson's disease.

**1968:** Rebeiz described corticobasal degeneration (CBD).

**1969:** Graham and Oppenheimer published their classic paper in which they introduced the term "multiple system atrophy".

**1969:** The overlapping pathology of three disorders, namely striatonigral degeneration (SND), olivopontocerebellar atrophy (OPCA) and Shy–Drager syndrome (SDS) was recognized.

**1989:** Papp and colleagues strengthened the definition of MSA with the discovery of glial cytoplasmic inclusions (GCIs) in the brains of patients.

**1998:** Several researchers (Gai *et al.*, Spillantini *et al.*, Wakabayashi *et al.*) observed that the MSA- specific GCIs were mainly composed of misfolded and aggregated α-synuclein (α-syn).

**2014-16:** Several researchers studied the environmental and genetic factors undergirding MSA to understand the disease etiology (Sturm and Stefanova, Jellinger and Wenning). In addition, *COQ2* gene polymorphisms and genetic variants have been associated with MSA in East Asian population (Fujioka *et al.*, Ogaki *et al.*, Chen *et al.*). However, the same variants were not confirmed in MSA patients from Europe or North America (Sailer *et al.*).

-o-o-o-

## 28 February is 'Rare Disease Day'

Raising awareness and generating change for the 300 million people worldwide living with a rare disease, their families, and carers.

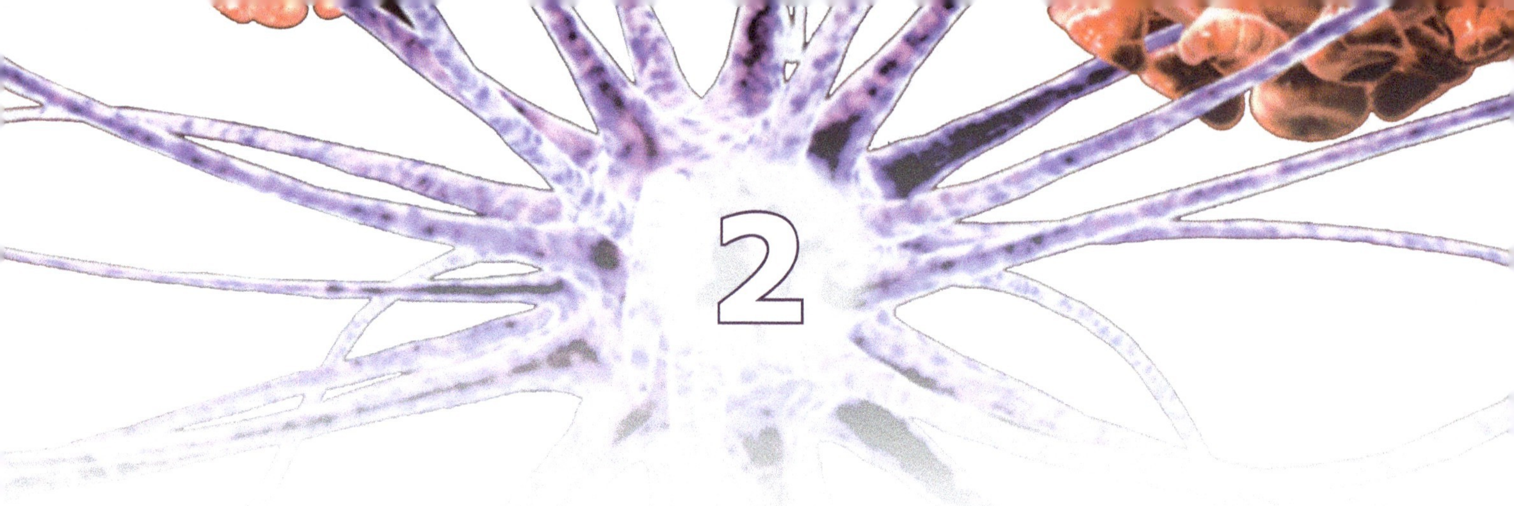

# 2

# Thomas Willis . . . the founder of clinical neuroscience

Thomas Willis, FRS (27 January 1621 – 11 November 1675) was an English doctor who played an important part in the history of anatomy, neurology, and psychiatry and was one of the founding members of the Royal Society.

**Figure 2.1 - Thomas Willis (1621 - 1675)**

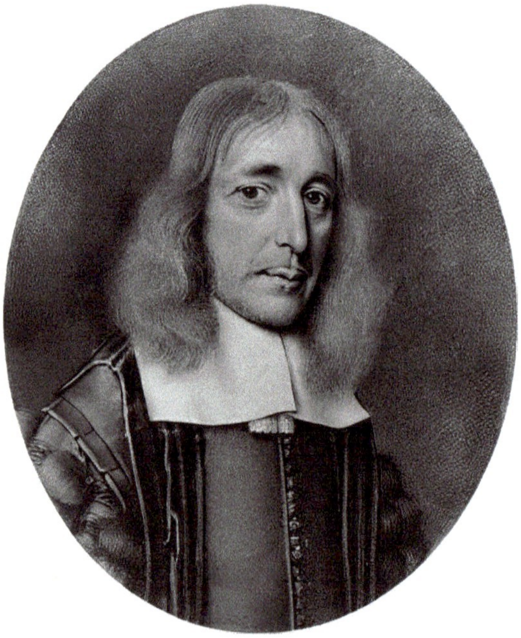

*Source: David Loggan - http://www.oxforddnb.com/view/article/29587*

## The early years

Thomas Willis was born the eldest of three sons in his parents' small farm in Great Bedwyn, Wiltshire, where his father held the stewardship of the Manor. He was a kinsman of the Willys baronets of Fen Ditton, Cambridgeshire and a staunch Royalist. He married Mary Fell whose brother would later be his biographer. He was dispossessed of the family farm at North Hinksey by parliamentary forces. During the Civil War, both Willises (father and son) would serve King Charles I of England in the auxiliary regiment of the Earl of Dover.

Willis went to Oxford as a servitor intending to follow a career in the church, graduating M.A. in 1642. When the Civil War made that intention appear chancy, he turned to medicine. While it is unclear whether or not he actually participated in any battles, Willis' loyalty and service to the King were rewarded by the early conferral of his medical degree, despite the fact that he was seven years away from graduating from the fourteen-year program. In the 1640s, Willis was one of the royal physicians to Charles I. Less grandly, once qualified B. Med. in 1646, he began as an active physician by regularly attending the market at Abingdon.

During the period 1656–1658, he employed Robert Hooke (1635-1703) as an assistant. Hooke later became in his own right a well-known polymath (scientist, natural philosopher, and architect). In addition to Hooke, other scientists grew up around Willis, including Nathaniel Hodges, John Locke, Richard Lower, Henry Stubbe, and John Ward.

## The Revival of Anne Green

Willis' breakthrough as a physician came about with the revival of Anne Green on December 14, 1650. Green, a 22 year old servant, was a prisoner of the state who was convicted of the infanticide of her newborn child, and was sentenced to be hanged. At the time, obtaining corpses for anatomical dissection was difficult, so the bodies of executed individuals were typically donated to universities. After being hanged in Oxford's Cattle Yard, Green's body was donated for scientific study to Oxford. Thus, she was delivered to the home of William Petty, a colleague of Willis and a lecturer in anatomy at Oxford. When the coffin was opened, an audible gagging was heard and Green started to breath. Together, Petty and Willis resuscitated the 'corpse' using unorthodox but ultimately successful techniques.

## The Oxford Club

While in Oxford, conform to his early religious vocation, Willis made his chambers available for Anglican services during the Puritan interregnum. One of several Oxford cliques of those interested in science grew up around Willis and Christ Church. Besides Robert

Hooke, who would become Willis' leading rival, and who both politically and medically held some incompatible views, others in the group were Nathaniel Hodges, John Locke, Richard Lower, Henry Stubbe, and John Ward as cited previously. In the broader Oxford scene, Willis was a member of the "Oxford club" of experimentalists with Ralph Bathurst, Robert Boyle, William Petty, John Wilkins, and Christopher Wren.

## Contributions to clinical neuroscience

In 1656 and 1659, Willis published two significant medical works, *De Fermentatione* and *De Febribus*. These were followed by his 1664 volume on the brain, *Cerebri Anatome, cui accessit Nervorum descriptio et usus* (*Anatomy of the brain, with a description of the nerves and their function*). It was actually a record of close collaborative experimental work with Christopher Wren and Richard Lower. This latter work was considered to be the most complete and accurate account of the nervous system at that time. Willis is credited with coining the term neurology, which first appears in *Cerebri Anatome*. He was also the first to number the cranial nerves in the order in which they are now usually enumerated by anatomists.

The *Cerebri Anatome* was the main reason why the arterial circle found at the base of the human brain is now called the "Circle of Willis". Though he was not the first one who discovered and described it, he was the only one who was able to discuss it in great detail, describing in depth each part and vascular pattern. Willis, therefore, is regarded by modern physicians and anatomists as the founder of clinical neuroscience, neurology, comparative anatomy, and neuroanatomy.

## Neurological research activities

Willis was a pioneer in research into the anatomy of the brain, nervous system, and muscles. His most notable discovery was the "Circle of Willis", as described in his 1664 *Cerebri anatome.* This work abounds in minutely detailed new information in enormous contrast with the vaguer efforts of his predecessors.

In his 1667 *Pathologicae cerebri, et nervosi generis specimen*, an important work on the pathology and neurophysiology of the brain, Willis developed a new theory of the cause of epilepsy and other convulsive diseases, and contributed to the development of psychiatry.

More particularly, Willis was:

1. First to number the cranial nerves in the order in which they are now usually enumerated by anatomists.
2. Noted the parallel lines of the mesolobe (corpus callosum), which were afterwards minutely described by Félix Vicq-d'Azyr.

3. Recognized the communication of the convoluted surface of the brain and that between the lateral cavities beneath the fornix.
4. Described the corpora striata and optic thalami. Also, the four orbicular eminences with the bridge, which he first named annular protuberance, and the white mammillary eminences behind the infundibulum.
5. Remarked in the cerebellum the arborescent arrangement of the white and grey matters.
6. Gave a good account of the internal carotids and the communications they make with the branches of the basilar artery.
7. Replaced the Nemesius' doctrine, deducing that the ventricles contained cerebrospinal fluid which collected waste products from effluents.
8. Recognized the cortex as the substrate of cognition and claimed that the gyrencephalia was related to a progressive increase in the complexity of cognition.
9. Placed the origin of voluntary movements at the cerebral cortex while involuntary movements came from the cerebellum.

## Other research activities

In 1672, Willis published the earliest English work on medical psychology with two discourses concerning the Soul of Brutes, which is that of the Vital and Sensitive of Man. He could also be seen as an early pioneer of the mind-brain supervenience claim prominent in present-day neuropsychiatry and philosophy of mind. Further:

- He coined the term 'mellitus' in diabetes mellitus. An old name for the condition is "Willis's disease".
- He observed, what had been known for many centuries elsewhere, that the urine is sweet in patients (glycosuria).
- His observations on diabetes formed a chapter of *Pharmaceutice rationalis* (1674).

In addition, Willis made significant original contributions to cardiology, endocrinology, and gastroenterology.

Willis's work gained currency in France through the writings of Daniel Duncan.

## The Royal Society and later years

From 1660 until his death, Willis was Sedleian Professor of Natural Philosophy at Oxford. At the time, he was one of the founders of the Royal Society of which he became a Fellow in 1661. He later worked as a physician in Westminster, London and built a successful medical practice in which he applied and integrated both his understanding of anatomy and known remedies, mixing both iatrochemical and mechanical views.

## Published works

- 1663: *Diatribae duae medico-philosophicae – quarum prior agit de fermentatione.*
- 1664: *Cerebri anatome: cui accessit nervorum descriptio et usus.*
- 1667: *Pathologiae Cerebri et Nervosi Generis Specimen.*

**Figure 2.2 – Frontispiece of Willis' 1663 book**

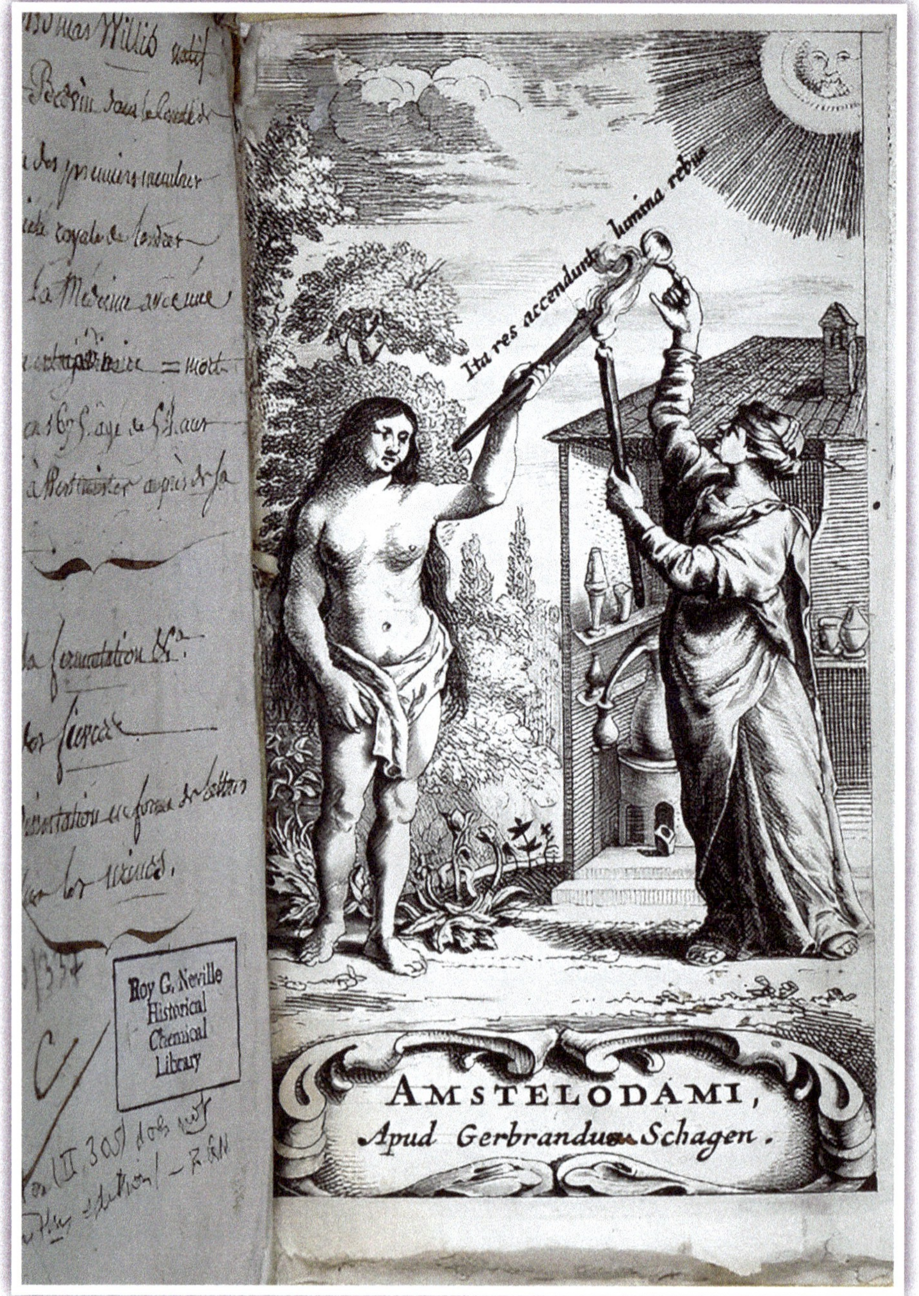


*Diatribae duae medico-philosophicae – quarum prior agit de fermentatione,* engraved and published by Gerbrandus Schagen in Amsterdam

- 1672: *De Anima Brutorum.*
- 1675-7: *Pharmaceutice rationalis. Sive Diatriba de medicamentorum operationibus in humano corpore.*
- 1681: *Clarissimi Viri Thomae Willis, Medicinae Doctoris, Naturalis Philosophiae Professoris Oxoniensis ... Opera Omnia : Cum Elenchis Rerum Et Indicibus necessariis, ut & multis Figuris aeneis.*
- 1683 *Dissertation sur les urines tirée des ouvrages de Willis* (in French)..

And so, we leave this great physician, father of clinical neuroscience, neurology, comparative anatomy, and neuroanatomy with the frontispiece to his 1663 book "*Diatribae duae medico-philosophicae – quarum prior agit de fermentatione*".

# B. THE DISEASE AND ITS PARTICULARS

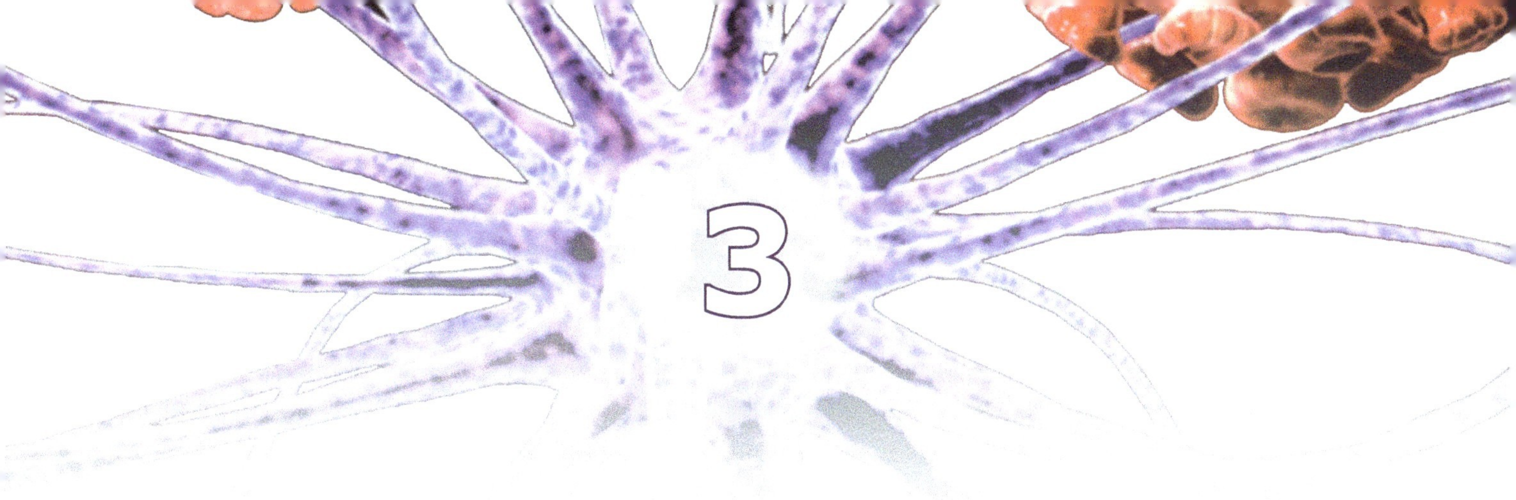


# Understanding the autonomic nervous system

Multiple system atrophy (MSA) affects both the autonomic nervous system (ANS) and the motor system (MS). It behooves us, therefore, to understand these two systems. For this purpose, two brief primers are provided in this and the following chapter, respectively.

## What is the nervous system (NS)?

The brain is made up of many networks of communicating cells that allow different parts of the brain to "talk" to each other and "work" together to control body functions, emotions, thinking, behavior, and other activities. In this context, the NS is a network of neurons whose main feature is to generate, modulate, and transmit information between the brain and all the different parts of the body, including internal organs. This property enables many important functions, such as the regulation of vital body functions (heartbeat, breathing, digestion), sensation, and body movements. It presides over everything that makes us human: our consciousness, cognition, behavior, and memories.

As the command center of the body, the NS guides, controls, and regulates almost every aspect of health, including:

- Thoughts, memory, learning, and feelings.
- Movements, such as balance and coordination.
- Senses, including how the brain interprets what we see, hear, taste, touch, and feel.
- Sleep, healing, and aging.
- Heartbeat and breathing patterns.
- Response to stressful situations.

- Digestion, as well as how hungry and thirsty we feel.
- Body processes, such as puberty.
- Things done without thinking, such as breathing, blushing, and blinking.
- Experiencing the environment.

## The parts of NS

NS has two main parts, each containing billions of cells called neurons or nerve cells. These parts are (Figure 3.1):

**Figure 3.1 – Parts of the nervous system**

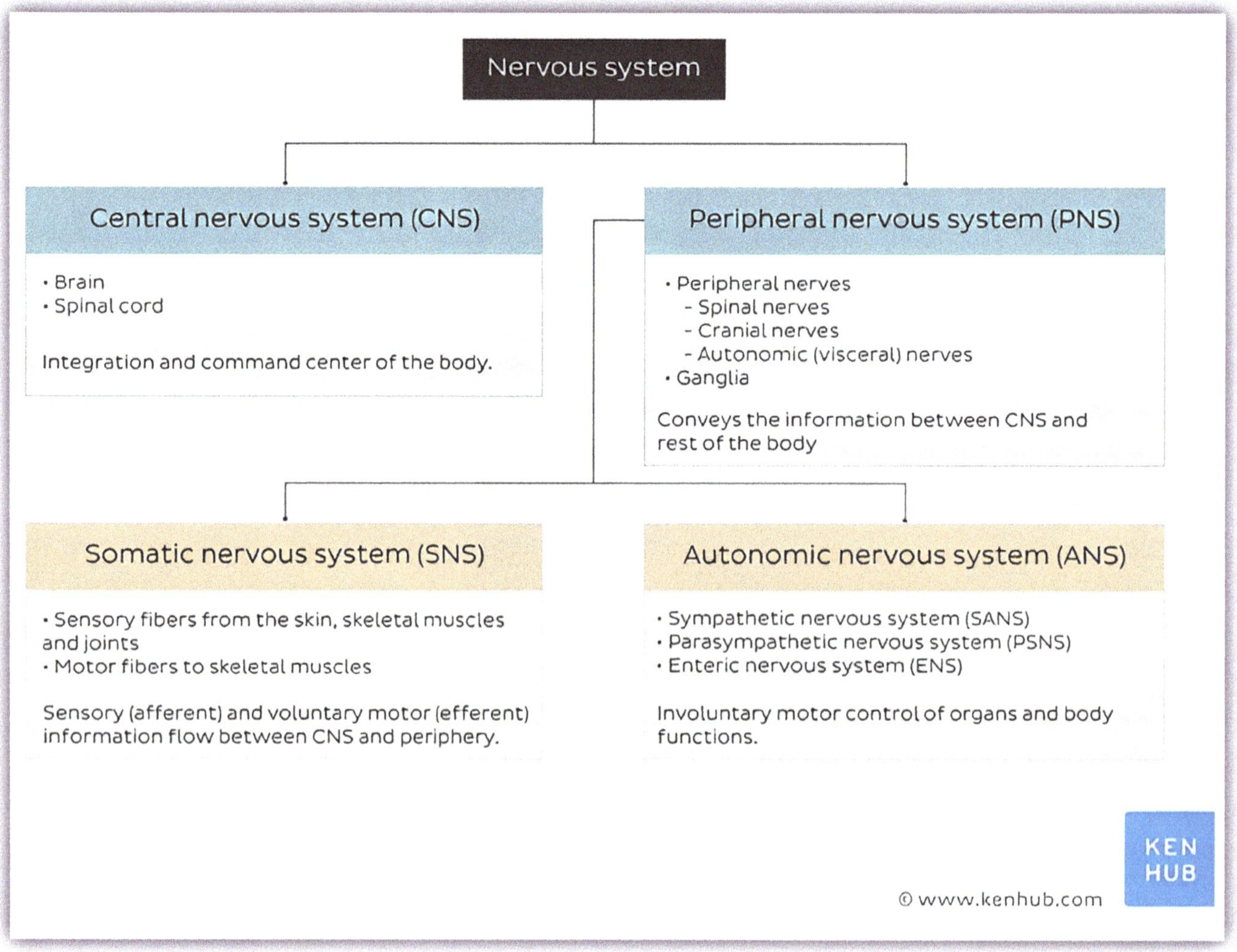


- The **central nervous system** (CNS): Made up of the brain and spinal cord, it is the integration and command & control center of the body. The brain uses the nerves to send messages to the rest of the body. Each nerve has a protective outer layer called **myelin**. Myelin insulates the nerve and helps the messages get through.

- The **peripheral nervous system** (PNS): Made up of nerves that branch off from the spinal cord and extend to all parts of the body, it is the conduit between the CNS and the body. It relays information from the brain and spinal cord to the organs, arms, legs, fingers, and toes. It is further subdivided into:
    - The **somatic nervous system (SNS):** To guide voluntary movements.
    - The **autonomic nervous system (ANS):** To control the activities done without thinking about them.

Understanding the nervous system requires knowledge of its various parts. Further, understanding the MSA disease additionally requires understanding the ANS and, as we shall see in the next chapter, also the motor system (MS).

## The autonomic nervous system (ANS)

Formerly referred to as the involuntary (or vegetative) nervous system, the ANS is a division of the peripheral nervous system (PNS) that supplies internal organs, smooth muscles, and glands.

### Structure

The ANS has four branches, namely the:

1. **Sympathetic nervous system (SNS):** It is often considered as the "fight-or-flight" system. It emerges from the spinal cord in the thoracic and lumbar areas, terminating around lumbar L2-3.
2. **Parasympathetic nervous system (PNS):** It is often considered as the "rest-and-digest" or "feed-and-breed" system. It has craniosacral "outflow", meaning that the neurons begin at the cranial nerves (specifically the oculomotor nerve, facial nerve, glossopharyngeal nerve, and vagus nerve) and sacral (S2-S4) spinal cord.
3. **Enteric nervous system (ENS):** Here, non-noradrenergic, non-cholinergic transmitters (so-referred to because they use nitric oxide as a neurotransmitter) are integral in autonomic function, in particular in the gut and the lungs.
4. **Visceral sensory nervous system (VSNS):** Although the ANS is also known as the visceral nervous system and although most of its fibers carry non-somatic information to the CNS, many authors still consider it is only connected with the motor side. Most autonomous functions are involuntary, but they can often work in conjunction with the somatic nervous system which provides voluntary control.

In many cases, it should be noted that both the SNS and PNS have "opposite" actions wherein one system activates a physiological response and the other inhibits it. The older simplification in which SNS is "excitatory" and PNS is "inhibitory" was overturned due to the many exceptions found. A more modern characterization is that the SNS is a "quick response mobilizing system" and the PNS is a "more slowly activated dampening system", but even this other distinction has its own exceptions, such as in sexual arousal and orgasm, wherein both play a role. There are inhibitory and excitatory synapses between neurons.

## Internal regulation

The ANS is internally regulated by integrated reflexes through the brainstem to the spinal cord and organs. It is unique in that it requires a sequential, two-neuron efferent pathway; the preganglionic neuron must first synapse onto a postganglionic neuron before innervating the target organ. The preganglionic (or first) neuron will begin at the "outflow" and will synapse at the postganglionic (or second) neuron's cell body. The postganglionic neuron will then synapse at the target organ.

Autonomic functions include:

- Control of respiration.
- Cardiac regulation (the cardiac control center).
- Vasomotor activity (the vasomotor center).
- Certain reflex actions such as coughing, sneezing, swallowing, and vomiting. Those functions are then subdivided into other areas and are also linked to autonomic subsystems and the PNS. The hypothalamus, just above the brain stem, acts as an integrator for autonomic functions, receiving autonomic regulatory input from the limbic system.

## External regulation

The ANS is a control system that acts largely unconsciously and regulates bodily functions, such as the heart rate, its force of contraction, digestion, respiratory rate, pupillary response, urination, and sexual arousal. It is the primary mechanism in control of the 'fight-or-flight' response.

## Innervation

Autonomic nerves travel to organs throughout the body. Most organs receive parasympathetic supply by the vagus nerve and sympathetic supply by splanchnic nerves. The sensory part of the latter reaches the spinal column at certain spinal segments. Pain in any internal organ is perceived as referred pain, more specifically as pain from the dermatome corresponding to the spinal segment. Table 3.1 identifies the autonomous nervous supply to organs in the human body.

**Table 3.1 - Autonomic nervous supply to organs in the human body**

| Organ | Nerves | Spinal column origin |
|---|---|---|
| **Appendix** | Nerves to superior mesenteric plexus | T10 |
| **Colon** | **PS:** Vagus nerves & pelvic splanchnic nerves<br>**S:** Lesser & least splanchnic nerves | T10, T11 (proximal colon)<br>L1, L2, L3 (distal colon) |
| **Duodenum** | **PS:** Vagus nerves<br>**S:** Greater splanchnic nerves | T5, T6, T7, T8, T9, T10 (sometimes) |
| **Gallbladder & Liver** | **PS:** Vagus nerves<br>**S:** Celiac plexus<br>Right phrenic nerve | T6, T7, T8, T9 |
| **Jejunum & Ileum** | **PS:** Posterior vagus trunks<br>**S:** Greater splanchnic nerves | T5, T6, T7, T8, T9 |
| **Kidneys & Ureters** | **PS:** Vagus nerves<br>**S:** Thoracic & lumbar splanchnic nerves | T11, T12 |
| **Pancreatic head** | **PS:** Vagus nerves<br>**S:** Thoracic splanchnic nerves | T8, T9 |
| **Spleen** | **S:** Greater splanchnic nerve | T6, T7, T8 |
| **Stomach** | **PS:** Anterior & posterior vagal trunks<br>**S:** Greater splanchnic nerve | T5, T6, T7, T8, T9, T10 (sometimes) |

*Reference: Wikipedia*

(PS = Parasympathetic; S = Sympathetic; L: Lumbar; T = Thoracic)

These are further illustrated in Figure 3.2.

## Function

Sympathetic and parasympathetic divisions typically function complementarily rather than antagonistically to each other. For an analogy, one may think of the sympathetic division as the accelerator and the parasympathetic division as the brake. The sympathetic division typically functions in actions requiring quick responses. The parasympathetic division functions with actions that do not require immediate reaction.

**Figure 3.2 – Autonomic nervous system innervation**

Illustration from Anatomy & Physiology, Connexions Web site. http://cnx.org/content/col11496/1.6/

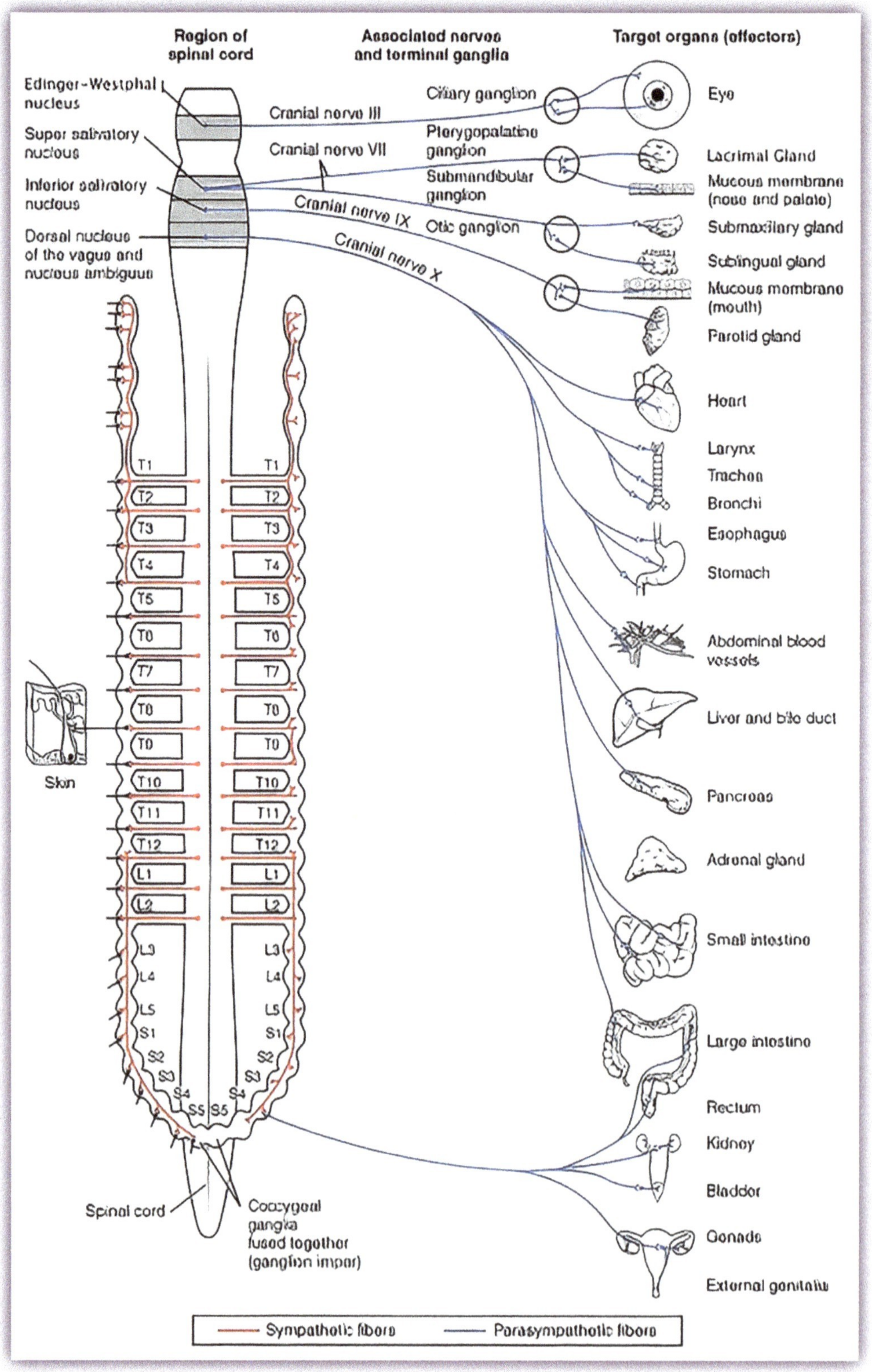

However, many instances of sympathetic and parasympathetic activity cannot be ascribed to "fight" or "rest" situations. For example, standing up from a reclining or sitting position would entail an unsustainable drop in blood pressure if not for a compensatory increase in the arterial sympathetic tonus. Another example is the constant, second-to-second, modulation of heart rate by sympathetic and parasympathetic influences, as a function of the respiratory cycles. In general, these two systems should be seen as permanently modulating vital functions in a usually antagonistic fashion to achieve homeostasis. Higher organisms maintain their integrity via homeostasis that relies on negative feedback regulation which, in turn, typically depends on the ANS.

## The sympathetic nervous system (SNS)

The SNS promotes a 'fight-or-flight' response, corresponds with arousal and energy generation, and inhibits digestion:

- Blood flow is diverted away from the gastro-intestinal (GI) tract and skin via vasoconstriction.
- Blood flow to skeletal muscles and the lungs is enhanced (by as much as 1200% in the case of skeletal muscles).
- Bronchioles of the lung are dilated through circulating epinephrine, which allows for greater alveolar oxygen exchange.
- Heart rate and the contractility of cardiac cells (myocytes) are increased, thereby providing a mechanism for enhanced blood flow to skeletal muscles.
- Pupils are dilated and the ciliary muscle to the lens are relaxed, allowing more light to enter the eye to enhance far vision.
- Vasodilation of the coronary vessels of the heart is provided.

## The parasympathetic nervous system (PNS)

The parasympathetic nervous system promotes calming of the nerves, returning to regular function, and enhancing digestion. Functions of nerves within the parasympathetic nervous system include:

- Dilating blood vessels leading to the GI tract, increasing the blood flow.
- Constricting the bronchiolar diameter when the need for oxygen has diminished.
- Imparting parasympathetic control of the heart (myocardium) through dedicated cardiac branches of the vagus and thoracic spinal accessory nerves.

- Facilitating accommodation and allowing for closer vision through constriction of the pupil and contraction of the ciliary muscles,
- Stimulating salivary gland secretion and accelerating peristalsis, mediating digestion of food and, indirectly, the absorption of nutrients.
- Stimulating sexual arousal trough nerves of the PNS that are involved in the erection of genital tissues via the pelvic splanchnic nerves 2–4.

Some typical actions of the SNS and PNS are shown in Table **3**.2.

**Table 3.2 – Typical actions of the sympathetic & parasympathetic nervous systems**

| Target/organism | Sympathetic | Parasympathetic |
|---|---|---|
| **Adrenal medulla** | Stimulates medulla cells to secrete epinephrine and norepinephrine | No effect |
| **Blood vessels** | o Constricts blood vessels on viscera<br>o Increases blood pressure | No effect on most blood vessels |
| **Digestive system** | Decreases activity | Increases peristalsis and amount of secretion by digestive glands |
| **Eye (iris)** | o Stimulates dilator muscles<br>o Dilates pupils | o Stimulates constrictor muscles<br>o Constricts pupils |
| **Eye (ciliary muscles)** | o Inhibits/decreases bulging of lens<br>o Prepares for distant vision | o Stimulates/increases bulging of lens for clear vision |
| **Heart** | Increases rate | Decreases rate |
| **Kidneys** | Decreases urine output | No effect |
| **Liver** | Causes glucose to be released in blood | No effect |
| **Lungs** | Dilates bronchioles | Constricts bronchioles |
| **Urinary bladder/ Urethra** | Constricts sphincter | Relaxes sphincter |
| **Salivary and lacrimal glands** | o Inhibits<br>o Results in dry mouth and dry eyes | o Stimulates<br>o Increases production of saliva and tears |
| **Skin's sweat gland** | o Stimulates sudmotor function to produce perspiration | o No effect |

*Reference: Wikipedia*

### The enteric nervous system (ENS)

The ENS is the intrinsic nervous system of the gastrointestinal system. It has been described as "the second brain of the human body". Its functions include:

- Sensing chemical and mechanical changes in the gut.
- Regulating secretions in the gut.
- Controlling peristalsis and some other movements.

### ANS and the immune system

Recent studies indicate that ANS activation is critical for regulating the local and systemic immune-inflammatory responses and may influence acute stroke outcomes. Therapeutic approaches modulating the activation of the ANS or the immune-inflammatory response could promote neurologic recovery after stroke.

## Neurons

Two basic types of cells are present in the nervous system: Neurons and glial cells that will now be considered.

### Basic description

Neurons (or nerve cells) are the main structural and functional units of the NS. Every neuron consists of a body (**soma**), which contains a nucleus and special extensions or neural processes called **axons** and neurites (**called** dendrites). Bundles of axons, called **nerves,** are found throughout the body. Axons and dendrites allow neurons to communicate, even across long distances. The nerve cell body containing the cellular organelles is where neural impulses ('action potentials') are generated. The processes stem from the body and connect neurons with each other and with other body cells, enabling the flow of neural impulses (Figure 3.3).

Neural processes exist in two types that differ in structure and function:

- **Axons:** They are long and conduct impulses away from the neuronal body.
- **Dendrites:** They are short and act to receive impulses from other neurons, conducting the electrical signal towards the nerve cell body.

**Figure 3.3 – Structure of a neuron**

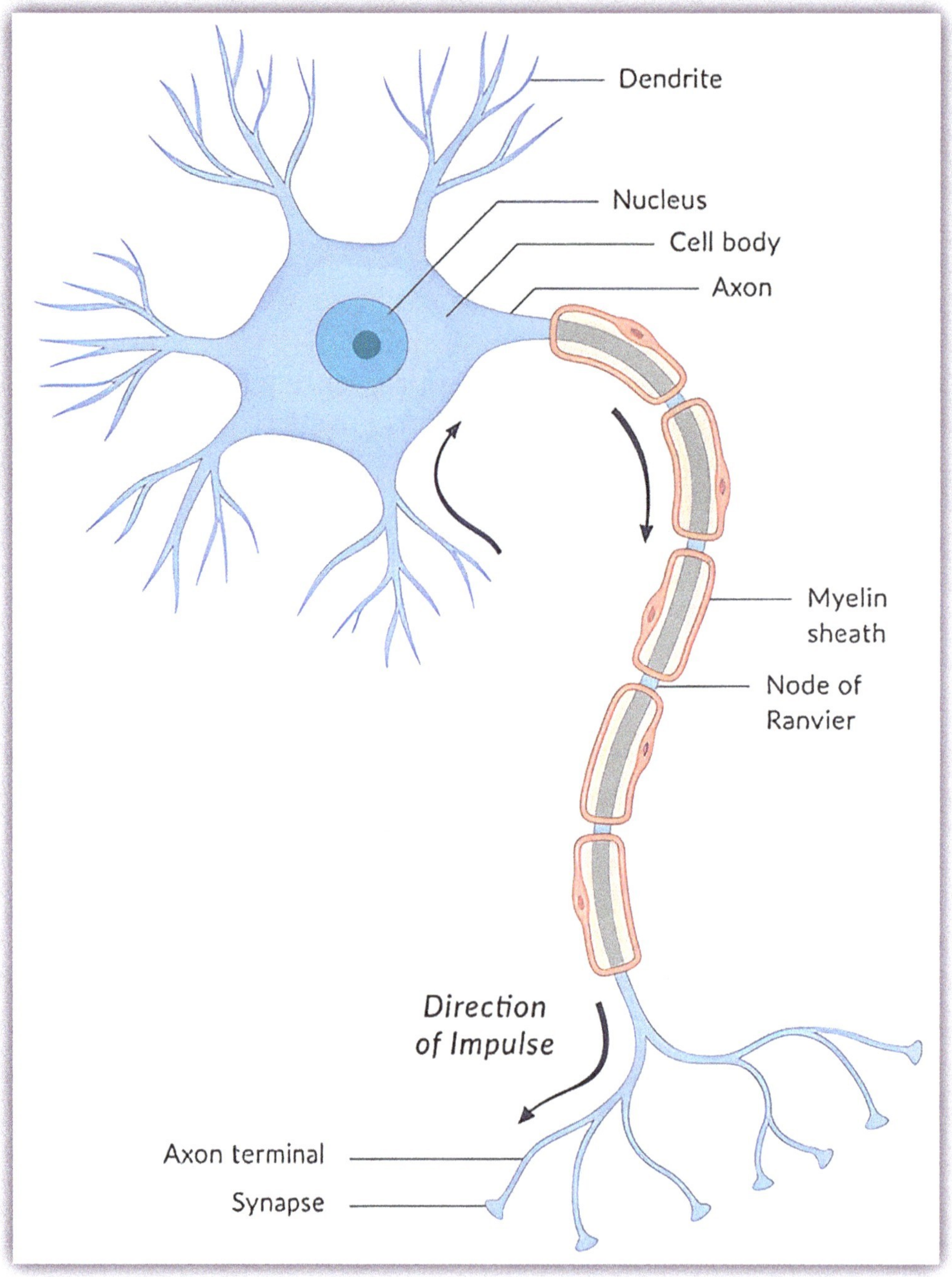


*Source: National Institute of Child Health and Human Development (NICHHF)*

## Neuron types

### Structural

Every neuron has a single axon, while the number of dendrites varies. Based on that number, there are four structural **types of neurons:**

- **Unipolar.**
- **Pseudounipolar.**
- **Bipolar.**
- **Multipolar.**

**Functional**

Different types of neurons control or perform different activities. For instance:

- **Motor neurons:** They transmit messages from the brain to the muscles to generate movement.
- **Sensory neurons:** They detect light, sound, odor, taste, pressure, and heat, and send messages about those things to the brain.
- **Other neurons:** They control involuntary processes, including keeping a regular heartbeat, releasing hormones like adrenaline, opening the pupil in response to light, and regulating the digestive system.

**Directional**

There are two types of neurons, named according to whether they send an electrical signal towards or away from the central nervous system (CNS):

- **Efferent neurons** (motor or descending): They send neural impulses from the CNS to the peripheral tissues, instructing them how to function.
- **Afferent neurons** (sensory or ascending): They conduct impulses from the peripheral tissues to the CNS. These impulses contain sensory information, describing the tissue's environment.

## Morphology

The morphology of neurons makes them highly specialized to work with neural impulses. They generate, receive, and send these impulses onto other neurons and non-neural tissues.

The site where an axon connects to another cell to pass the neural impulse is called a synapse. The synapse does not connect to the next cell directly. Instead, the impulse triggers the release of chemicals called **neurotransmitters** from the very end of an axon. These neurotransmitters bind to the effector cell's membrane, causing biochemical events to occur within that cell according to the orders sent by the CNS.

## White and gray matter

The white-colored myelinated axons are distinguished from the gray-colored neuronal bodies and dendrites. Based on this, nervous tissue is divided into white matter and gray matter, both of which having a specific distribution:

- **White matter:** It comprises the outermost layer of the spinal cord and the inner part of the brain.
- **Gray matter:** It is located in the central part of the spinal cord, the outermost layer of the brain (cerebral cortex), and in several subcortical nuclei of the brain deep to the cerebral cortex.

## Neurotransmitters

At the effector organs, sympathetic ganglionic neurons release noradrenaline (norepinephrine), along with other co-transmitters such as adenosine triphosphate (ATP), to act on adrenergic receptors, with the exception of the sweat glands and the adrenal medulla:

- **Acetylcholine:** This is the pre-ganglionic neurotransmitter for both divisions of the ANS, as well as the post-ganglionic neurotransmitter of parasympathetic neurons. Nerves that release acetylcholine are said to be cholinergic. In the parasympathetic system, ganglionic neurons use acetylcholine as a neurotransmitter to stimulate muscarinic receptors.
- **Adrenaline:** At the adrenal medulla, there is no postsynaptic neuron. Instead, the presynaptic neuron releases acetylcholine to act on nicotinic receptors. Stimulation of the adrenal medulla releases adrenaline (epinephrine) into the bloodstream, which acts on adrenoceptors, thereby indirectly mediating or mimicking sympathetic activity.

(Note: Complete tables of neurotransmitter actions in the ANS are available in the published literature, but will not be provided here.)

## How do neurons function?

Most axons are wrapped by a white insulating substance called the **myelin sheath** produced by oligodendrocytes and Schwann's cells. Myelin encloses an axon segmentally, leaving unmyelinated gaps between the segments called the ***nodes of Ranvier*** **(Figure 3,1)**. The neural impulses propagate through the Ranvier nodes only, skipping the myelin sheath. This significantly increases the speed of neural impulse propagation.

When a neuron sends a message to another neuron, it sends an electrical signal down the length of its axon. At the end of the axon, the electrical signal changes to a chemical signal. The axon then releases the chemical signal with chemical messengers called **neurotransmitters** (see section above) into the synapse - the space between the end of an axon and the tip of a dendrite from another neuron. The neurotransmitters move the signal through the synapse to the neighboring dendrite, which converts the chemical signal back into an electrical signal. The electrical signal then travels through the neuron and goes through the same conversion processes as it moves to neighboring neurons. Different kinds of neurons send different signals. Thus, motor neurons tell the muscles to move. On the other hand, sensory neurons take information from the senses and send signals to the brain. Other types of neurons control the things the body does automatically, like breathing, shivering, having a regular heartbeat, and digesting food.

- All the intestinal sphincters and the urinary sphincter are constricted.
- Peristalsis is inhibited.
- Orgasm is stimulated.

The pattern of innervation of the sweat gland—namely, the postganglionic sympathetic nerve fibers—allows clinicians and researchers to use sudomotor function testing to assess dysfunction of the ANS through electrochemical skin conductance.

## Glial cells

The NS also includes smaller cells, called **glia**, **gliocytes**, or **neuroglia.**

In the CNS, glial cells include:

- **Oligodendrocytes.**
- **Astrocytes** (also called **astroglia**).
- **Ependymal cells.**
- **Microglia**.

In the peripheral nervous system (PNS), glial cells include **Schwann's cells** and satellite cells.

### Basic description

Glial cells are non-neuronal cells in the central nervous system (brain and spinal cord) and the peripheral nervous system (PNS) **that act to support neurons, but** do not produce electrical impulses. **Instead, throughout the nervous system, they maintain homeostatic balance, myelinate neurons, provide structural support, and protect and nourish neurons They** perform many other important functions that keep the NS working properly, including:

- Help support and hold neurons in place.
- Protect neurons.
- Create insulation called **myelin,** which helps move nerve impulses.

- Repair neurons and help restore neuron function.
- Trim out dead neurons.
- Regulate neurotransmitters.

### Types

The above functions are performed by different types of glial cells:

- **Myelinating glia:** They produce the axon-insulating myelin sheath. These are called **oligodendrocytes** in the CNS and **Schwann's cells** in the PNS. [Remember these easily with the mnemonic "**COPS**" (Central - Oligodendrocytes; Peripheral – Schwann).]
- **Astrocytes** (CNS) and **satellite glial cells** (PNS): They both share the function of supporting and protecting neurons. [Mnemonic "**CAPS**" (Central – Astrocytes; Peripheral – Satellite).]
- Two other glial cell types are found in CNS exclusively as the PNS does not have a glial equivalent to microglia as the phagocytic role is performed by macrophages:
  - **Microglia:** These are the phagocytes of the CNS.
  - **Ependymal cells:** They line the ventricular system of the CNS.

## Take-away points

- Multiple system atrophy affects both the autonomic nervous system and the motor system. It behooves us therefore to understand these two systems.
- The nervous system is a network of neurons whose main feature is to generate, modulate, and transmit information between all the different parts of the human body. This property enables many important functions, such as the regulation of vital body functions, sensation, and body movements.
- The nervous system transmits signals between the brain and the rest of the body, including internal organs. In this way, its activity controls the ability to move, breathe, see, think, and more.
- The autonomic nervous system is internally regulated by integrated reflexes through the brainstem to the spinal cord and organs. It is unique in that it requires a sequential two-neuron efferent pathway. It is also externally regulated by a control system that acts largely unconsciously and regulates bodily functions.
- The autonomic nervous system is innervated by autonomic nerves that travel to organs throughout the body. Most organs receive parasympathetic supply by the vagus nerve and sympathetic supply by splanchnic nerves.
- Sympathetic and parasympathetic divisions of the autonomous nervous system typically function complementarily rather than antagonistically to each other. In

general, these two systems permanently modulate vital functions, in a usually semi-antagonistic fashion, to achieve homeostasis.

- The sympathetic nervous system promotes a 'fight-or-flight' response whereas the parasympathetic one promotes a 'rest-and digest' response. The enteric nervous system is the intrinsic nervous system of the gastrointestinal system. It has been described as "the second brain of the human body".
- Activation of the autonomous nervous system is critical for regulating the local and systemic immune-inflammatory responses and may influence acute stroke outcomes, offering therapeutic approaches for neurologic recovery after stroke.
- Two basic types of cells are present in the nervous system: neurons and glial cells.
- There are two types of neural processes that differ in structure and function: Axons and dendrites. In addition, every neuron has a single axon, while the number of dendrites varies. Accordingly, there are four structural **types of neurons: U**nipolar; pseudounipolar; bipolar; and multipolar.
- Different types of neurons control or perform different activities, including: motor neurons, sensory neurons, and others.
- The morphology of neurons makes them highly specialized to work with neural impulses. They generate, receive, and send these impulses onto other neurons and non-neural tissues.
- There are two types of neurons, named according to whether they send an electrical signal towards or away from the CNS: **Efferent** (motor or descending) and **afferent** (sensory or ascending).
- The site where an axon connects to another cell to pass the neural impulse is called a **synapse**. The synapse does not connect to the next cell directly. Instead, the impulse trigger the release of chemicals called neurotransmitters from the very end of an axon. These neurotransmitters bind to the effector cell's membrane, causing biochemical events to occur within that cell according to the orders sent by the central nervous system.
- White matter comprises the outermost layer of the spinal cord and the inner part of the brain whereas gray matter makes up the central part of the spinal cord, the outermost layer of the brain (cerebral cortex), and several subcortical nuclei of the brain deep in the cerebral cortex.
- When a neuron sends a message to another neuron, it sends an electrical signal down the length of its axon. At the end of the axon, the electrical signal changes to a chemical signal. The axon then releases the chemical signal with chemical messengers called **neurotransmitters** into the **synapse** - the space between the end of an axon and the tip of a dendrite from another neuron. The neurotransmitters move the signal through the synapse to the neighboring dendrite, which converts the chemical signal back into an electrical signal. The electrical signal then travels through the neuron and goes through the same conversion processes as it moves to neighboring neurons. Different kinds of neurons send different signals.

- A sidebar lists some of the most frequent conditions and disorders affecting the nervous system and their frequency of occurrence.

## Sidebar 3.1 - Conditions and disorders affecting the nervous system

Thousands of disorders and conditions can affect the nerves. An injured nerve has trouble sending or receiving a message. Nerve damage can happen in several ways, the most important causes include:

- **Accidental injury:** Nerves can be crushed, stretched, or cut in an accident. Car crashes and falls are common injuries that can damage nerves anywhere in the body.
- **Aging process:** In older individuals, neurons' signals may not travel as fast as they used to causing feelings of weakness and slower reflexes. Some people may lose sensation in their fingers, toes or other parts of their body.
- **Disease:** Many infections, cancers, and autoimmune diseases (diabetes, lupus, rheumatoid arthritis, etc.) can cause nervous system problems. This author has suggested that Alzheimer's disease and other neurological diseases are but autoimmune diseases. Diabetes can lead to diabetes-related neuropathy, causing tingling and pain in the legs and feet. A condition called multiple sclerosis attacks the myelin around nerves in the CNS.
- **Pressure:** If a nerve is pinched or compressed, it cannot get enough blood to do its job. Nerves can be pinched or trapped for many reasons, such as overuse (as in carpal tunnel syndrome), a tumor, structural problems like sciatica, and implant dentistry.
- **Stroke:** A stroke happens when one of the brain's blood vessels becomes blocked or suddenly bursts. Without enough blood, part of the brain dies and can no longer send messages via nerves. A stroke can cause nerve damage ranging from mild to severe.
- **Toxic substances:** Chemotherapy medicines, illegal drugs, excessive alcohol and poisonous substances can cause peripheral neuropathy or nerve damage. People with kidney disease are more likely to develop nerve damage because their kidneys have a hard time filtering out toxins.

Some causes of nerve damage occur more frequently than others. They include:

- **Diabetes:** This disorder of the endocrine system causes nerve damage called diabetes-related neuropathy. Around 30 million Americans have diabetes and nearly 50% of them have some nerve damage. Neuropathy of diabetes usually affects the arms, legs, hands, feet, fingers and toes.
- **Lupus:** About 1.5 million Americans live with lupus, and 15% of them have experienced nerve damage.
- **Rheumatoid arthritis:** People with rheumatoid arthritis can also develop neuropathy. Rheumatoid arthritis affects more than 1.3 million people in the U.S. It is one of the most common forms of arthritis.
- **Stroke:** Around 800,000 Americans have a stroke every year. Strokes occur more often in people over age 65.

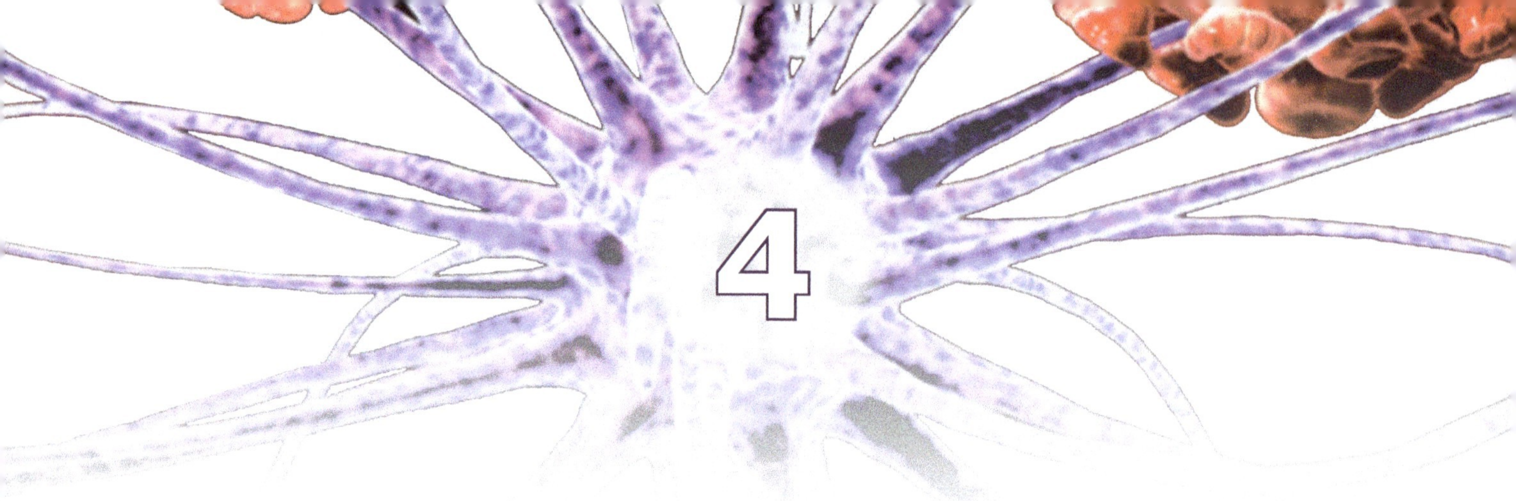

# 4

# Understanding the motor system

The motor system (MS) is a broad term used to describe all the central and peripheral structures that support motor functions, i.e. movement. Central structures include the cerebral cortex, brainstem, spinal cord, pyramidal system including the upper motor neurons, extrapyramidal system, cerebellum, and the lower motor neurons in the brainstem and the spinal cord. Peripheral structures may include skeletal muscles and neural connections with muscle tissues.

The MS is a biological system with close ties to the muscular system and the circulatory system. To achieve motor skill, it must accommodate the working state of the muscles, whether hot or cold, stiff or loose, as well as physiological fatigue.

## The pyramidal motor system (PMS)

### Structure and function

The pyramidal tracts are so named because they pass through the pyramids of the medulla oblongata. They include both the corticobulbar tract and the corticospinal tract. These are aggregations of efferent nerve fibers from the upper motor neurons involved in the control of motor functions (Figure 4.1):

- **Corticobulbar tract:** It conducts impulses from the brain to the cranial nerves. The nerves within this tract are involved in movement in muscles of the head. They are involved in swallowing, phonation, and movements of the tongue. By virtue of involvement with the facial nerve, this tract is also responsible for transmitting facial expression. With the exception of lower muscles of facial expression, all functions of the corticobulbar tract involve inputs from both sides of the brain.[
- **Corticospinal tract:** The nerves within this tract are involved in movement of muscles of the body. Because of the crossing-over of fibers, muscles are supplied by the side of the brain opposite to that of the muscle. This tract conducts impulses from the brain to the spinal cord. It

## Figure 4.1 – Motor and sensory pathways

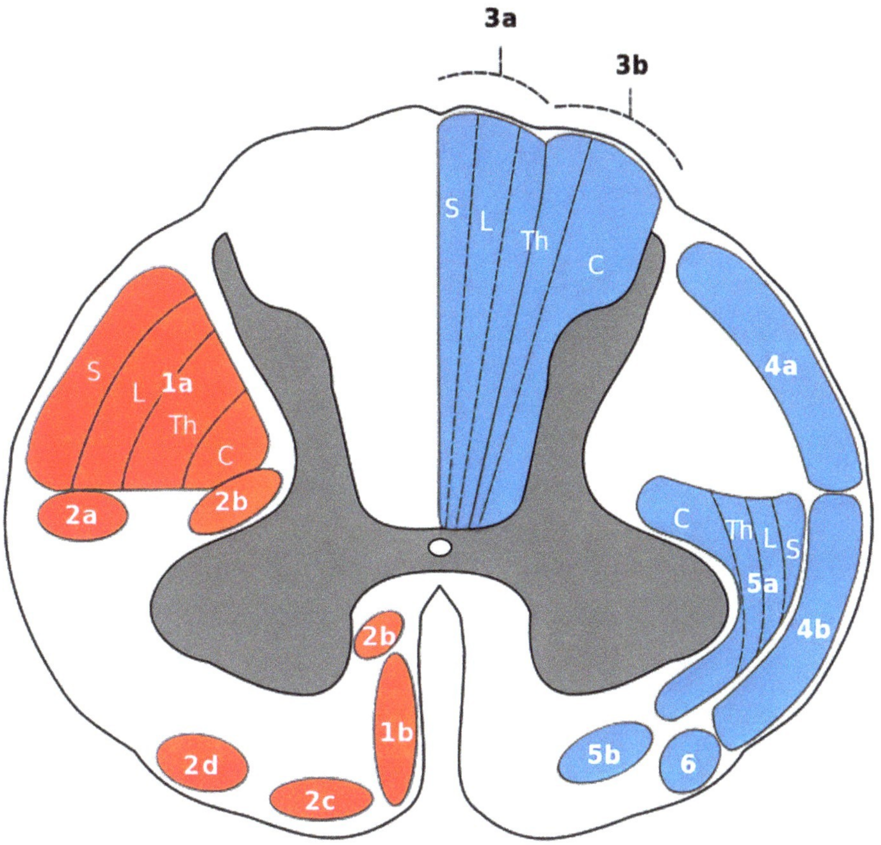


| **Motor and decending (efferent) pathways (left, red)** | **Sensory and ascending (afferent) pathways (right, blue)** |
|---|---|
| **1. Pyramidal Tracts** | **3. Dorsal Column Medial Lemniscus System** |
| 1a. Lateral corticospinal tract | 3a. Gracile fasciculus |
| 1b. Anterior corticospinal tract | 3b. Cuneate fasciculus |
| **2. Extrapyramidal Tracts** | **4. Spinocerebellar Tracts** |
| 2a. Rubrospinal tract | 4a. Posterior spinocerebellar tract |
| 2b. Reticulospinal tract | 4b. Anterior spinocerebellar tract |
| 2c. Vestibulospinal tract | **5. Anterolateral System** |
| 2d. Olivospinal tract | 5a. Lateral spinothalamic tract |
| | 5b. Anterior spinothalamic tract |
| Somatotopy Abbreviations: | |
| **S:** Sacral, **L: Lumbar** | 6. Spino-olivary fibers |
| **Th:** Thoracic, **C: Cervical** | |

**Figure 4.2 - The motor tract**

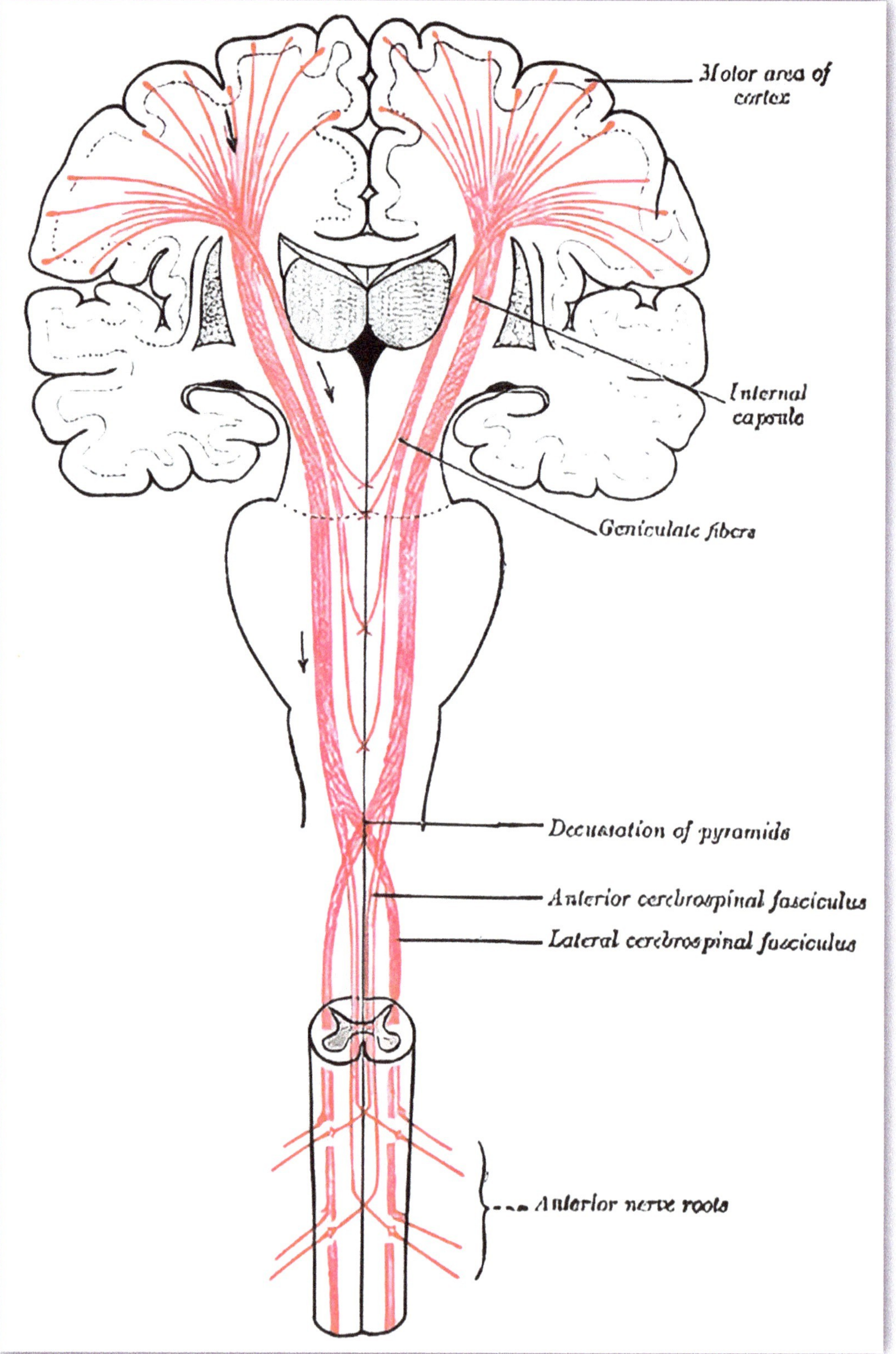


*Source: Gray Anatomy (plate 674)*

contains the axons of the pyramidal cells, the largest of which are the Betz cells located in the cerebral cortex.

**Figure 4.3 - Deep dissection of the brain-stem** (lateral view)

("pyramidal tract" visible in red, and "pyramidal decussation" labeled at lower right.)

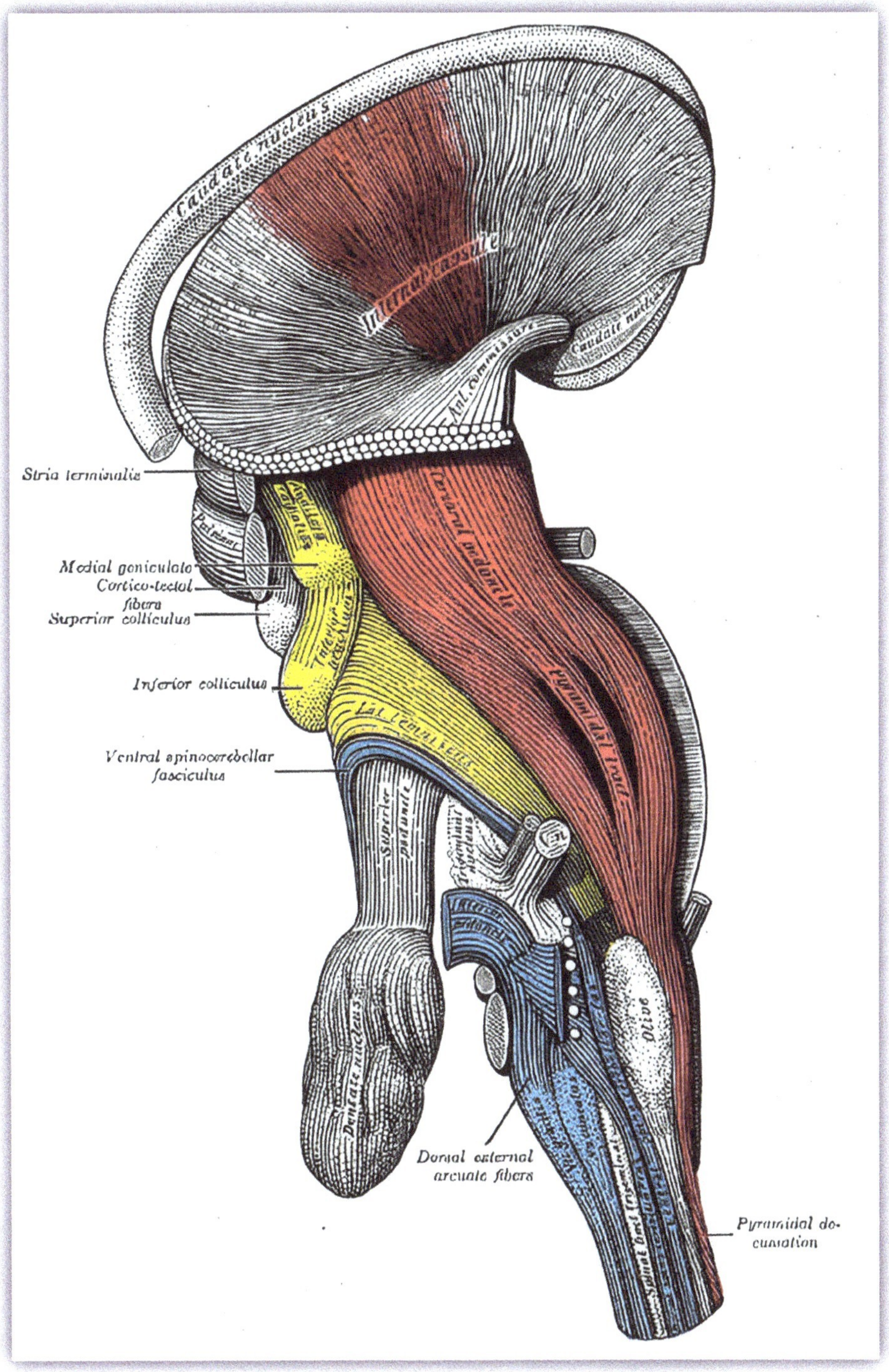


*Source: Gray Anatomy (plate 684)*

There are two types of neurons in the corticospinal tract:

- **Upper motor neurons (UMN):** The axons of these cells pass in the depth of the cerebral cortex to the corona radiata and then to the internal capsule, passing through the posterior branch of internal capsule and continuing to descend in the midbrain and the medulla oblongata.
- **Lower motor neurons (LMN):** They are located where the fibers of the corticospinal tract terminate and carry the motor impulses from the anterior horn to the voluntary muscles.

## The extrapyramidal motor system (ePMS)

The system is called extrapyramidal to distinguish it from the tracts of the motor cortex that reach their targets by traveling through the pyramids of the medulla. It refers specifically to tracts within the spinal cord that are involved in involuntary movement but not part of the pyramidal tracts. In anatomy, the ePMS is a part of the motor system network causing involuntary actions. The ePMS consists of motor-modulation systems, particularly the basal ganglia and cerebellum. The tracts include parts of the following (Figures 4.1-2):

- Rubrospinal tract.
- Pontine reticulospinal tract.
- Medullary reticulospinal tract.
- Lateral vestibulospinal tract.
- Tectospinal tract.

Their functions include the control of posture and muscle tone.

## Clinical significance

The clinical significance of the MS devolves from the following:

- **Signs and symptoms:** A few days after the injury to the upper motor neurons, a pattern of motor signs and symptoms appears, including spasticity, hyperactive reflexes, a loss of the ability to perform fine movements, and an extensor plantar response known as the Babinski sign. Symptoms generally occur alongside other sensory problems.
- **Motor neuron syndrome:** Damage to the fibers of the corticospinal tracts (anywhere along their course from the cerebral cortex to the lower end of the spinal cord) can cause an upper motor neuron syndrome.

- **Causes:** They may include disorders such as strokes, cerebral palsy, subdural hemorrhage, abscesses and tumors, neurodegenerative diseases such as MSA, inflammation such as meningitis and multiple sclerosis (MS), and trauma to the spinal cord including from slipped discs.
- **Hemiballismus or severe chorea:** These other severe disabling involuntary movements might exhaust the patient and become a life-threatening situation.
- **Pseudobulbar palsy:** If the corticobulbar tract is damaged on only one side, then only the lower face will be affected. However, if there is involvement of both the left and right tracts, then the result is pseudobulbar palsy. This causes problems with swallowing, speaking, and emotional lability.
- **Treatment:** In the past, this condition was treated by partial resection of the pyramidal tract either at the primary motor cortex or at the cerebral crus (pedunculotomy).

## Schwab & England Activities of Daily Living (ADL) Scale

**Schwab & England ADL scale is an** estimation of a person's abilities to carry-out daily living activities, that is the person's degree of independence. The person (or a family member) can self-assess this as:

**Table 4.1 -** Schwab & England Activities Daily Scale (ADL) scale

| | Performance | Notes |
|---|---|---|
| 10 | 100% | Completely independent. Able to do all chores without slowness, difficulty or impairment |
| 9 | 90% | Completely independent. Able to do all chores with some slowness, difficulty or impairment. May take twice as long to complete |
| 8 | 80% | Independent in most chores. Takes twice as long. Conscious of difficulty |
| 7 | 70% | Not completely independent. More difficulty with chores. 3 to 4 times longer to complete chores for some. May take large part of day for chores. slowing |
| 6 | 60% | Some dependency. Can do most chores, but very slowly and with much effort. Errors, some impossible |
| 5 | 50% | More dependent. Help with 1/2 of chores. Difficulty with everything |

| | | |
|---|---|---|
| **4** | **40%** | Very dependent. Can assist with all chores but few alone. |
| **3** | **30%** | With effort, now and then does a few chores alone or begins alone. Much help needed |
| **2** | **20%** | Nothing alone. Can do some slight help with some chores. Severe invalid state |
| **1** | **10%** | Totally dependent, helpless |
| **0** | **9%** | Vegetative functions such as swallowing, bladder/bowel function are not functioning. Bedridden |

## Take-away points

- The motor system describes all the peripheral and central structures that support motor functions. Peripheral structures may include skeletal muscles and neural connections with muscle tissues. Central structures include cerebral cortex, brainstem, spinal cord, pyramidal system including the upper motor neurons, extrapyramidal system, cerebellum, and the lower motor neurons in the brainstem and the spinal cord.

- The motor system is a biological system with close ties to the muscular system and the circulatory system.

- The pyramidal tracts include both the corticobulbar tract and the corticospinal tract. These are aggregations of efferent nerve fibers from the upper motor neurons that are involved in the control of motor functions of the body.

- The corticobulbar tract conducts impulses from the brain to the cranial nerves. It involves inputs from both sides of the brain.[

- The corticospinal tract conducts impulses from the brain to the spinal cord and is involved in movement of muscles of the body.

- There are two types of neurons in the corticospinal tract: Upper and lower motor neurons.

- The extrapyramidal system refers to tracts within the spinal cord and is involved in involuntary movement. It includes parts of the rubrospinal tract, pontine reticulospinal tract, medullary reticulospinal tract, lateral vestibulospinal tract, and tectospinal tract.

- The clinical significance of the motor system devolves from damage to the fibers of the corticospinal tracts. Motor signs and symptoms include spasticity, hyperactive reflexes, a loss of the ability to perform fine movements, and an extensor plantar response known as the Babinski sign. Symptoms generally occur alongside other sensory problems.

- Damage to the fibers of the corticospinal tracts can cause an upper motor neuron syndrome.
- Causes may include disorders such as strokes, cerebral palsy, subdural hemorrhage, abscesses and tumors, neurodegenerative diseases such as multiple system atrophy, inflammation such as meningitis and multiple sclerosis, and trauma to the spinal cord, including from slipped discs.
- Involvement of both the left and right tracts may result is pseudobulbar palsy.
- **Schwab & England ADL scale is an** estimation of a person's abilities to carry-out daily living activities. The person (or a family member) can self-assess it in a scale of 0% to 100%.

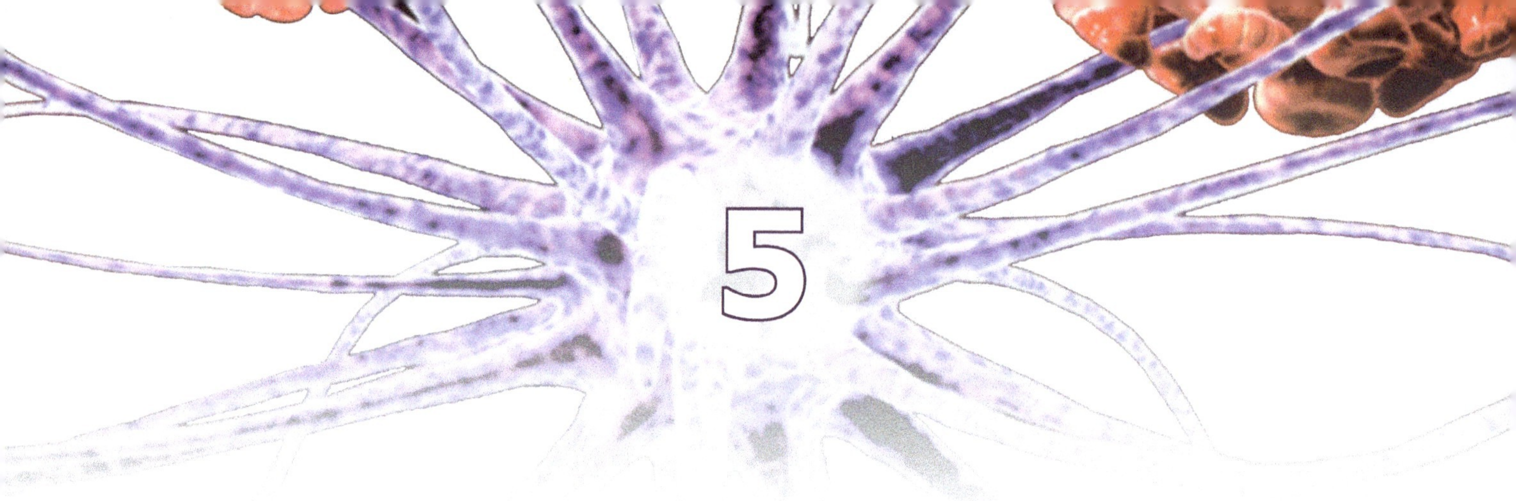

# 5

# What is MSA?

Multiple system atrophy (MSA) is a sporadic, progressive, and fatal neurodegenerative disorder characterized by autonomic failure (cardiovascular and/or urinary), parkinsonism, cerebellar impairment, and corticospinal signs with a median survival of 6-9 years. The combination of its symptoms shows that it affects both the (involuntary) autonomic nervous system (ANS) and the motor system (MS). ANS is that part of the nervous system that controls the body's automatic or regulating functions whereas, as its name implies, MS controls movement (see Chapters 3 and 4 for more details).

MSA causes the loss of nerve cells (neurons) in several parts of the brain, thus affecting the associated brain functions. It impacts the basal ganglia (Figure 5.1), the cerebellum (Figure 5.2) which is involved in controlling movement and some emotions as well as certain types of learning and memory, and the inferior olivary nucleus (Figure 5.3). Sidebar 5.1 provides more details on these several structures.

MSA is distinct from multiple system proteinopathy (MSP), a more common muscle-wasting syndrome. It is also different from multiple organ dysfunction (MOD) syndrome, and from multiple organ system (MOS) failure, an often-fatal complication of septic shock and other severe illnesses.

## Clinical description

MSA is an adult-onset disorder (>30 years, mean age 55-60 years). Clinical manifestations include autonomic failure (orthostatic hypotension, syncope), respiratory disturbances (sleep apnea, stridor, and inspiratory sighs), constipation, bladder dysfunction (early urinary incontinence), erectile dysfunction in males, and Raynaud's syndrome. In some cases, pyramidal signs (generalized hyper-reflexia and positive Babinski sign) are observed.

Neuropsychiatric features, oculomotor dysfunction, and sleep disturbances are also observed. They include apathy, anxiety, depression, rapid eye movement/sleep behavior disorder (REM/SBD), and periodic limb movements in sleep.

The disease was formerly called by such other names as:

- **Shy-Drager syndrome (SDS):** This term was used to describe MSA with predominant autonomic dysfunction. Now, it is no longer used as almost every patient is affected by autonomic or urinary dysfunction;
- **Olivopontocerebellar atrophy (OPCA):** This atrophy relates to the olivary nucleus, the basis pontis, and the cerebellum; and
- **Striatonigral degeneration (SND):** This degeneration refers to the efferent connection of the striatum with the substantia nigra.

## Symptoms

The varied symptoms of MSA reflect the death of different types of nerve cells in the brain and spinal cord and the progressive loss of associated functions. The symptoms caused by dysfunction of the ANS include, for example, bladder control, blood pressure, digestion, and temperature. On the other hand, the symptoms caused by the MS dysfunction cause motor control problems, rigidity of muscles, loss of coordination, and malfunction of internal body processes; which are commonly manifest as orthostatic hypotension, impotence, loss of sweating, dry mouth, and urinary retention and incontinence.

**Figure 5.1 – Brain structures affected by MSA: Basal ganglia and related structures**

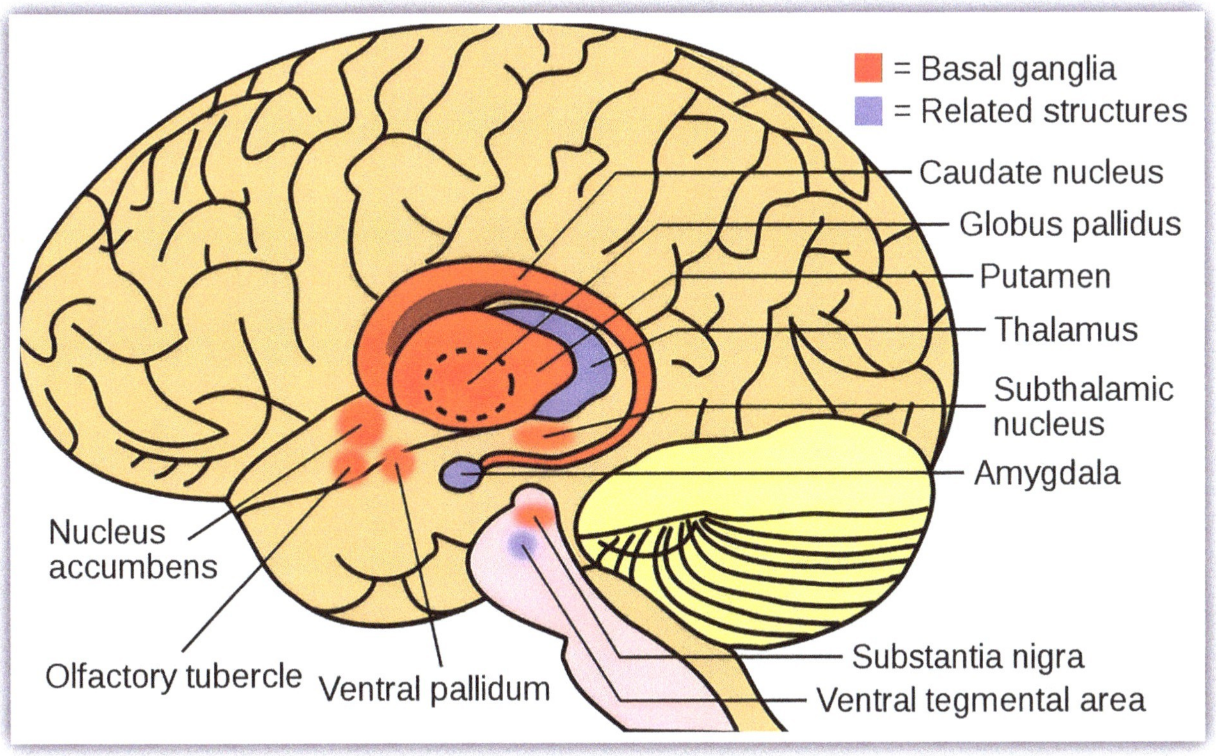


*Source: BrainCaudatePutamen.svg*

The initial symptoms are often difficult to distinguish from the symptoms of Parkinson's disease (PD). They may include:

- **Slowness of movement.**
- **Tremor or rigidity (stiffness).**
- **Clumsiness or coordination problems.**

**Figure 5.2 – Brain structures affected by MSA: Cerebellum**

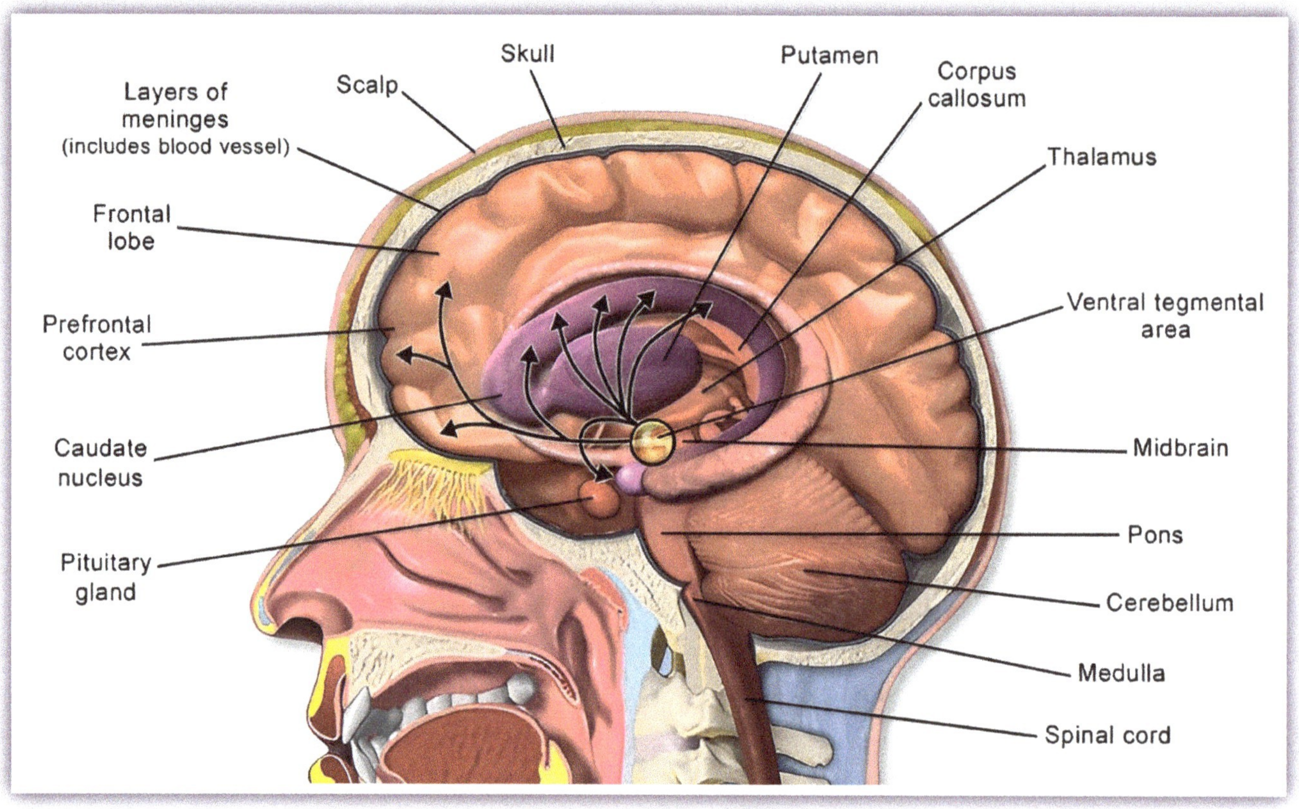


*Source: Bruce Baus*

- **Impaired speech.**
- **Croaky, quivering voice.**
- **Fainting or light-headedness due to orthostatic hypotension** (a condition in which blood pressure drops when rising from a seated or lying down position).

- **Bladder control problems:**, such as a sudden urge to urinate or difficulty emptying the bladder.

Additional symptoms of MSA may include:

- **Muscle contractures:** A chronic shortening of muscles or tendons around joints in the hands or limbs, which prevents the joints from moving freely.
- **Pisa syndrome:** An abnormal posture in which the body appears to be leaning to one side like the Leaning Tower of Pisa;
- **Antecollis:** A condition in which the neck bends forward and the head drops down.
- **Palsy of the vocal cords.**
- **Involuntary, uncontrollable sighing or gasping.**
- **Sleep disorders:** Including a tendency to act out dreams called REM/SBD (rapid eye movement/ sleep behavior disorder).
- **Emotional problems:** Such as feelings of anxiety or depression experienced by some.

## Presentation

The initial symptoms of MSA start around age 50-60 and affect about twice as many men as women. They advance rapidly over the course of five to ten years, with progressive loss of motor function and eventual confinement to bed. People with MSA often develop breathing problems while sleeping (sleep apnea), irregular heart rhythms, and pneumonia in later stages of the disease.

- The first symptoms are often autonomic and may predate recognition of motor manifestations. Orthostatic hypotension and, in men, erectile failure are among the first symptoms.
- The most common first sign of MSA is the appearance of an "akinetic-rigid syndrome" (i.e. slowness of initiation of movement resembling Parkinson's disease - PD) found in 62% at first presentation. Other common signs at onset include problems with balance (cerebellar ataxia) found in 22% at first presentation, followed by genito-urinary symptoms (9%): both men and women often experience urgency, frequency, incomplete bladder emptying, or an inability to pass urine (retention). About 1 in 5 MSA patients experience a fall in their first year of disease. For men, the first sign can be erectile dysfunction. Women have also reported reduced genital sensitivity.
- Patients may also present with parkinsonian symptoms, often with a poor or temporary response to *Levodopa* therapy, or cerebellar dysfunction.

- Corticospinal tract dysfunction may occur but is not usually a major presentation.
- When the disorder presents with non-autonomic features, imbalance caused by cerebellar or extrapyramidal abnormalities is the most common feature.
- Constipation may also occur.

**Figure 5.3 - Brain structures affected by MSA: Olivary nucleus**

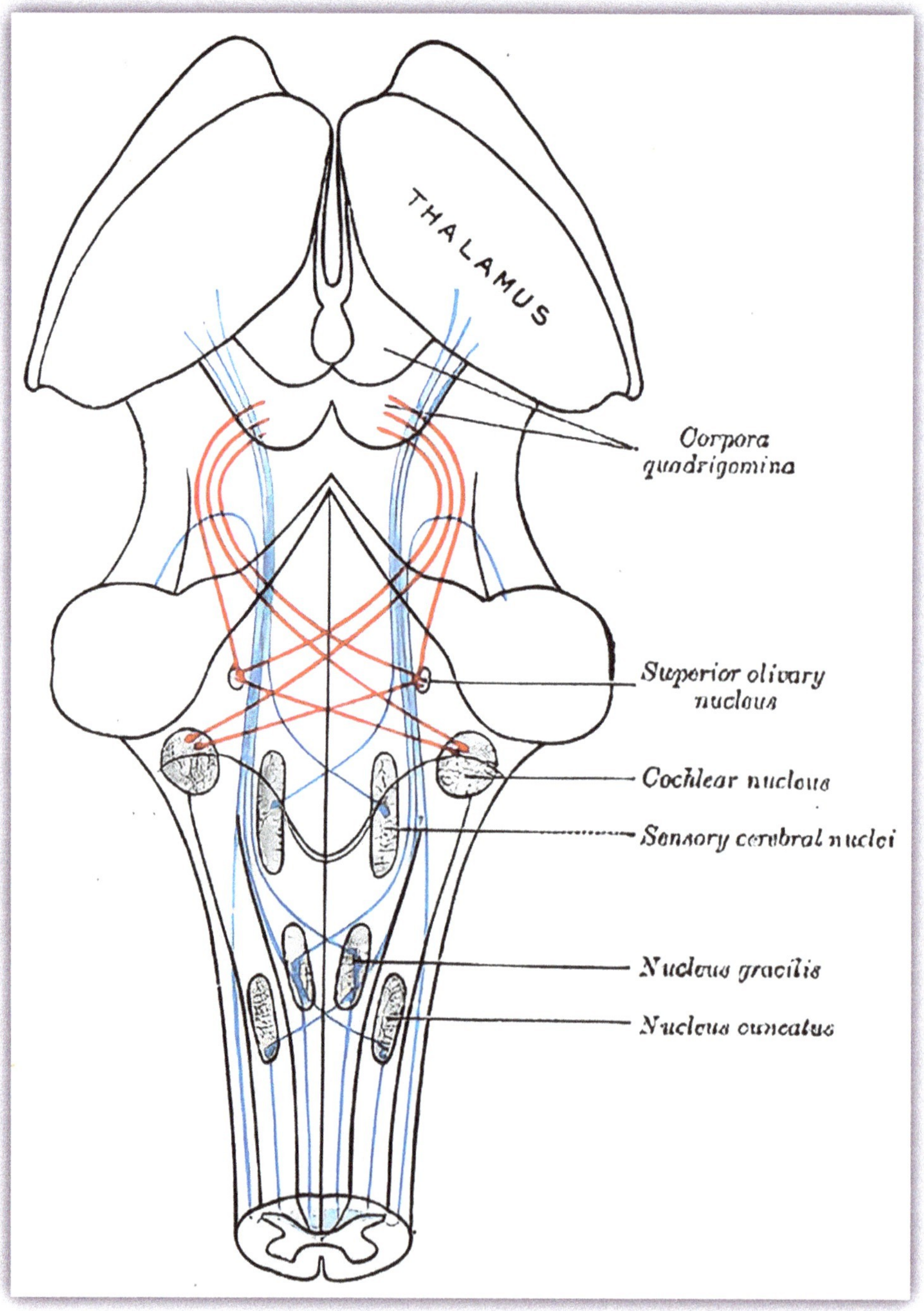


*Source: Gray Anatomy Plate – Gray713.png*

1. There may possibly be mild intellectual impairment. This is particularly so in older patients with greater physical disability.
2. Other neuropsychiatric problems may include depression, insomnia, daytime sleepiness, restless legs, hallucinations, and dementia.

## Progression

MSA tends to progress more rapidly than PD, and most people with MSA will require an aid for walking, such as a cane or walker, within a few years after symptoms begin.

As the disease progresses one of three groups of symptoms predominates. These are:

- **Parkinsonism:** Slow and stiff movement; writing becomes small and spidery.
- **Cerebellar dysfunction:** Difficulty coordinating movement and balance.
- **Autonomic nervous system dysfunction:** Impaired automatic body functions, including one, some, or all of the following:
    - Postural or orthostatic hypotension, resulting in dizziness or fainting upon standing up.
    - Urinary incontinence or urinary retention.
    - Impotence.
    - Constipation.
    - Vocal cord paralysis.
    - Dry mouth and dry skin.
    - Trouble regulating body temperature due to sweating deficiency in all parts of the body.
    - Loud snoring, abnormal breathing or inspiratory stridor during sleep.
    - Other sleep disorders including sleep apnea, REM/SBD.
    - Double vision.
    - Muscle twitches.
    - Cognitive impairment.

## Take-away points

- Multiple system atrophy (MSA) is a sporadic, progressive, and fatal neurodegenerative disorder characterized by a combination of symptoms that affect both the (involuntary) autonomic nervous system that controls the body's automatic or regulating functions and the motor system that controls movement.
- MSA causes the loss of nerve cells (neurons) in several parts of the brain, thus affecting the associated brain functions. It impacts the basal ganglia, the cerebellum, and the inferior olivary nucleus.
- MSA is distinct from multiple system proteinopathy, multiple organ dysfunction, and multiple organ system failure.
- MSA was formerly known as Shy-Drager syndrome, olivopontocerebellar atrophy, and striatonigral degeneration, but these other names are either not used any longer or rarely used.
- The varied symptoms of MSA reflect the death of different types of nerve cells in the brain and spinal cord and the progressive loss of associated functions. The initial symptoms are often difficult to distinguish from the initial symptoms of Parkinson's disease. Additional symptoms may include: Muscle contractures; the Pisa syndrome; antecollis; palsy of the vocal cords; involuntary, uncontrollable sighing or gasping; sleep disorders; sleep behavior disorder; and emotional problems such as feelings of anxiety or depression.
- The initial symptoms of MSA start around age 50-60 and affect about twice as many men as women. They advance rapidly over the course of five to ten years. They tend to progress more rapidly than Parkinson's disease.
- Sidebars 5.1 – 5.4 will present, respectively, the brain structures affected by MSA, What is a rare disease?, pure autonomic failure phenoconversion to other alpha-synucleopathies, and the European Union Orphanet

### Sidebar 5.1 –Brain structures affected by MSA

#### The basal ganglia (BG) or basal nuclei (BN)

The BG or BN (in red color in Figure 5.1) are a group of subcortical nuclei of varied origin situated between the forebrain and the midbrain. They are strongly interconnected with the cerebral cortex (in beige color), the thalamus (blue/purple color), and the brainstem as well as several other brain areas. They are associated with a variety of functions, including control of voluntary motor movements, learning (procedural, habit, conditional), eye movements, cognition, and emotion.

Defined functionally, the main BG components are the:

- **Striatum:** Consisting of both the dorsal striatum (caudate nucleus and putamen) and the ventral striatum (nucleus accumbens and olfactory tubercle).
- **Globus pallidus.**
- **Ventral pallidum.**
- **Substantia nigra.**
- **Subthalamic nucleus.**

(See all these brain components in the different red areas of Figure 5.1).

Each of these components has a complex internal anatomical and neurochemical organization. Thus, the:

- **Striatum (dorsal and ventral):** It is the largest component, receiving input from many brain areas beyond the BG, but only sending output to other components of the BG.
- **Globus pallidus:** It receives input from the striatum and sends inhibitory output to a number of motor-related areas.
- **Substantia nigra:** It is the source of the striatal input of the neurotransmitter dopamine, which plays an important role in basal ganglia function.
- **Subthalamic nucleus:** It receives input mainly from the striatum and cerebral cortex and projects to the globus pallidus.

It has been hypothesized that the BG are not only responsible for motor action selection (that is helping to decide which of several possible behaviors to execute at any given time) but also for the selection of more cognitive actions.

The BG are of major importance for normal brain function and behavior. Their dysfunction results in a wide range of neurological conditions including disorders of behavior control and movement, as well as cognitive deficits that are similar to those that result from damage to the prefrontal cortex.

Behavioral disorders include:

- Tourette's syndrome (TS).
- Obsessive–compulsive disorder (OCD).
- Addiction.

Movement disorders include:

- PD, which involves degeneration of the dopamine-producing cells in the substantia nigra.
- Huntington's disease (HD), which primarily involves damage to the striatum.
- Dystonia. More rarely:
- Hemiballismus.

The BG have a limbic sector whose components are assigned distinct names, including the:

- **Nucleus accumbens (NA).**
- **Ventral pallidum (VP).**
- **Ventral tegmental area (VTA):** This limbic part plays a central role in reward-learning as well as cognition. There is also evidence implicating overactivity of the VTA dopaminergic projection in schizophrenia.

## The cerebellum

The cerebellum (Latin for "little brain") is a major feature of the hindbrain (see Figure 5.2). It appears as a separate structure attached to the bottom of the brain, tucked underneath the cerebral hemispheres. It includes several types of neurons with a highly regular arrangement, the most important being Purkinje cells and granule cells. This complex neural organization gives rise to a massive signal-processing capability.

Although usually smaller than the cerebrum, the cerebellum plays an important role in motor control. While definitely associated with movement-related functions, it may also be involved in some cognitive functions (such as attention and language) as well as emotional control (such as regulating fear and pleasure responses). It does not initiate movement, but contributes to coordination, precision, and accurate timing. Cerebellar damage produces disorders in fine movement, equilibrium, posture, and motor learning. In addition to its direct role in motor control, the cerebellum is necessary for several types of motor learning, most notably learning to adjust to changes in sensorimotor relationships.

# The olivary nucleus (ON)

The ON is an oval shaped prominence (olive) in the medulla (see Figure 5.3). It is divided into two parts with two different functions. The superior olive complex (SOC) is a part of the pons in the cerebellum; it functions in the auditory pathway. The inferior olive complex (IOC) rests below that structure, and functions as a part of the cerebellar motor learning pathway.

## Superior olivary complex (SOC)

The SOC can be further divided into the medial and lateral superior olive, which serve slightly different functions in auditory processing. They are both paired structures, meaning one exists on each half of the spinal cord. Collectively, the medial and lateral superior olive serve to help the person identify which direction an auditory stimulus is coming from, the left or the right side of the head. The medial superior olive determines the direction of an incoming sound whereas the lateral superior olive identifies the origin of a sound.

## Inferior olivary complex (IOC)

The IOC is located close to the cerebellum and functions as a relay between the spinal cord and cerebellum. it is a structure found in the medulla oblongata underneath the SOC. It coordinates signals from the spinal cord to the cerebellum to regulate motor coordination and learning. These connections have been shown to be tightly associated, as degeneration of either the cerebellum or the IOC results in degeneration of the other.

Injury to the cerebellum almost always results in inferior olive injury, and inferior olive injury likewise results in cerebellar injury. Such lesions lead to a difficulty with learning complex coordination tasks. On the level of neural circuitry, the inferior olive receives GABA-ergic projections from various other structures, including the deep cerebellar nuclei and the parasolitary nucleus (adaptive balance in posterior cerebellum).

Some disorders affect the inferior olive and cerebellum along with other brain structures. For instance, progressive supranuclear palsy (PSP) is a disease associated with a problem in the tau-protein that normally functions to maintain the microtubule structure of cells. In PSP, a person experiences bradykinesia (slowed movements) and difficulty with gait and posture during locomotion. Sometimes, they may also exhibit psychological symptoms such as dementia or difficulty with speech. Because the symptoms may appear similar to other neurodegenerative disorders such as PD and Alzheimer's disease (AD), PSP may be under-diagnosed. It also is involved heavily in signaling of the spino-olivary tract, which carries information about proprioception from the muscles up the spinal cord. This pathway is sometimes also called Helwig's tract.

Another important feature of the inferior olivary nucleus is related to the production of sex hormones in the body. For example, the inferior olive produces the enzyme aromatase, which is the primary enzyme that converts testosterone into estradiol.

## Sidebar 5.2 – What is a rare disease?

Over 6,000 - 7,**000** different rare diseases have been identified to date of which MSA is but one.

### What is a rare disease?

In the U.S., a rare disorder has been arbitrarily defined as a disease or condition that affects fewer than 200,000 Americans. By contrast, the European Union (EU) considers a disease as rare when it affects **less than 1 in 2,000** citizens.Cumulatively, they affect more than 30 million Americans and **3.5% – 5.9%** of the worldwide population. **72%** of rare diseases are genetic whilst others are the result of infections, allergies, and environmental causes.

Rare diseases are characterized by a wide diversity of symptoms and **signs that vary not only from disease to disease but also from patient to patient** suffering from the same disease.

Due to the low prevalence of each disease, medical expertise is rare, knowledge is scarce, care offerings inadequate, and research limited. Despite their great overall number, **rare disease patients are the orphans of health systems**, often denied diagnosis, treatment, and the benefits of research.

Relatively common symptoms can hide underlying rare diseases, leading to **misdiagnosis and delaying treatment**. Typically disabling, the quality of life of a person living with a rare disease is affected by the lack or loss of autonomy due to the chronic, progressive, degenerative, and frequently life-threatening aspects of the disease.

The fact that there are often no existing effective cures adds to the **high level of pain and suffering** endured by patients and their families.

Rare diseases not only affect the person diagnosed – they also **impact families, friends, care takers, and society as a whole**.

### The NORD rare disease database

The National Organization for Rare Disorders (NORD) is committed to the identification, treatment, and cure of rare diseases through education, advocacy, research, and service programs. It has developed a database covering more than 1,200 rare disorders. There, rare disease reports can be explored, including: Information on symptoms, causes, treatments, clinical trials, and sources of help such as patient advocacy organizations. Each report has a list of references, such as textbooks, articles, and government agency reports.

## Sidebar 5.3 – Pure autonomic failure conversion to other alpha-synucleopathies

Pure autonomic failure (PAF) is a disorder of the autonomic system. In a study of 74 subjects at five U.S. medical centers (Harvard University, Mayo Clinic in Rochester, the National Institutes of Health, New York University, and Vanderbilt University), about one-third (34%) developed dementia with Lewy bodies (DLB) (n=13), Parkinson's disease (PD) (n=6), or multiple system atrophy (MSA) (n=6) over four years. Overall, 14% of people converted from PAF to one of these three alpha-synculein disorders each year. Many of those who converted had REM sleep behavior disorder (RBD).

Other symptoms were associated with who converted to MSA, DLB, or PD:

### Phenoconversion

#### To MSA

On average, patients who phenoconverted from PAF to MSA had PAF symptoms for fewer than five years, a younger age at onset of autonomic failure, severe bladder/bowel dysfunction, preserved olfaction, and a cardiac chronotropic response upon tilt > 10 beats per minute.

#### To PD or DLB

On average, patients who phenoconverted to PD or DLB had PAF symptoms for nearly ten years, decreased olfaction, and a lesser chronotropic response to tilt. Those who retained the PAF phenotype had very low plasma norepinephrine levels, slow resting heart rate, no RBD, and preserved smell.

## Sidebar 5.4 - The European Union Orphanet nomenclature of rare diseases

### Nomenclature

The EU maintains the Orphanet nomenclature of rare diseases, which is essential in improving the visibility of rare diseases in health and research information systems. Each disease in Orphanet is attributed a unique and stable identifier (called the **ORPHAcode**).

Orphanet uses the European definition of a rare disease, as defined by the European Union Regulation on Orphan Medicinal Products (1999), that being "a disease that affects not more than 1 person per 2000 in the European population".

The Orphanet rare disease nomenclature is comprised of a heterogeneous typology of entities of decreasing extension, including:

- **Groups of disorders.**
- **Disorders:** A disorder in the database can be a disease, a malformation syndrome, a clinical syndrome, a morphological or a biological anomaly, or a particular clinical situation (in the course of a disorder).
- **Sub-types:** The disorders are further divided into clinical, etiological or histopathological sub-types.

### Orphadata

**Orphadata is a database using the Orphanet Nomenclature, its Files for Coding in a range of languages, and the EU Classification of Rare Diseases. One can access aggregated datasets from Orphanet. For this purpose, one has to enter a** requested disease name, ORPHAcode, a gene symbol/name, and an MIM (online Mendelian Inheritance in Man) number or ICD-10 ($10^{th}$ edition of WHO's International Classification of Diseases).

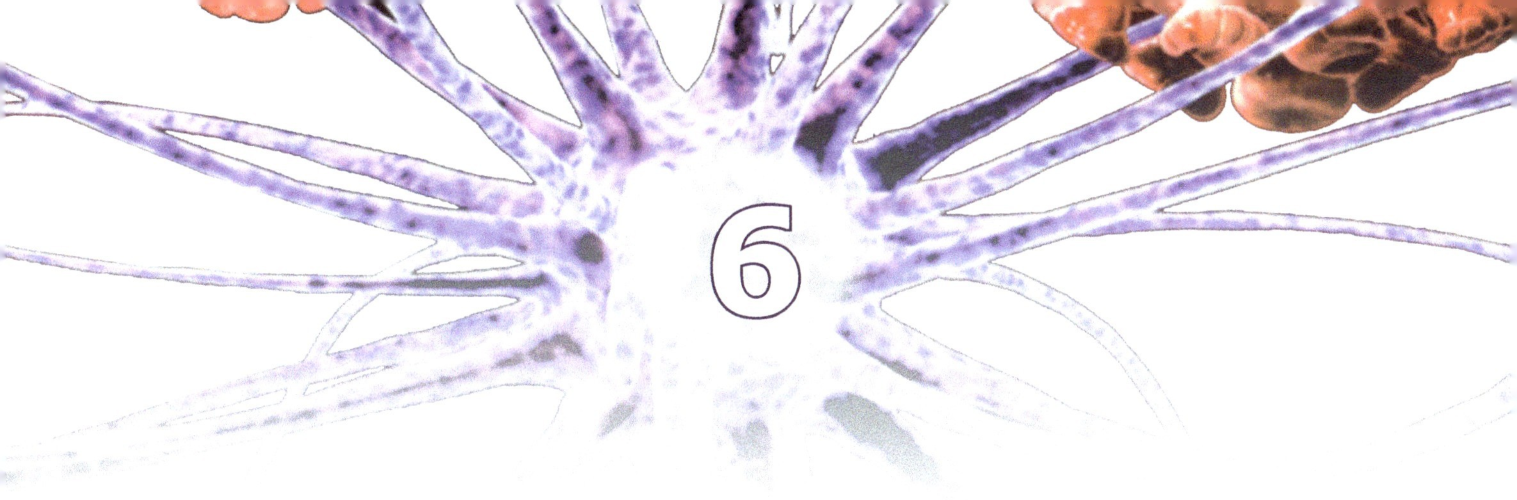

# 6

# Types and variants of MSA

MSA is one of several neurodegenerative diseases known as synucleinopathies (Figure 6.1). They have in common an abnormal accumulation of the α(alpha)-synuclein protein in various parts of the brain. Other synucleinopathies include Parkinson's disease (PD), the Lewy body dementias (LBD), and other rarer conditions.

**Figure 6.1 - Alpha synuclein immunohistochemistry showing many glial inclusions seen in MSA**

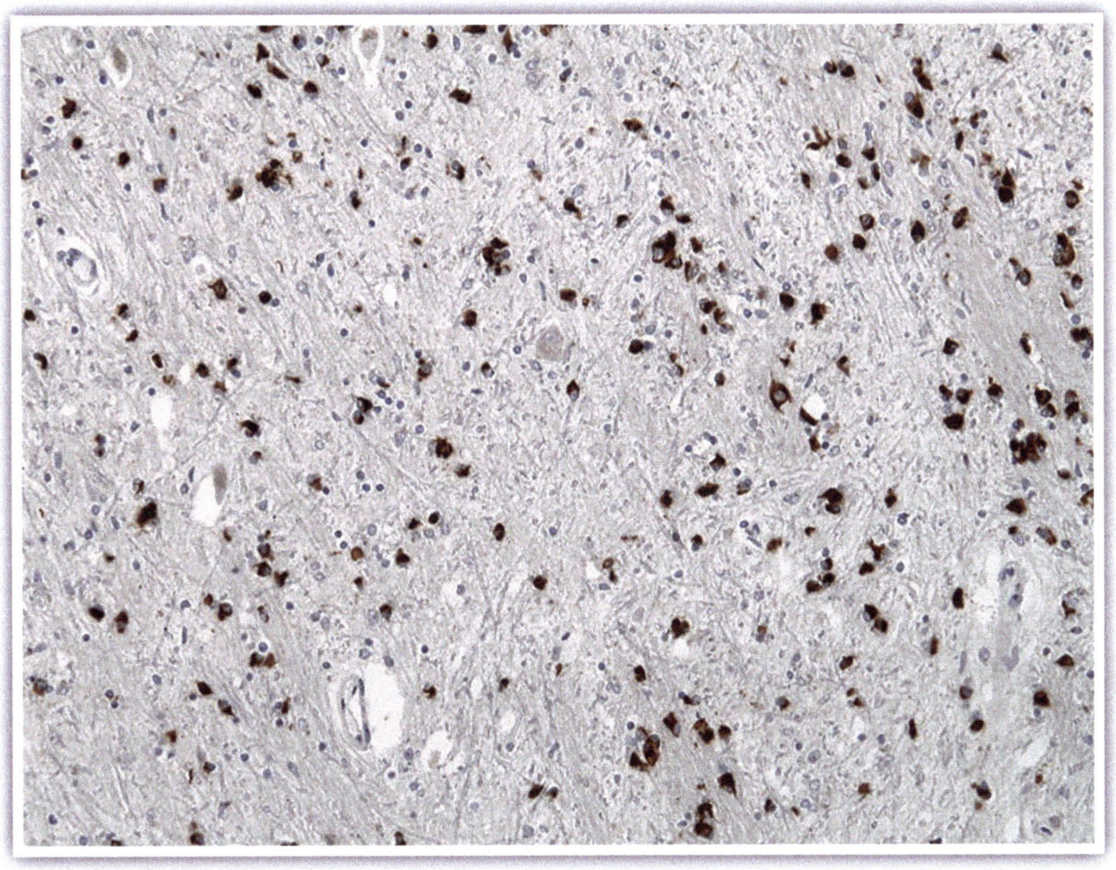

*Reference: Jensflorian*

## Old terminology

Historically, many terms were used to refer to this disorder based on the predominant symptoms presented, including striatonigral degeneration (SND), olivopontocerebellar atrophy (OPCA), and Shy–Drager syndrome (SDS). These terms were discontinued by consensus in 1996 and replaced with MSA and its subtypes. Awareness of these older terms and their definitions is nonetheless helpful to understanding the relevant literature prior to 1996.

Table 6.1 describes the characteristics and modern names of these conditions:

**Table 6.1 – Characteristics and modern names of synucleinopathies**

| Historical name | Characteristics | Modern name & Abbreviations |
| --- | --- | --- |
| **Striatonigral degeneration** | Predominating Parkinson's-like symptoms | MSA-P<br>"P" = Parkinsonian subtype |
| **Sporadic olivopontocerebellar atrophy** | o Progressive ataxia of the gait and arms<br>o Dysarthria | MSA-C<br>"C" = Cerebellar dysfunction type |
| **Shy-Drager syndrome** | o Parkinsonism<br>o More pronounced failure of the autonomic nervous system | No modern equivalent<br>Before 1998, consensus referred to it as MSA-A<br>"A" = Autonomic dysfunction subtype |

## MSA types and variants

The current terminology and diagnostic criteria for the disease were established at the 2007 Second Consensus Statement, which defined two categories of MSA based on the predominant symptoms at the time of evaluation. Although the disease begins as one of these types, symptoms of the other type eventually develop. After about 5 years, symptoms tend to be similar regardless of which disorder developed first. They are:

### MSA-P

MSA is referred to as of the *MSA-P type* (indicated by the 'P') if parkinsonian features predominate (so-called parkinsonism: Bradykinesia, rigidity, irregular jerky postural tremor, and postural instability). It is defined as MSA where extrapyramidal features predominate. It is a rare condition that causes symptoms similar to Parkinson's disease (PD) except that tremor often does not develop. However, people with MSA-P have more widespread damage to the part of the nervous system that controls important functions such as heart rate, blood pressure, and sweating. Only about 9% of MSA patients with tremor exhibit a true parkinsonian pill-rolling tremor. The symptoms include slow movement, rigid muscles (stiffness), tremor, postural instability, low blood pressure when a person stands (orthostatic hypotension), problems with urination, and constipation. Other symptoms may include problems of balance, coordination, and ANS dysfunction. Those with MSA generally show little response to medications used to treat PD (such as *Levodopa*).

## Clinical description

The mean age of disease onset is 55 to 60 years. MSA-P is characterized by a number of the following symptoms:

- **Parkinsonism:** Bradykinesia, rigidity, irregular jerky tremor, and postural instability.
- **Autonomic failure:** In the form of bladder dysfunction (including early urinary incontinence) and/or orthostatic hypotension. The presence of autonomic failure is mandatory for the diagnosis of MSA-P.
- **Other autonomic features:** Dysphonia, dysphagia, respiratory disturbances such as sleep apnea, stridor and inspiratory sighs, as well as constipation and sexual dysfunction.
- **Some cerebellar signs:** Gait and limb ataxia, oculomotor dysfunction, and dysarthria.
- **Abnormal postures:** Camptocormia, Pisa syndrome, and disproportionate antecollis are frequently observed.
- **Neuropsychiatric features:** Rapid eye movement/sleep behavior disorder (REM/SBD), periodic limb movements in sleep (PLMS), depression, apathy and anxiety.
- **Pyramidal signs:** Generalized hyper-reflexia with a positive Babinski sign may also be observed in some cases.
- **Early-onset Levodopa-induced effects:** Orofacial and craniocervical dystonia.

## MSA-C

MSA is referred to as of the *MSA-C type* (indicated by the 'C') if features of cerebellar dysfunction (such as gait and limb ataxia, oculomotor dysfunction, and dysarthria) predominate. It used to be known as olivopontocerebellar atrophy (OPCA). It is a rare disease that causes areas deep in the brain, just above the spinal cord, to shrink. "Cerebellar" reflects a part of the brain involved with coordination. MSA-C features primary symptoms like ataxia (problems with balance and coordination), difficulty swallowing, speech abnormalities or a quivering voice, and abnormal eye movements. It is characterized by loss of coordination and difficulty maintaining balance. The loss of muscular coordination results from a disease in the cerebellum, that part of the brain that is responsible for movement coordination such as problems with balance and coordination, difficulty swallowing and speaking, and abnormal eye movements.

The predominant motor feature can change with time and patients with cerebellar ataxia can develop increasingly severe parkinsonian features which dominate the clinical presentation.

## Clinical description

The mean age of disease onset is 55 to 60 years. MSA-C is characterized by a number of the following symptoms:

- **Gait ataxia:** The most typical early symptom.
- **Autonomic dysfunction:** Bladder dysfunction including early urinary incontinence, orthostatic hypotension, and constipation. Raynaud's syndrome occurs early and is mandatory for the diagnosis of MSA-C.
- **Additional features:** They include dysphonia and other cerebellar features such as limb ataxia and occulomotor dysfunction (sustained gaze-evoked nystagmus, positional down-beat nystagmus).
- **Parkinsonism:** All patients develop at least some parkinsonian signs (bradykinesia, rigidity, irregular jerky postural tremor) in the course of the disease.
- **Pyramidal signs:** Generalized hyper-reflexia and, in some cases, positive Babinski sign may be observed. Respiratory disturbances (sleep apnea, stridor and inspiratory sighs) and night time sleep disturbances, including REM/SBD) and PLMS are frequently observed.

## MSA variants

MSA-P and MSA-C can be present in any combination. A variant with combined features of MSA and Lewy bodies dementia (LBD) may also exist. There have been occasional instances of frontotemporal lobar degeneration (FTLD) associated with MSA.

There may also be other autonomic dysfunctions, particularly urogenital, and corticospinal features along the axis connecting the cortex and the spine.

## Take-away points

- MSA is one of several neurodegenerative diseases known as synucleinopathies, having in common an abnormal accumulation of the α(alpha)-synuclein protein in various parts of the brain.
- Historically, many terms were used to refer to MSA, including striatonigral degeneration, olivopontocerebellar atrophy, and Shy–Drager syndrome. While they were discontinued

by consensus in 1996 and replaced with MSA and its subtypes, awareness of these older terms is helpful to understanding the relevant literature prior to 1996.

- There are two main variants of the disease based on which symptoms occur first: MSA-P ("P" = parkinsonism) if parkinsonian features predominate (so-called parkinsonism) and MSA-C ("C" = Cerebellar) if features of cerebellar dysfunction or ataxia predominate. There may also be other autonomic dysfunctions, particularly urogenital, and corticospinal features.
- A variant with combined features of MSA and Lewy bodies dementia may also exist. There have also been occasional instances of frontotemporal lobar degeneration associated with MSA.

### Sidebar 6.1 – The constellation of brain diseases

To provide a perspective, Tables 6.2 through 6.5 below are a synoptic overview of the brain diseases/disorders. They are for a proper contextual clinical background of the contributions reported in this book. Pathologies due to inflammation, encephalopathy (degenerative, demyelinating, episodic/paroxysmal, cerebrospinal fluid, and other causes), spinal cord/myelopathy, and/or degenerative encephalopathy and spinal cord/myelopathy have been tabulated. (Those diseases mentioned in this volume appear as black-boldfaced whereas multiple system atrophy appears as red-boldfaced.)

## Diseases of the central nervous system due to inflammation

These are shown in Table 6.2.

**Table 6.2 – Diseases of the central nervous system: Inflammation**

| Pathology | Organ | Disorders/diseases |
|---|---|---|
| **Inflammation** | **Brain** | o Amoebic<br>o Brain abscess<br>o Cavernous sinus thrombosis<br>**o Encephalitis:**<br>- Herpes viral<br>- *Lethargica*<br>- Limbic<br>- Viral |
| | **Spinal cord** | o Epidural abscess<br>o Myelitis:<br>- Polio<br>- Transverse<br>o Tropical spastic paraparesis |

| | | |
|---|---|---|
| | **Either/both** | o Acute/disseminated<br>o Myalgic<br>o Myelitis:<br>- Encephalo-Meningo<br>**o Myeloneuritis** |

*Source: A. L. Fymat (2017)*

## Diseases of the central nervous system due to brain encephalopathy

Likewise, Table 6.3 lists the disorders/diseases due to encephalopathy whether degenerative, demyelinating, episodic/paroxysmal, cerebrospinal fluid, and other causes. Further, Table 6.4 indicates similarly the disorders/diseases due to spinal cord/myelopathy. Lastly, Table 6.5 shows the similar pathologies due to degenerative encephalopathy and/or spinal cord/myelopathy.

**Table 6.3 - Diseases of the central nervous system: Brain encephalopathy**

| Pathology | Characteristics | Disease category | Disorders/diseases |
|---|---|---|---|
| **Encephalopathy** | **Degenerative** | **Extrapyramidal & movement disorders** | o Akathisia<br>o Athetosis<br>o Basal ganglia disease<br>o Blepharospasm<br>**o Chorea**<br>o Choreoathetosis<br>**o Dyskinesia**<br>**o Dystonia**<br>o Epilepsy<br>- Myoclonic<br>o **Hemiballismus**<br>o Huntington's disease<br>o Meige's syndrome<br>o Myoclonus<br>o NMS<br>o OA<br>**o Parkinson's disease**<br>**- Parkinsonism**<br>o PKAN<br>o Postencephalitic<br>**o Palsy: Progressive supranuclear (PSP)**<br>o Restless legs<br>o Spasmodic torticollis<br>o Status dystonicus<br>o Stiff person<br>**o Striatonigral degeneration**<br>**o Tauopathy**<br>**o Tremor**<br>**- Essential**<br>- Intentional |

| | | | |
|---|---|---|---|
| | | **Dementia** | **o Alzheimer's disease (AD)**<br>o Aphasia: Primary progressive (PPA)<br>**o Frontotemporal lobar degeneration: (FLD)**<br>**o Dementia:**<br>- Early onset<br>**- Frontotemporal**<br>- Juvenile<br>**- Lewy body dementias**<br>**- with Lewy bodies**<br>- Late onset<br>- Pugilistica<br>**- Vascular**<br>**o Parkinson's disease (PD)**<br>**o Pick's disease**<br>**o Synucleinopathy**<br>**o Tauopathy** |
| | | **Mitochondrial disease** | o Leigh's syndrome |
| | **Demyelinating** | o Alpers' disease<br>o Autoimmune:<br>**- Multiple sclerosis**<br>**- Neuromyelitis optica**<br>- Schilder's disease<br>o Hereditary:<br>- Adrenoleukodystrophy<br>- Alexander's disease<br>- CAMFAK syndrome<br>- Canavan's disease<br>- Krabbe's disease<br>- Marchiafava–Bignami disease<br>- MFC<br>- ML<br>- Myelinolysis: central pontine<br>- PMD<br>- VWM | |
| | **Episodic/ paroxysmal** | **Seizure/epilepsy** | o Dravet's syndrome<br>- Focal<br>- Generalized<br>o Epilepsy:<br>- Myoclonic<br>- Status *epilepticus*<br>o Lennox-Gastaut syndrome |

| | | | |
|---|---|---|---|
| | | **Headache** | o Migraine<br>- Cluster<br>- Familial<br>- Tension |
| | | **Cerebrovascular** | o ACA<br>o Aphasia: acute<br>o Amaurosis: *fugax*<br>o Foville's syndrome<br>o MCA<br>o Medullary:<br>- Lateral<br>- Medial<br>o Millard–Gubler<br>o PCA<br>o Stroke<br>- Lacunar<br>o Transient global amnesia (TGA)<br>o Transient ischemic attack (TIA)<br>o Weber's disease |
| | | **Sleep disorders** | o Cataplexy<br>o Circadian rythm<br>o Insomnia<br>- Hyper<br>- Hypo<br>o Klein-Levin disease<br>o Narcolepsy<br>o Sleep apnea<br>- Hypoventilation syndrome: Congenital Central<br>**o Sleep disorder:**<br>- Advanced phase<br>- Delayed phase<br>- Non-24 hour wake<br>- Jet lag |
| | **Cerebrospinal fluid** | o Cerebral edema<br>1. o Choroid plexus papilloma<br>2. o Hydrocephalus: Normal pressure (NPH)<br>o Hyper/hypotension: Intracranial idiopathic | |
| | **Other** | o Brain herniation<br>o Encephalopathy:<br>- Hashimoto's<br>- Hepatic<br>- Toxic<br>o Reyes' syndrome | |

*Source: A. L. Fymat (2017)*

## Diseases of the central nervous system due to the spinal cord

Diseases of the central nervous system due to the spinal cord are charted in Table 6.4.

**Table 6.4 - Diseases of the central nervous system: Spinal cord**

| Organ | Disorders/diseases |
|---|---|
| **Spinal cord/Myelopathy** | 1. o Foix-Alajouanine syndrome<br>2. o Morvan's syndrome<br>3. o Spinal cord compressiom<br>4. o Syringobulbia<br>o o Syringomyelia<br>o a o Vascular myelopathy |

*Source: A. L. Fymat (2017)*

## Diseases of the central nervous system due to either/both encephalopathy or spinal cord/myelopathy

These are summarized in Table 6.5.

**Table 6.5 - Diseases of the central nervous system: (Either/both) Encephalopathy/ Spinal cord myelopathy**

| Characteristic | Disease category | Diseases |
|---|---|---|
| **Degenerative** | **SA** | **o Ataxia telangectasia**<br>o Friedreich's ataxia<br>*LMN only*:<br>o Atrophy:<br>- Progressive muscular PMA)<br>- Spinal Muscular (SMA)<br>- Congenital DSMA<br>- DSMA1<br>- SMA-LED<br>- SMA-PCH<br>- SMA-PME<br>- SMAX1<br>- SMAX2 |

| | | |
|---|---|---|
| | **MND** | o Distal hereditary neuropathies<br>*UMN only*:<br>o **Palsy:**<br>**- Progressive bulbar**<br>- Fazio-Lande infantile (IPBP)<br>**- Pseudobulbar**<br>o Paraplegia:<br>- Hereditary spastic (HSP)<br>o Sclerosis: Primary lateral<br>Both LMN, UMN:<br>o Amyotrophic lateral sclerosis (ALS) |

*Source: A. L. Fymat (2017)*

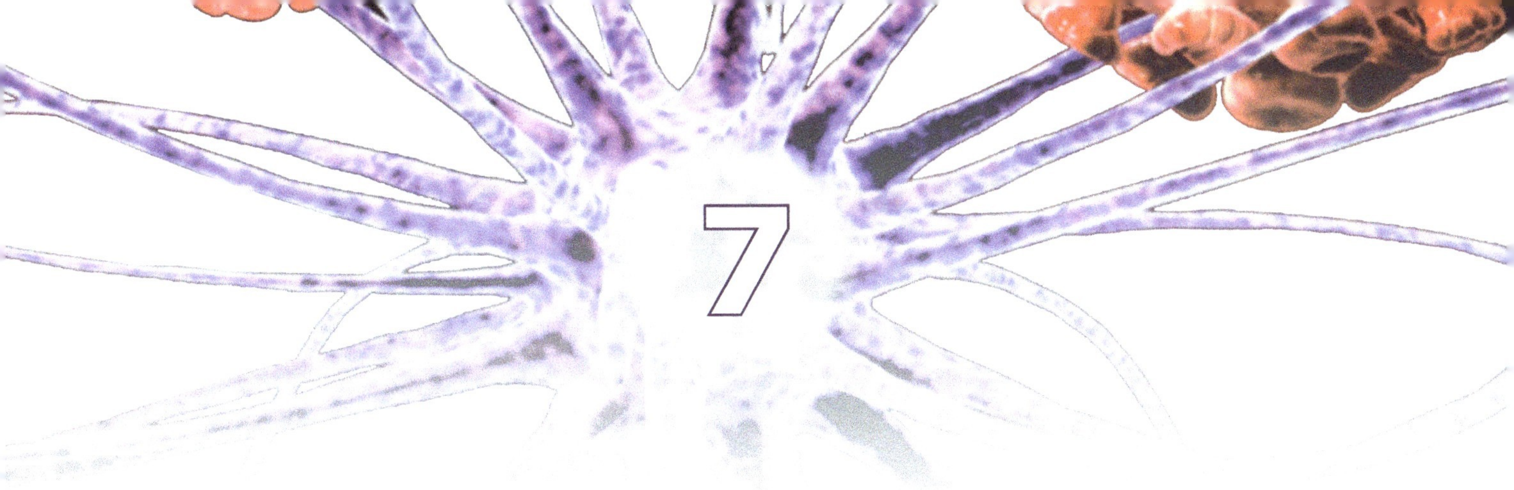

7

# Signs and symptoms of MSA

Non-specific symptoms can precede the occurrence of the disease by several years including erectile dysfunction, orthostatic hypotension, sleep apnea, urinary dysfunctions, etc. At this stage, there are no important disruptions of superior functions but cognitive deficits or memory losses may be noted. While simple measures and drugs can help lessen symptoms, the disorder is progressive and ultimately fatal.

## Spectrum of dysfunctions and associated symptoms

The primary sign of MSA is autonomic failure, which may cause problems with body functions that cannot be controlled. The originating dysfunctions and associated symptoms are summarized in Table 7.1:

**Table 7.1 – Dysfunctions and associated symptoms**

| Dysfunction | Symptom(s) |
|---|---|
| **Cardiovascular problems** | o Color changes in hands and feet caused by pooling of blood |
| **Postural (orthostatic) hypotension** | o Form of low blood pressure causing dizziness or lightheadedness or even fainting when standing up from a sitting or lying down position |
| **Psychiatric problems** | o Difficulty controlling emotions (e.g., laughing or crying inappropriately) |
| **Sexual dysfunction** | o Inability to achieve or maintain an erection (impotence)<br>o Loss of libido |
| **Sleep disorders** | o Agitated sleep due to "acting out" dreams<br>o Abnormal breathing at night or harsh breathing sound (stridor) |

| | |
|---|---|
| **Supine hypertension** | o Dangerously high blood pressure levels while lying down |
| **Sweat production changes** | o Producing less sweat<br>o Heat intolerance due to reduced sweating<br>o Impaired body temperature control often causing cold hands or feet |
| **Urinary and bowel dysfunction** | o Incontinence (loss of bladder or bowel control)<br>o Constipation |

Table 7.2 lists most symptoms and ranks them on a scale of 0 (common) to 100 (always). All presentations below are ~ 50 (frequent):

**Table 7.2 – Symptoms, description, and severity: Autonomic and motor dysfunctions**

| Symptom | Synonym | Description |
|---|---|---|
| **Anorgasmia, female** | Female orgasmic disorder | o Persistent, recurrent difficulty, delay in, or absence of attaining orgasm following sufficient sexual stimulation and arousal |
| **Apnea, central sleep** | Central sleep apnea | o Results from transient abolition of central drive to ventilatory muscles |
| **Ataxia, gait** | Inability to coordinate movements when walking | o Impairment of ability to coordinate movements required for normal walking with tendency to fall |
| **Ataxia, progressive cerebellar** | Progressive ataxia | o Mobility-impairment condition marked by loss of balance and decreased coordination.<br>o Inability to coordinate the muscles in the execution of voluntary movement |
| **Bladder, autonomic dysfunction** | Autonomic bladder dysfunction | o Abnormal bladder function (increased urge or frequency of urination or urge incontinence) |
| **Bradykinesia** | Slowness of movements | o Slowness in execution of movements |
| **Camptocormia** | Forward-flexed posture | o Abnormal forward-flexed posture noticeable when standing or walking |
| **Constipation** | Dyschezia | o Infrequent or difficult evacuation of feces |
| **Dysarthria** | Slurred or impaired speech | o Neurological speech disorder characterized by poor articulation, further classified as spastic, flaccid, ataxic, hyper/hypokinetic, or mixed |

| | | |
|---|---|---|
| **Dysautonomia** | Dysautonomia | o Functional abnormality of the autonomic nervous system |
| **Dyskinesia, orofacial** | Orofacial dyskinesia | o Involuntary, uncontrollable, and often excessive orofacial movement |
| **Dystonia, axial** | Truncal dystonia | o Dystonia affecting the midline muscles (chest, abdomen, and back muscles) |
| **Erectile, autonomic dysfunction** | Impotence | o Inability to develop or maintain an erection resulting from abnormal functioning of the autonomic nervous system. |
| **Falls, frequent** | Frequent falls | o Frequent falls |
| **Hypokinesia** | Hypokinesia | o Reduced number of movements<br>o Slowness in initiation of movements |
| **Hypotension, orthostatic** | Orthostatic hypotension | o **S**udden drop in blood pressure (>20 mm Hg systolic) upon standing and accompanied by symptoms such as dizziness, fatigue, and syncope |
| **Instability, postural** | Imbalance | o Tendency to fall or inability to keep oneself from falling |
| **Nystagmus, gaze-evoked** | Nystagmus | o Made apparent by looking to the right or to the left |
| **Parkinsonism** | Parkinsonian disease | o Characteristic neurologic anomaly resulting from degeneration of dopamine-generating cells in the substantia nigra |
| **Pyramidal sign, abnormal** | Pyramidal tract signs | o Functional neurological abnormalities related to dysfunction of the pyramidal tract |
| **Rapid eye movement (REM), abnormal** | Abnormal REM sleep | o Desynchronization of EEG patterns<br>o Increased heart rate, blood pressure, sympathetic activation<br>o Profound loss of muscle tonus (except for the eye and middle-ear muscles) |
| **Raynaud's phenomenon** | Raynaud phenomenon or disease | o Spasm of the digital arteries with blanching and numbness of the fingers |
| **Rigidity** | Rigidity | o Continuous involuntary sustained muscle contraction as distinguished from muscle spasticity |

| | | |
|---|---|---|
| **Stridor** | Noisy breathing | o High pitched sound resulting from turbulent air flow in the upper airway |
| **Sweating, decreased** | Anhydrosis | |
| **Syncope, orthostatic** | Orthostatic syncope | o Syncope following a quick change in position from lying down to standing. |
| **Tremor, resting** | Tremor at rest | o Occurs when muscles are at rest. Less noticeable or disappears when affected muscles are moved. Often slow and coarse |
| **Tremor, postural** | Postural tremor | o Triggered by holding a limb in a fixed position |

## Autonomic symptoms

Autonomic symptoms usually start in adulthood, usually in the 50s or 60s. The age of onset can vary for different variants and may be different from person to person. In 50%-70% of cases, they appear months or even years ahead of motor (movement-related) symptoms. Some people may have more symptoms than others and symptoms can range from mild to severe. Early symptoms vary, depending on which part and how much of the brain is affected first. Many people are confined to a wheelchair or are otherwise severely disabled within 5 years after symptoms begin. The disorder results in death 9 to 10 years after symptoms begin.

Symptoms of autonomic dysfunctions are classified into three groups:

- **Parkinsonism:** MSA-P symptoms resembling those of Parkinson's disease (PD) often start on one side of the body and then spread to both sides. They result from degeneration in the basal ganglia. Muscles are stiff (rigid), and movements become slow, shaky, and difficult to initiate. When walking, people may shuffle and not swing their arms. People feel unsteady and off balance, making them more likely to fall. Posture may be stooped. Limbs may tremble jerkily, usually when they are held in one position. Articulating words is difficult, and the voice may become high-pitched and quiver. People with MSA are less likely to have tremors during rest than people with PD.
- **Loss of coordination:** It results from degeneration in the cerebellum. People lose their balance. Later, they may be unable to control movements of their arms and legs. Consequently, they have difficulty walking and take wide, irregular steps. When reaching for an item, they may reach beyond it. When sitting, they may feel unstable. People may have difficulty focusing their eyes on, and following, objects. Tasks that require rapidly alternating movements, such as turning a door knob or screwing in a light bulb, also become difficult.

- **Malfunction of internal body processes:** Functions controlled by the autonomic nervous system may also be impacted. Blood pressure may decrease dramatically when a person stands up, causing dizziness, light-headedness, or fainting—a condition called orthostatic hypotension. Blood pressure may increase when a person lies down. People may need to urinate urgently or frequently or may pass urine involuntarily (urinary incontinence). They may have difficulty emptying the bladder (urinary retention). Constipation is common. Vision becomes poor. Men may have difficulty initiating and maintaining an erection (erectile dysfunction).

Other symptoms of autonomic malfunction are among those listed in Table 6.3.

## Movement-related symptoms

The cerebellum – that part of the brain that plays a major role in controlling muscle movements is affected. Cerebellar symptoms of MSA-C usually take the form of ataxia. That loss of coordination can cause the following:

1. **Limb movements:** They are are clumsy or poorly controlled.
2. **Action tremor:** Shaking gets worse when trying to use the affected body part.
3. **Walking steps:** Unusually wide.
4. **Eye movements:** They are jerky and uncontrolled (nystagmus).

## Cognitive and emotional symptoms

In about one-third of MSA cases, people experience disruptions in their ability to think, concentrate, and control their own emotions. That often leads to mental health issues such as:

- **Anxiety.**
- **Depression.**
- **Emotional instability:** It leads to inappropriately exaggerated crying or laughing that do not fit the situation.
- **Panic attacks.**
- **Thoughts of self-harm or suicide.**

## Take-away points

- Non-specific symptoms can precede the occurrence of the disease by several years. The primary sign is autonomic failure, which may cause problems with body functions that cannot be controlled.
- The age of onset of autonomic symptoms can vary for different variants of the disease and may be different from person to person. Many of the autonomic symptoms appear months or even years ahead of motor symptoms.
- Autonomic dysfunctions (MSA-P) cause three groups of symptoms: Parkinsonism, loss of coordination, and malfunction of internal body processes.
- Movement-related symptoms (MSA-C) involve the loss of coordination that can cause limb movements, action tremor, and uncontrolled eye movements (nystagmus)
- Cognitive and emotional symptoms cause disruptions in the ability to think and concentrate, and with controlling emotions (anxiety, depression, and emotional instability).

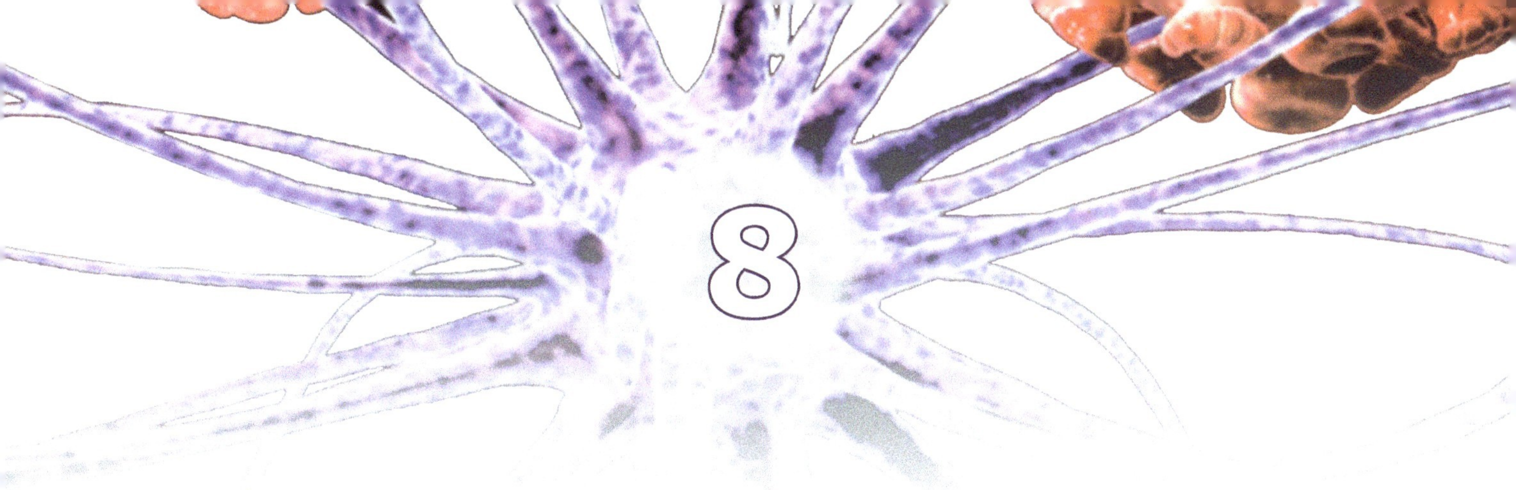


# Etiology, neuropathophysiology, and potential causes of MSA

MSA autopsy studies show olivopontecerebellar atrophy and degeneration of the striatum with typical inclusions in the cytoplasm of oligodendrocytes (Papp-Lantos bodies) that consist of misfolded α (alpha)-synuclein proteins. These proteins are a vital chemical for how the body operates, assisting with communication between different body systems, carrying different chemical compounds throughout the body, and more. But when proteins build up in the wrong places, they can cause damage. Damage is the culprit for the progressive deterioration of brain tissue with MSA.

## Etiology

The exact etiology of MSA-P is still unknown but the presence of cytoplasmic aggregates of α-synuclein, primarily in oligodendroglia, in combination with predominant neurodegeneration of the striatonigral pathway are the pathological hallmark features of MSA-P.

Likewise, the exact etiology of MSC-C is unknown while the presence of cytoplasmic aggregates of α-synuclein, primarily in the oligodendroglia, in combination with predominant neurodegeneration of the olivopontocerebellar structures are pathological hallmark features of MSA-C.

## Neuropathophysiology

MSA is characterized by widespread **glial cytoplasmic inclusions** (GCI), which are the hallmark of the disease (see Figure 6.1). Their main component has more recently been identified as **misfolded, hyperphosphorylated, fibrillary α-synuclein protein** – the same protein that is involved in Parkinson's disease (PD). The presence of GCIs is associated with neuronal loss in the basal ganglia, cerebellum, pons, inferior olivary nuclei and the spinal cord, hence giving rise to the spectrum of symptoms and clinical findings.

Whereas the disease is often defined at the time of initial manifestation of any motor or autonomic features, subclinical neuropathology is likely to have started several years before overt disease. The density of GCI containing α-synuclein also correlates significantly with neuronal deterioration and disease duration. Another important protein, p25α has been found to stimulate α-synuclein *in vitro*.

MSA can be explained as cell loss and gliosis or a proliferation of astrocytes in damaged areas of the central nervous system, forming a scar termed a 'glial scar'. The presence of the Papp-Lantos inclusion bodies in the movement, balance, and autonomic control centers of the brain are the defining histopathologic hallmark of MSA. Their major filamentous component - the glial and neuronal cytoplasmic inclusions, is α-synuclein. Mutations in this substance may play a role in the disease. The conformation of the α-synuclein is different from that of α-synuclein in Lewy bodies. The disease starts with an oligodendrogliopathy. Also, tau proteins have been found in some GCI bodies.

**Figure 8.1 – Brain areas degenerated by MSA**

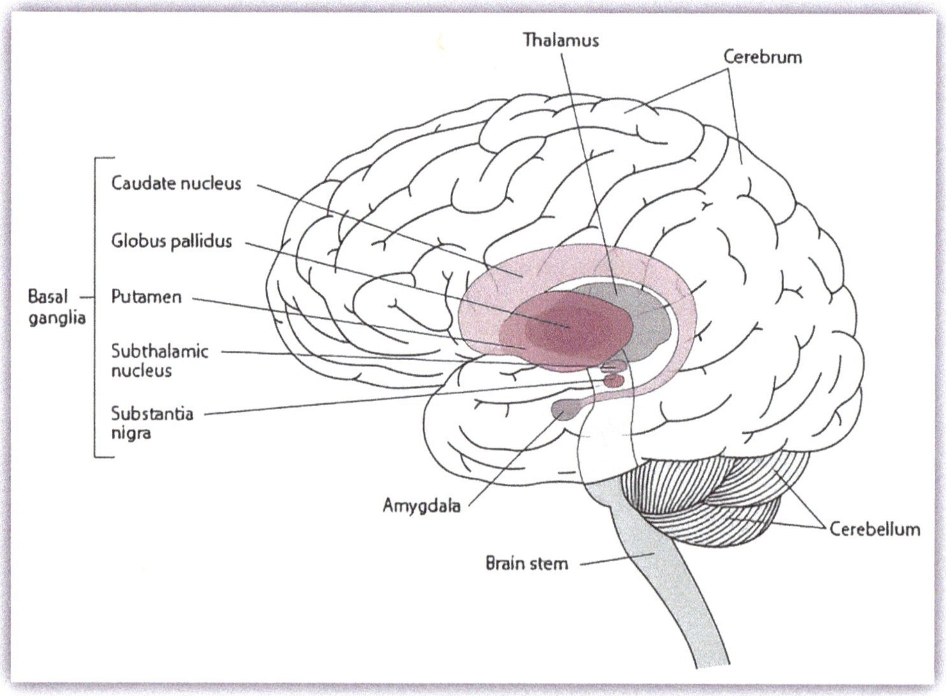


*Source: Merck Manual*

## Causes of MSA

MSA results from degeneration of several parts of the brain and spinal cord (Figure 8.1):

- **The basal ganglia:** These are collections of nerve cells at the base of the cerebrum, deep within the brain. They help control voluntary muscle movements by balancing the actions of muscle groups that move the same muscles in opposite ways (for example, a group that bends an arm and a group that straightens the arm)

- **The cerebellum:** It coordinates voluntary movements (particularly complex movements done simultaneously) and helps maintain balance.
- **The autonomic nervous system:** It regulates involuntary body processes, such as how blood pressure changes in response to changes in posture.

The cause of the degeneration is unknown, but probably results when α-synuclein changes shape (misfolds) and accumulates in support cells in the brain. Synuclein is a protein in the brain that helps nerve cells communicate, but whose function is not yet fully understood. Abnormal synuclein can also accumulate in people with pure autonomic failure, PD or dementia with Lewy bodies (DLB). A modified form of the α-synuclein protein within affected neurons may cause MSA.

The causes of MSA are unknown, although genetics, environmental processes (toxins), and lifestyle factors (trauma) may contribute to the pathological processes underlying MSA. Most cases occur at random, without any other cases in the family.

## MSA-P

The cause of MSA-P is unknown. The affected areas of the brain overlap with areas affected by PD, with similar symptoms. Evidence that it is passed within families has not been found.

## MSA-C

The cause of MSA-C in people with the sporadic form is also not known. The disease slowly gets worse (it is progressive) and can be passed down through families (inherited form). It can also affect people without a known family history (sporadic form).

## Genetics

Researchers have identified certain genes that are involved in the inherited form of this condition. The gene mutations (COQ2, SHC2, and SNCA1) may be involved. Mutations in the *COQ2* gene (4q21.23) (encoding an enzyme involved in the biosynthesis of coenzyme Q10) have been shown in multiplex families with MSA, while some variants were associated with an increased risk for sporadic MSA.

One study, involving a group of Japanese patients, found a correlation between the deletion of genes in a specific genetic region and the development of MSA. The region in question includes the SHC2 gene which, in mice and rats, appears to have some function in the nervous system. The authors of this study hypothesized that there may be a link between the deletion of SHC2 and the development of MSA.

A follow-up study was unable to replicate this finding in American MSA patients. Its authors concluded that "... SHC2 gene deletions underlie few, if any, cases of well-characterized MSA in the U.S. population. This is in contrast to the Japanese experience reported by Sasaki *et al.*, likely reflecting heterogeneity of the disease in different genetic backgrounds".

Another study investigated the frequency of RFC1 intronic repeat expansions, a phenomenon implicated in a disease with a diagnostic overlap with MSA. It concluded that these repeats were absent in pathologically confirmed MSA, suggesting an alternative genetic cause.

The presence of mutations, duplications, and triplications of the SNCA gene, encoding α-syn, in familial cases showing features of MSA or Parkinson's disease (PD) gave rise to the question whether SNCA was associated with MSA. Polymorphisms of the SNCA locus were identified in some European MSA patients; however, such observations were not replicated in larger cohorts of pathologically confirmed MSA cases (Al-Chalabi *et al.,* 2009; Scholz *et al.,* 2009).

A genome-wide association study (GWAS) reported in 2016 no association of COQ2 and SNCA with MSA, but several potential interesting candidates were identified, highlighting the need for further genome studies with larger and well-characterized MSA samples to understand the genetics of this disorder (Sailer et al. 2016). Recently, a GWAS summary statistics study of MSA and seven autoimmune diseases identified a shared genetic etiology between MSA and inflammatory bowel disease (Shadrin *et al.,* 2020). These findings reinforced the role of neuroinflammation and the gut-brain axis in association with a possible polygenic predisposition in the pathophysiology MSA.

## Take-away points

1. MSA autopsy studies show olivopontecerebellar atrophy and degeneration of the striatum with typical inclusions in the cytoplasm of oligodendrocytes (Papp-Lantos bodies) that consist of misfolded α-synuclein.
2. MSA is characterized by widespread glial cytoplasmic inclusions, which are the hallmark of the disease. Their main component is misfolded, hyperphosphorylated fibrillary α-synuclein – the same protein that is involved in Parkinson's disease.
3. Whereas the disease is often defined at the time of initial manifestation of any motor or autonomic features, subclinical neuropathology is likely to have started several years before overt disease.
4. MSA can be explained as cell loss and gliosis (a proliferation of astrocytes in damaged areas of the central nervous system forming a scar called a glial scar). The Papp-Lantos inclusion bodies in the movement, balance, and autonomic control centers of the brain are the defining histopathologic hallmark of MSA.
5. MSA results from the degeneration of several parts of the brain (basal ganglia, cerebellum, autonomic nervous system) and spinal cord.
6. The cause of the degeneration is unknown, but probably results when the α-synuclein protein misfolds and accumulates in support cells in the brain. Abnormal synuclein can also accumulate in cases of pure autonomic failure, Parkinson's disease, or dementia with Lewy bodies.
7. The causes of MSA are unknown, although genetics, environmental processes (toxins), and lifestyle factors (trauma) may contribute to the pathological processes

underlying MSA. Most cases occur at random, without any other cases in the family.

8. The gene mutations (COQ2, SHC2, and SNCA1) may be involved in MSA. Conflicting results indicate the possibility of heterogeneity of the disease in different genetic backgrounds.
9. Sidebar 8.1 will succinctly describe the animal models employed to unravel the processes underlying MSA.

## Sidebar 8.1 - Animal models of multiple system atrophy

The currently available models include toxicant-induced animal models, α-synuclein-overexpressing cellular models, and mouse models that express α-synuclein specifically in oligodendrocytes through cell type-specific promoters.

### Toxicant-induced models

*In vitro* and *in vivo* toxicant-induced models involve the systemic administration and local stereotaxic injection of toxins (E.G., 6-hydroxydopamine, quinolinic acid, 3-nitropropionic acid, and 1-methyl-4-phenylpyridinium ion) to induce lesions in specific anatomical areas so as to reproduce MSA symptoms. However, these approaches only partially mimic MSA neuropathology, result in symptoms only within the area of administration, fail to spread outside the basal ganglia, and do not induce GCI pathology, which is one of the essential hallmarks of MSA.

### In vitro genetic models

Because one of the main components of GCIs in MSA is α-synuclein, many studies have used *in vitro* expression of α-synuclein to investigate the disease mechanism.

#### U-373 MG cell line and primary mixed rat glial cultures

In a study conducted by Stefanova *et al.,* it was shown that upon treatment with TNFα, a pro-inflammatory cytokine released by microglia in MSA, significant cytotoxic changes were observed in α-synuclein-expressing cells. This suggested that a toxic environment, along with high levels of α-synuclein in glia, might represent a severe risk for the development of MSA.

#### OLN-93 cell line

OLN-93 cells, primary oligodendrocytic cells derived from Wistar rat brain cultures, have been used to study MSA pathology by co-expressing α-synuclein and p25α in the OLN-93 cell line.

### CG4 cell line

The central glia 4 (CG4) cell line, a rodent oligodendroglial cell line, has been used to stably express α-synuclein. The overexpression of the protein impaired the maturation of cells into oligodendrocytes.

### iPSCs from human MSA patients

The advancement of stem cell technologies has allowed the culturing of patient-derived cells and their differentiation into various cell types, including oligodendrocytes. However, there is no difference between patient-derived and healthy control iPSC.

## In vivo genetic models

The transgenic expression of the α-synuclein gene under oligodendrocyte-specific promoters has been used to create mouse models of MSA. However, transgenic mouse lines overexpressing α-synuclein displayed different pathological features of MSA under different oligodendroglial promoters. Nonetheless, the various symptoms described in each of these models and the pattern and degree of degeneration in the nervous system did not precisely correlate with disease pathology.

### PLP-hαSyn transgenic mice

PLP promoter-driven α-synuclein (PLP-hαSyn) transgenic mice bred on a C57/BL6 background exhibited phosphorylation of α-synuclein at Ser129 and aggregation of α-synuclein along with GCI-like inclusions. Mitochondrial inhibition by 3-NP in these mice induced the degeneration of the striatonigral system and gliosis. The loss of dopaminergic neurons in the SNpc, Purkinje cells, and neurons in the pons and medulla oblongata, as in the human MSA-C subtype, was also observed. Gliosis and increased levels of cytokines were also reported.

### MBP-hαSyn transgenic mice

Mice with MBP promoter-driven α-synuclein expression in oligodendrocytes exhibited somewhat different pathological features of MSA that those exhibited by PLP-hαsyn and CNP-hαsyn tg mice. These mice displayed demyelination along with axonal degeneration in the cerebellum, basal ganglia, brain stem, corpus callosum, and neocortex.

### CNP-hαSyn transgenic mice

CNP promoter-hαSyn mice exhibited the accumulation of fibrillary human α-synuclein in oligodendrocytes, a loss and demyelination of these cells, and severe gliosis in the brain and spinal cord.

### Viral-mediated oligodendroglial α-synuclein expression models

The viral expression of α-synuclein in animals has advantages over genetic models in that expression can be manipulated temporally. The recombinant virus can be injected at an early stage or later in development. The cell specificity of viral infection has significantly improved over the years. However, more studies of such models in rodents and nonhuman primates are still needed for the development of MSA models.

## Transmission models

Numerous studies have reported little to no α-synuclein expression in mature oligodendrocytes *in vitro* and *in vivo*. The mechanisms of the accumulation of α-synuclein aggregates in the oligodendrocytes and astrocytes of MSA patients are still largely unknown. However, recent reports of the transfer of α-synuclein from one cell to another, particularly from neurons to glia, have led to the hypothesis that toxic α-synuclein aggregates secreted from neurons are taken up by oligodendrocytes and disrupts their function. Based on this hypothesis, several groups have developed transmission models.

## Stereotaxic injection of recombinant proteins or MSA brain extracts into animal models

Brain extracts from 14 MSA patients were inoculated into the brains of TgM83+/− hemizygous mice expressing the A53T α-synuclein mutant under the prion promoter. All mice showed neurodegeneration and accumulation of α-synuclein aggregates in neuronal cell bodies and axons at 4 months postinjection, whereas control injections did not induce neurodegeneration at the same age. Interestingly, PD brain extracts did not promote the aggregation of α-synuclein in TgM83 mice, indicating that pathogenic α-synuclein species may differ in MSA and PD. These injection models support the α-synuclein transmission hypothesis, as pathological α-synuclein from diseased patients was transferred to nonsymptomatic mice and induced pathology.

## In summary

Various models have been generated over the years to study the mechanism of MSA development and progression. The main goal of the genetic models is to generate oligodendrocytes with GCI-like α-synuclein pathology, thereby allowing the study of the roles of α-synuclein in MSA pathogenesis. More recent efforts to develop MSA models have utilized the fact that α-synuclein can be transferred between cells. However, none of these models present *bona fide* MSA pathology. Recent studies have suggested that GCIs are generated through the transfer of α-synuclein from neurons to oligodendrocytes. To test this hypothesis, we will have to understand more about the biology of oligodendrocytes in MSA. Critical questions include how oligodendrocytes respond to and process neuron-derived α-synuclein and how normal oligodendrocytes and MSA oligodendrocytes respond differently to α-synuclein.

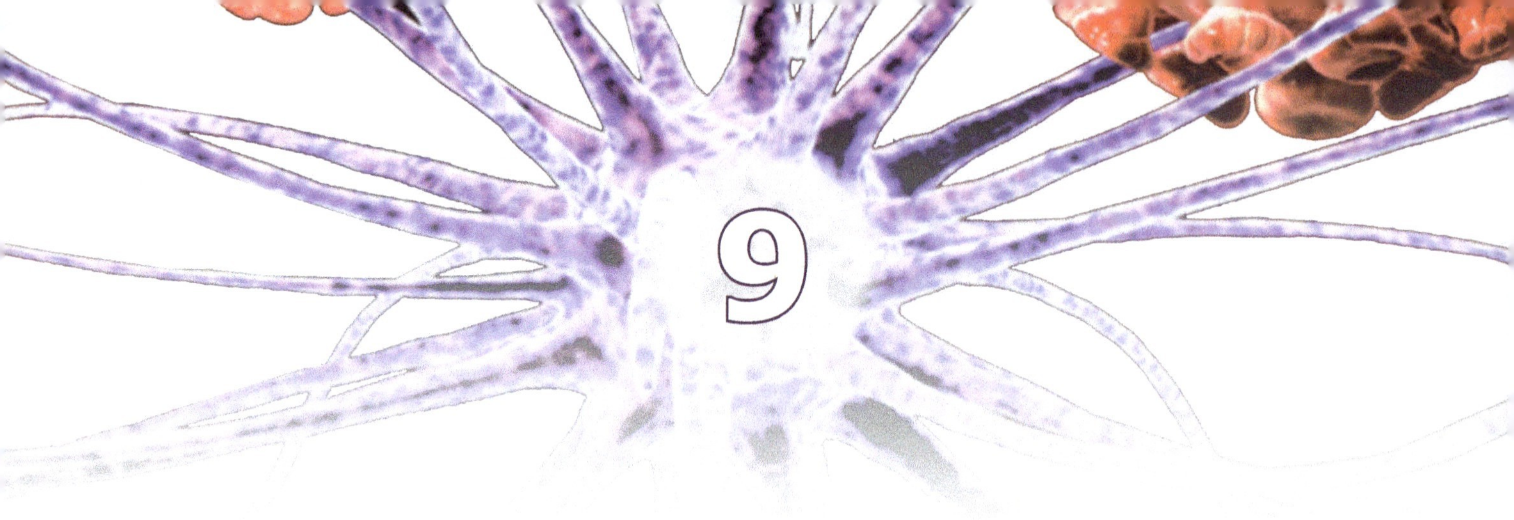

# 9

# Epidemiology

The epidemiology of MSA is extremely sketchy as indicated by the shortness of this chapter. There are approximately 6-7,000 (10,000 according to certain authors) rare diseases, depending on the definition of their frequency of occurrence in a given population (in the U.S., for example, this means. each one affects fewer than 200,000 people). While individually each disease is rare, collectively rare diseases are common: They affect nearly 400 million people worldwide. In the U.S., the prevalence of rare diseases (over 30 million people) rivals or exceeds that of common diseases such as diabetes (37.3 million people), Alzheimer's disease (6.5 million people), and heart failure (6.2 million people). They diminish the quality of life and threaten health. Moreover, they have significantly higher medical expenses, with medical care costing three to five times more for individuals with rare diseases than for individuals without rare diseases.

Many rare diseases have limited information. Regarding MSA, it is estimated to affect approximately 5 per 100,000 people in the general population with the mean age of 50-55 as the approximate age of onset. In Europe, prevalence ranges from 1/50,000-1/20,000. The condition most commonly presents in persons aged 50–60.

At autopsy, many patients diagnosed during life with PD are found actually to have MSA, suggesting that the actual incidence of MSA is higher than that estimate. While some suggest that MSA affects slightly more men than women (1.3:1), others suggest that the two sexes are equally likely to be affected.

MSA-parkinsonian type (MSA-P) predominates in the Western Hemisphere (Europe and North America) with 68% of cases whereas one-third of all MSA patients have MSA-C. In Japan, MSA-C is more common. However, MSA-P is more common than MSA-C in Korea, indicating that the subtypes of MSA vary among Asian countries.

MSA-cerebellar type (MSA-C) predominates in the Eastern Hemisphere. A Japanese study reported a high percentage of patients (83.8%) exhibiting MSA-C features with only 16.2% of patients being categorized as MSA-P. This is not strictly rigorous as Korea does not follow the same pattern as Japan.

Genders are equally distributed.

## Take-away points

1. MSA-P predominates in the Western Hemisphere.
2. MSA-C predominates in the Eastern Hemisphere; however, the subtypes of MSA vary among Asian countries..
3. Genders are equally distributed.

# C. DIAGNOSIS, TREATMENT, AND PROGNOSIS

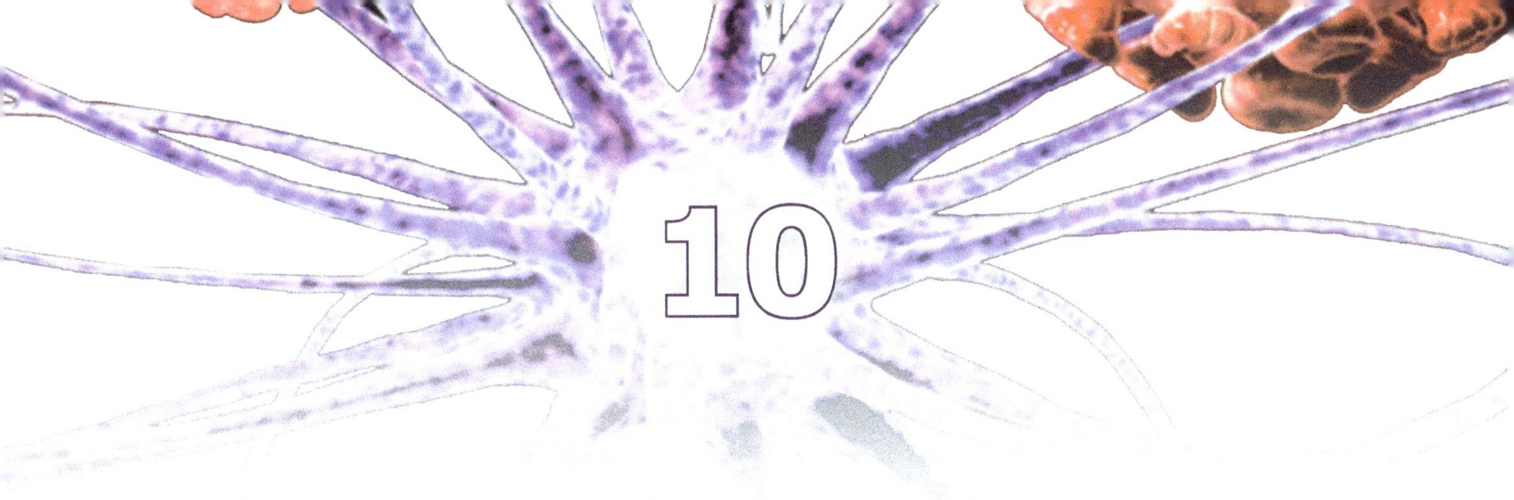


# How is MSA diagnosed?

Diagnosis of MSA is clinically based on the combination of signs and symptoms, medical history, physical examination, laboratory test results, various autonomic insufficiency tests, neuroradiological imaging studies, and response to certain treatments. The tests can help determine whether the diagnosis is 'probable MSA' or 'possible MSA'.

''Probable'' MSA requires the presence of parkinsonism with poor Levodopa response or cerebellar signs together with severe autonomic failure (otherwise unexplained urinary incontinence or an orthostatic decrease of blood pressure within 3 min of standing-up by at least 30 mm Hg systolic or 15 mm Hg diastolic). MRI findings include atrophy of putamen and middle cerebellar peduncles, as well as putaminal and cerebellar hypometabolism on [18F]-fluorodeoxyglucose positron emission tomography (PET).

''Definite'' MSA requires *post-mortem* demonstration of α-synuclein positive glial cytoplasmic inclusions with neurodegeneration of striatonigral and olivopontocerebellar structures.

However, reaching a diagnosis can be challenging and difficult, particularly in the early stages, in part because many of its features are similar to those observed in Parkinson's disease (PD), parkinsonism, and a number of other confounding diseases (detailed below). Because of this difficulty, some people are actually never properly diagnosed.

It must be noted that no laboratory or imaging studies are able to definitively confirm the diagnosis. Further, it is necessarily differential as MSA may be confused with other diseases. In addition, the histologic proof can only be obtained *post mortem* as it is impossible to identify a buildup of α-synuclein in areas of the brain (a hallmark of the disease) while the person is alive. The diagnosis, therefore, remains essentially clinical and differential.

It is common for healthcare providers to initially diagnose a person as having PD or another form of parkinsonism, and then to revise the diagnosis when other symptoms appear or when certain treatments do not work.

## Main differential diagnoses

In addition to pure autonomic failure, autonomic neuropathies, multiple cerebral infarcts, drug-induced parkinsonism, cerebellar symptoms, and response to certain medications, the main differential diagnoses seek to rule-out any one or more of the following diseases:

- **Alzheimer 's disease (AD).** (See this author's textbook on the subject, Fymat, 2019 in the list of references for AD at the end of the book.)
- **Corticobasal degeneration (CBD):** Manifested by obvious signs of cortical dysfunction, e.g., apraxia, dementia, and aphasia.
- **Creutzfeldt-Jakob disease (CJD):** Dementia is usually apparent with myoclonic jerking, ataxia, and common pyramidal signs.
- **Dementias:** (See this author's textbook on the subject, Fymat, 2020a in the list of references for dementias at the end of the book.)
    1. **Lewy bodies dementia (LBD):** Often mimics Parkinsonian features.
    2. **Multi-infarct dementia (MID):** Characterized by cognitive impairment, spasticity, and extrapyramidal signs.

- **Frontotemporal degeneration (FTD)**, including **Pick's disease (PD),** which affects the frontal and/or temporal lobes. The level of consciousness is not affected (unlike in AD) and Parkinsonism is usually mild.
- **Guam disease (GD)** or **Lytico-Bodig syndrome (LBS)**.
- **Huntington's disease (HD):** Can present earlier with rigidity instead of chorea when parkinsonism is not expected. Normally, there is a family history.
- **Parkinson's disease** (PD): MSA may also present with parkinsonian symptoms, often with a poor or temporary response to Levodopa therapy. (See this author's textbook on the subject, Fymat, 2020c in the list of references for PD at the end of the book.)
- **Parkinsonism:** (See this author's textbook on the subject, Fymat, 2020c in the list of references for PD at the end of the book.)
    1. **Atypical parkinsonism syndromes:** A group which looks like PD, but are much more severe. Median survival is only seven years compared with the normal lifespan in PD.

- **Progressive supranuclear palsy (PSP)** or **Steele-Richardson-Olszewski disease (SROD):** It is characterized by paresis of conjugate gaze with initially problems looking up and down on request, advancing to difficulty in following objects up and down.

- **Tremors:** The variety of confounding tremors includes:
  - **Benign essential tremor:** It is far more common and worse on movement (e.g., while trying to hold a cup of tea), and rare while at rest.
  - **Cerebellar tremor:** It presents as a unilateral or bilateral, low-frequency intention tremor. It may be caused by stroke, brain stem tumor, or multiple sclerosis.
  - **Drug- or toxin-induced tremor:** Numerous drugs or toxins may cause tremor, notably selective serotonin reuptake inhibitors (SSRIs), caffeine, amphetamines, beta-adrenergic blockers, tricyclics, and lithium. Neuroleptics (e.g., Haloperidol, Chlorpromazine) and anti-emetics (e.g., Prochlorperazine) can cause parkinsonian features that look identical to Parkinson's disease.
  - **Pyschogenic tremor:** The tremor is variable, increases under direct observation, decreases with distraction.

- **Wilson's disease (WD):** It has an earlier onset with characteristic Kayser-Fleischer rings and hepatitis.

The above long list of confounding diseases will preclude their in-depth treatment here. Therefore, only PD and parkinsonism will be considered below as they are the main differentials. (For more details, se this author's textbook on the subject (Fymat, 2020c.)

## Parkinson's disease (PD) – A digest

### Epidemiology

- PD is the second most common neurodegenerative disorder after Alzheimer's disease (AD).
- The prevalence increases with age: 4–5 per 100,000 in people aged 30-39 years; 1,700 per 100,000 in people aged 80-84 years.
- About 0.3% of the general population is affected, and the prevalence is higher among men than women, with a ratio of 1.5 to 1.
- PD may be more common among white people than those of Asian or African descent, but the data are conflicting.

### Signs & symptoms

PD is a slowly progressing neurodegenerative disorder, causing impaired motor and non-motor functions. Motor symptoms include: slow movements, tremor, and gait and balance disturbances. Non-motor symptoms are common and include: Disturbed autonomic function with orthostatic hypotension, constipation and urinary disturbances, sleep disorders, and neuropsychiatric symptoms.

Onset is insidious with peak age of onset at 55-65 years. It commonly presents with impairment of dexterity or, less commonly, with a slight dragging of one foot. A fixed facial expression is characteristic with infrequent blinking. There may also be saliva drooling from the mouth, often due to impaired swallowing, and a quiet voice.

Main features are resting tremor, rigidity, bradykinesia, and gait disturbance (mnemonic: **TRBG**):

- **Tremor:** At a frequency of 4-6 Hz, it is seen at rest and, if not immediately apparent, may be induced by concentration (e.g., asking the patient to recite months of the year backwards). It is absent during activity (e.g., tipping water from cup to cup). Tremor is usually apparent in one limb or the limbs on one side for months or even years before becoming generalized.
- **Rigidity:** It presents as an increase in resistance to passive movement that can produce a characteristic flexed posture in many patients. It may be increased by asking the patient to perform an action in the opposite limb - contralateral synkinesis.
- **Bradykinesia:** It presents as a slowness of voluntary movement and reduced automatic movements. It is particularly noticeable in a reduced arm swing whilst walking. It can also be seen as a progressive reduction in the amplitude of repetitive movements (e.g., asking the patient to repeatedly oppose middle finger and thumb). Patients may still retain the ability to move quickly in an emergency situation. Typically, muscles are of normal strength if given time to develop power. There is no alteration in tendon reflexes or plantar responses.
- **Gait disturbance:** The patient may have difficulty in rising from a sitting position and starting to walk. Gait is characterized by small shuffling steps with unsteadiness on turning and difficulty in stopping ('festination'). There may be a tendency to fall. When patients have a gait disorder without other parkinsonian features, the most likely diagnosis is gait apraxia, which is more common and usually caused by small-vessel cerebrovascular disease.

Gait disorders and postural instability are the leading causes of falls and disability in PD. Cognition plays an important role in postural control and may interfere with gait and posture. It is very important to recognize gait, posture, and balance dysfunction.

## Cause

Although PD is mainly caused by dysfunction of dopaminergic neurons, nondopaminergic systems are also involved, however, the exact cause is unknown. The majority of cases are thought to arise sporadically, but up to 20% of people with PD have a family history in a first-degree relative.

## Diagnostic criteria

PD is suspected in people presenting with tremor, stiffness, slowness, balance problems and/or gait disturbances. The approach to diagnosis usually follows the three steps below:

### Step 1: Diagnosis of Parkinsonian syndrome

Bradykinesia (the slowness of initiation of voluntary movement with progressive reduction in speed and amplitude or repetitive actions) and at least one of the following:

- **Muscular rigidity.**
- **Resting tremor:** 4- 6 Hz frquency.
- **Postural instability:** Not caused by primary visual, vestibular, cerebellar or proprioceptive dysfunction.

### Step 2: Exclusion criteria for Parkinson's disease

- **Strokes:** Repeated history with stepwise progression of Parkinsonian features.
- **Head injury:** Repeated history.
- **Encephalitis:** History of definite occurrence.
- **Oculogyric crises.**
- **Neurolepsy:** Treatment at onset of symptoms.
    - More than one affected relative.
    - Sustained remission.
    - Strictly unilateral features after three years.
- **Supranuclear palsy:** Gaze.
- **Cerebellar signs.**
- **Autonomic involvement:** Early severe.
- **Dementia:** Early severe with disturbances of memory, language, and praxis.
- **Babinski's sign.**

- **Cerebral tumor or communicating hydrocephalus:** Presence on a CT scan.
- **L-dopa response:** Negative to large doses of (if malabsorption excluded).
- **MPTP (N-Methyl-4-Phenyl-1,2,3,6- TetrahydroPyridine):** Exposure.

**Step 3: Supportive prospective positive criteria of Parkinson's disease**

Three or more from the following list are required for the diagnosis of definite Parkinson's disease:

- **Unilateral onset.**
- **Rest tremor present.**
- **Progressive disorder.**
- **Persistent asymmetry:** Affecting the side of onset most.
- **Excellent response (70%-100%) to L-dopa.**
- **Chorea:** Severe L-dopa-induced.
- **L-dopa response:** For five years or more.
- **Clinical course:** Ten years or more.
- **Hyposmia.**
- **Hallucinations:** Visual.

## Long-term problems

After an initial 'honeymoon period', the majority of people who have received L-dopa for 5-10 years may experience the following:

### Motor fluctuations

- **"On-off "health status:** When PD patients are moving well, they say they are 'on'. When they are stiff and bradykinetic, they say they are 'off'.
- **Treatment wearing-off**: Before the next dose is due. May start to occur as well as 'on-off' fluctuations, which occur randomly.

- **Involuntary movements:** Patients may experience them whilst 'on'. These are dyskinesias.

- **Motor fluctuations:** Difficult to treat and are best managed by a specialist.

### Axial problems not responding to treatment

- Axial problems are balance, speech and gait disturbance which do not respond to PD medication.
- They are thought to be a consequence of axonal degeneration outside the substantia nigra where dopamine is not the neurotransmitter.
- If a patient cannot walk or speak well but has no limb parkinsonism (i.e., is otherwise well medicated), they will not be improved by increasing their dose.
- Their treatment options include physiotherapy, occupational therapy and speech and language therapy (SALT).

### Parkinson's disease dementia

This is dementia occurring more than one year after a diagnosis of PD. It is similar to Alzheimer-type dementia but has three typical features:

- **Presence of parkinsonism in the limbs.**

- **Frequent visual hallucinations.**

- **Frequent fluctuations in lucidity.**

Sudden deteriorations may be mistaken for intercurrent illness (e.g., urinary tract infection), but the midstream specimen of urine is negative and the patient becomes better.

PD dementia is difficult to treat, as confusion and hallucinations may be worsened by the treatment of PD with dopamine agonists. Atypical antipsychotics (e.g., Quetiapine) are effective without worsening the Parkinsonism.

### Differential diagnosis between PD and MSA

PD is the main differential; about 10% of patients diagnosed with PD are actually found to have MSA on autopsy. Features that suggest MSA over PD include:

- **MSA progresses faster:** People with PD usually take years to develop autonomic dysfunction. With MSA, autonomic dysfunction can start within a year.
- **MSA symptoms develop differently:** Autonomic symptoms in particular (rigidity and bradykinesia) are usually more severe with MSA, while tremors are less severe or may not happen at all. The way the symptoms spread throughout the body can also happen differently.
- **MSA responds poorly to Levodopa – The main treatment option for PD. This is often a key way healthcare providers recognize that a person has MSA instead of PD.**

In 2020, researchers at The University of Texas Health Science Center at Houston concluded that **protein misfolding cyclic amplification could be used to distinguish between PD and MSA**, providing the first process to give an objective diagnosis of MSA instead of just a differential diagnosis.

## Parkinsonism

Parkinsonism is a general term for the clinical features of bradykinesia plus at least one of tremor, rigidity, and/or postural instability. PD is the most common form of parkinsonism. Other causes of parkinsonism include drug-induced parkinsonism, cerebrovascular disease, LBD, and PSP.

### Risk factors

- Increasing prevalence with age, and slightly more common in men.
- Pesticide exposure.
- Small-scale studies have suggested that patients born in the spring have a higher incidence.

### Pathogenesis

- The ventral tier of the zona compacta of the substantia nigra is particularly affected with reduction of dopamine in the striatum.
- PD is used to describe the idiopathic syndrome of parkinsonism.
- Drug-induced parkinsonism is caused by drugs that block the dopamine receptors or reduce storage of dopamine. These are mainly the major tranquilizers used to

treat psychosis, but the condition can also be seen with drugs used to treat nausea (e.g., Metoclopramide).

- Parkinsonism may also occur following encephalitis or exposure to certain toxins (e.g., manganese dust, carbon disulfide, and severe carbon monoxide poisoning).

### Differences between MSA and parkinsonism

MSA is suspected if parkinsonian symptoms are rapidly worsening and Levodopa (used to treat PD) has little or no effect on symptoms.

## MSA diagnostic tests

**Clinical diagnostic criteria were defined in 1998 and updated in 2007. Certain signs and symptoms of MSA also occur with other disorders (as listed earlier in this chapter), making the diagnosis even more difficult.** Diagnostic techniques include some or all of the following, as appropriate:

### Autonomic function testing

Tests to assess autonomic (body's involuntary) functions include:

- **Blood pressure test:** This test can be performed on a tilt table to help determine if there is a problem with blood pressure control. In this procedure, the person is placed on a motorized table and strapped in place. Then, the table is tilted upward so that the body is positioned at a 70-degree angle. **During the test, blood pressure and heart rate are monitored. The findings can document both the extent of blood pressure irregularities and whether they occur with a change in physical position.**
- **Thermoregulatory sweat test:** To evaluate areas of the body that sweat.
- **Bladder function test:** Bladder function assessment often detects early abnormalities consistent with neurogenic disturbance. Initially, detrusor hyper-reflexia and abnormal urethral sphincter function predominate; these are later followed by increased residual urinal volume (as detected by bladder ultrasound).
- **Bowel function test.**
- **Electrocardiogram:** To track the electrical signals of the heart.
- **Sleep test:** To evaluate sleep irregularities, especially interrupted breathing or snoring. It can help diagnose an underlying and treatable sleep disorder, such as sleep apnea.

Other autonomic abnormalities include:

- **Diminished respiratory sinus arrhythmia test.**
- **Olfactory testing:** To help differentiate PD from other parkinsonian disorders.
- **Skin biopsy:** Some types of skin biopsy can pick up signs of α-synuclein buildup in nerve tissue. However, more research is necessary before scientists could determine if it is useful enough to recommend making it a standard part of the diagnostic process.
- **Abnormal response to the Valsalva maneuver:** No blood pressure recovery in late phase II and/or no overshoot in phase IV.
- **Diminished response to isometric exercise:** Hand grip.
- **Diminished response to cold pressor stimuli.**

**Generalized failure of autonomic tests is helpful for the diagnosis.**

## Neuropathological testing

Pathological diagnosis can only be made at autopsy by finding abundant glial cytoplasmic inclusions (GCI) on histological specimens of the central nervous system.

Contrary to most other synucleinopathies, which develop α-synuclein inclusions primarily in neuronal cell populations, MSA differs in its pathological presentations such as:

- **Extensive pathological α-synuclein inclusions:** In the cytosol of oligodendrocytes with limited pathology in neurons.
- Regional differences: **α-synuclein positive inclusions detected predominantly in the striatum, midbrain, pons, medulla and cerebellum, rather than the brainstem, limbic and cortical regions typically affected in Lewy inclusion diseases. However, recent studies using novel, monoclonal antibodies specific for C-terminally truncated α-synuclein (αsyn-C) have now shown that neuronal α-synuclein pathology is more abundant than previously thought. One group revealed robust α-synuclein pathology in the pontine nuclei and medullary inferior olivary nucleus upon histological analysis of neurological tissue from MSA patients. Histopathological investigation on six cases of pathologically confirmed MSA, using antibodies directed at a variety of α-synuclein epitopes, revealed substantial variation in α-synuclein protein deposition across both cases and brain regions within cases, providing evidence for 'strains' of aggregated conformers that may differentially promote pathological prion-like spread.**
- **High density of glial cytoplasmic inclusions (GCI):** These are seen (see Figure 6.1) in association with degenerative changes in certain brain structures (e.g., putamen, caudate nucleus, globus pallidus, thalamus, pontine nuclei, cerebellar

Purkinje's cells and autonomic nuclei of the brain stem). **GCIs can be stained by the Gallyas silver technique. They are a hallmark of MSA.**

## Radiopharmaceutical imaging testing

### DaTscanTM

**This radiopharmaceutical can assess the dopamine transporter in a part of the brain called the striatum and can help physicians determine if the condition is caused by a dopamine system disorder. However, the test cannot differentiate between MSA and PD.**

### Iodine-123 (I-123) scintigraphy

- **MIBG scans show intact innervation of the heart (because the lesion is preganglionic in MSA).**
- Thought to be useful for differentiation between PD and MSA early after onset of autonomic dysfunction.
- Patients with PD have significantly lower cardiac uptake of I-123 than patients with MSA and controls.

## Neuroradiological imaging testing

**Brain imaging scans can show signs that may suggest MSA and also help determine if there are other causes that may be contributing to the observed symptoms. Both MRI and CT scanning may show a decrease in the size of the cerebellum and pons in those with cerebellar features (MSA-C).** The following scans may be considered for making the diagnosis of MSA. Regarding:

- **CT or MRI brain scan:** This test can sometimes show deterioration in areas of the brain, which can help narrow-down the diagnosis. It is also useful in diagnosing MSA-C, which can cause a part of the brain to show a criss-cross pattern (experts call this the "hot cross bun" sign). That sign appears as some areas of brain tissue deteriorate while others do not. However, that sign can appear with other conditions as well, so it alone is not enough to diagnose MSA.
    - MRI scanning is needed to exclude rare secondary causes (e.g., supratensorial tumors and normal pressure hydrocephalus) and extensive subcortical vascular pathology.
    - Functional MRI and CT imaging are useful research tools. Blood flow changes monitored by these methods and correlated with functional disability are providing useful clues as to the structural abnormalities which cause parkinsonism and PD.

- Structural MRI may be considered in the differential diagnosis of other parkinsonian syndromes.
- Brain imaging may be normal in MSA. Localized brain degeneration may be detected by MRI techniques.
- **MRI changes are not required to diagnose the disease as these features are often absent, especially early in the course of the disease. Additionally, the changes can be quite subtle and are usually missed by examiners who are not experienced with MSA. However, characteristic changes in the midbrain, pons, and cerebellum are helpful for the diagnosis.**
- The putamen is hypointense on T2-weighted MRI and may show an increased deposition of iron in the parkinsonian (MSA-P) form. In MSA-C, a "hot cross bun" sign is sometimes found, reflecting atrophy of the pontocerebellar tracts that give T2 hyper intense signal intensity in the atrophic pons.
- The slit hyper-intensity of the lateral margin of the putamen in T2-weighted MRI is a characteristic finding in patients with MSA, involving the extrapyramidal system.
- For patients who fail to respond to therapeutic doses of L-dopa (at least 600 mg/day) administered for 12 weeks.

* **Positron emission tomography (PET) scanning with fluorodopa: PET scans may demonstrate if metabolic function is reduced in specific parts of the brain:**
  - They can localize dopamine deficiency in the basal ganglia, while autonomic tests and sphincter electromyography may support a diagnosis of MSA.
  - **The caudate nucleus c**an be used for differentiation between MSA and PD.
  - The caudate-putamen index (difference in the uptakes in the caudate and putamen divided by the caudate uptake) is lower in patients with MSA than in patients with PD.
* **123I-FP-CIT single photon emission computerized tomography (SPECT):**
  - It should be considered for people with tremor if essential tremor cannot be clinically differentiated from Parkinsonism.
* **Transcranial sonography:**
  - Recommended for the early diagnosis of PD, for the detection of subjects at risk for PD, and for the differentiation of PD from atypical and secondary Parkinsonian disorders, However, the technique is not universally available and requires some expertise.

## Genetic testing

- This test can show if a person has a mutation that changes how their body processes α-synuclein. Genetic tests are more likely to identify mutations related to MSA-C in people of Japanese descent. Genetic testing may be required (e.g., Huntington's gene). Fewer than 5% of all PD cases are caused by known single-gene mutations.
- Further investigations for young-onset or atypical disease may include measurement of ceruloplasmin levels (Wilson's disease) and syphilis serology.

Table 10.1 summarizes the major features supporting the diagnosis of 'probable MSA' whereas Table 10.2 summarizes the additional features supporting a diagnosis of 'possible MSA'. Sporadic, progressive disease of onset after 30 years of age is therein characterized.

**Table 10.1 - Major features supporting the diagnosis of 'probable' MSA**

| System | Features | Notes |
|---|---|---|
| **Autonomic** | **o Severe (symptomatic or otherwise) orthostatic hypotension**<br>**o Commonly associated symptoms include light-headedness, dizziness, weakness of legs, fatigue, and syncope.**<br>**o Postprandial hypotension may be a major feature.** | **o Blood pressure fall by ≥30 mm Hg systolic and ≥15 mm Hg diastolic within 3-minutes of standing from a previous 3-minute supine position**<br>**o Associated supine hyper-tension is common, and is aggravated by medication used to reduce orthostatic hypotension.** |
| **Urogenital** | **o Urinary incontinence or incomplete emptying**<br>o Erectile dysfunction | **o Urinary dysfunction is the most frequent initial complaint in women**<br>o Erectile dysfunction is the most frequent initial complaint in men |
| **Extrapyramidal tracts** | **o Tremor (but not classic pill-rolling)**<br>**o Rigidity**<br>**o Bradykinesia**<br>o Gait postural instability | **o Check that postural instability is not caused by primary visual, vestibular, cerebellar, or proprioceptive dysfunction** |

| | | |
|---|---|---|
| **Cerebellar function** | **o Gait/limb ataxia**<br>o Ataxic dysarthria<br>o Oculomotor dysfunction (sustained gaze-evoked nystagmus) | |

**Table 10.2 – Additional features supporting the diagnosis of 'possible' MSA**

| System | Features | Notes |
|---|---|---|
| **Parkinsonism** | **Parkinsonism** | |
| **Cerebellar** | **Cerebellar signs** | |
| **Autonomic system** | **Autonomic dysfunction (at least one feature)** | **Features include:**<br>o **Urinary symptoms**<br>o **Erectile dysfunction**<br>o **Orthostatic hypotension that does not meet the level required in 'probable MSA' (see Table above10.1)** |
| **MSA-P or MSA-C** | o **Babinski's sign with hyper-reflexia.**<br>o **Stridor** | |
| **MSA-P** | o Rapidly progressive parkinsonism with poor response to Levodopa<br>o Postural instability within 3 years of motor onset<br>o Gait ataxia<br>o Cerebellar dysarthria<br>o Limb ataxia<br>o Cerebellar oculomotor dysfunction.<br>o Dysphagia within 5 years of motor onset. | |
| **MSA-C** | o Parkinsonism (bradykinesia and rigidity).<br>o Atrophy on MRI of putamen, middle cerebellar peduncle, or pons. | |

**Table 10.3 lists features suggestive of an alternative diagnosis.**

Table 10.3 - Features suggesting an alternative diagnosis

| Assessment | Feature |
|---|---|
| **History** | o Symptomatic onset at <30 years or >75 years<br>o Family history of ataxia or parkinsonism<br>o Known co-morbidity featuring symptoms and signs listed in Tables 10.1-2<br>o Hallucinations unrelated to medication<br>o Dementia |
| **Examination** | o Classical parkinsonian pill-rolling rest tremor<br>o Clinically significant neuropathy<br>o Prominent slowing of vertical saccades or vertical supranuclear gaze palsy<br>o Evidence of focal cortical dysfunction such as dysphasia, alien limb syndrome, and parietal dysfunction |

## Other diagnoses to consider

Other diagnoses to consider include:

- **Pure autonomic failure.**
- **Progressive supranuclear palsy (Steele-Richardson-Olszewski disease).**
- **Multi-infarct dementia.**
- **Multiple sclerosis. (**See this author's textbook on the subject, Fymat, 2022 in the list of references for multiple sclerosis at the end of the book.)
- **Neuroacanthocytosis.**
- **Neurosarcoidosis.**
- **Neurosyphilis.**

## Genetic counseling

MSA occurs sporadically. However, some familial cases have been described.

## Take-away points

- Diagnosis of MSA is clinically based on the combination of signs and symptoms, medical history, physical examination, laboratory test results, various autonomic insufficiency tests, neuroradiological imaging studies, and response to certain treatments. The tests can help determine whether the diagnosis is 'probable MSA' or 'possible MSA'. No laboratory or imaging studies are able to definitively confirm the diagnosis.
- Reaching a diagnosis can be challenging and difficult, particularly in the early stages, in part because many of its features are similar to those observed in Parkinson's disease (PD), parkinsonism, and a number of other confounding diseases. Because of this difficulty, some people are actually never properly diagnosed.
- The main differential diagnoses seek to rule-out any one or more of the following confounding diseases: Alzheimer's, corticobasal degeneration, Creutzfeldt-Jakob, dementias (Lewy bodies, multi-infarct), frontotemporal degeneration, Guam (Lytico-Bodig syndrome), Huntington's, Parkinson's, parkinsonism (including atypical syndromes), progressive supranuclear palsy (Steele-Richardson-Olszewski), tremors (benign essential, cerebellar, drug- or toxin-induced, psychogenic), and Wilson's disease.
- A brief primer on Parkinson's disease has been provided including its epidemiology, signs & symptoms, cause, diagnostic criteria, long-term problems, motor fluctuations, axial problems not responding to treatment, Parkinson's disease dementia, and differential diagnosis between PD and MSA wherein MSA **progresses faster, its symptoms develop differently, and it responds poorly to Levodopa.**
- A parkinsonism has likewise been provided, including its risk factors, pathogenesis, and differences between MSA and parkinsonism.
- MSA diagnostic tests reviewed included: **Autonomic function testing (blood** pressure, thermoregulatory sweat, bladder function, bowel function, electrocardiogram, sleep, diminished respiratory sinus arrhythmia, olfactory testing:, skin biopsy, abnormal response to the Valsalva maneuver, diminished response to isometric exercise, diminished response to cold pressor stimuli,

n**europathological testing, r**adiopharmaceutical imaging (**DaTscanTM, Iodine-123 (I-123) scintigraphy), n**euroradiological imaging (CT or MRI brain scan, positron emission tomography scanning with fluorodopa, 123I-FP-CIT single photon emission computerized tomography, transcranial sonography, and genetic testing.

- Further investigations for young-onset or atypical disease may include measurement of ceruloplasmin levels (Wilson's disease) and syphilis serology.
- The major features supporting the diagnosis of 'probable MSA' or 'possible MSA' have been provided for autonomic, urogenital, extrapyramidal tracts, cerebellar, Parkinson's, MSA-P, and MSA-C,
- Other diagnoses to consider include: Pure autonomic failure, progressive supranuclear palsy (Steele-Richardson-Olszewski disease), multi--infarct dementia, multiple sclerosis. neuroacanthocytosis. neurosarcoidosis, and neurosyphilis.

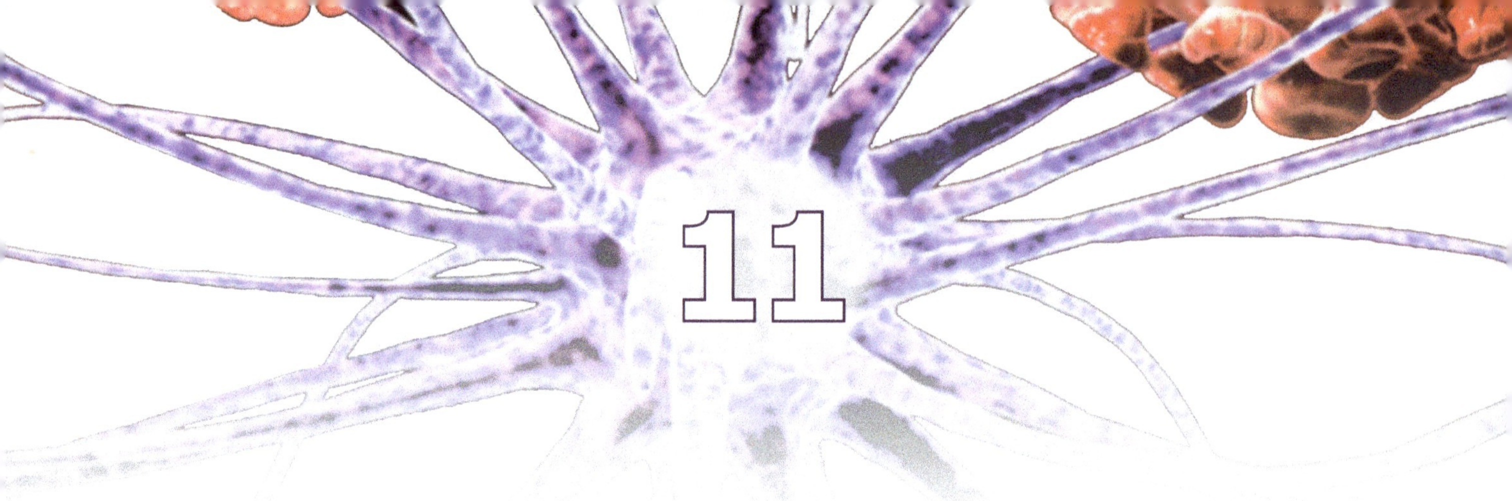


# Management of symptoms

Therapy mainly targets parkinsonism and autonomic failure. Levodopa may transiently improve parkinsonism (20%-30% of patients) but no effective neuroprotective therapy is available.

## Monitoring symptoms

Regulatory agencies have approved a few devices to help monitor symptoms. Kinesia 360, KinesiaU, PDMonitor, Personal KinetiGraph (PKG), STAT-ON, and possibly others are only conditionally recommended as options for the remote monitoring of PD.

## Symptoms relief

At present, no available treatment can cure MSA. However, a combination of simple measures and drugs may help relieve symptoms. These are summarized below for a few important symptoms:

- **Parkinsonism**
  - Continuing to do as many daily activities as possible helps maintain muscle strength and flexibility.
  - Stretching and exercising regularly may also help.
- **Orthostatic hypotension**

  Measures are taken to stabilize the sudden changes in blood pressure:
  - **Increasing blood pressure:** Consuming more salt and water may increase the volume of blood and, thus, help increase blood pressure.
  - **Preventing blood pressure from increasing:** Raising the head of the bed by about 4 inches (10 centimeters) can help prevent blood pressure from increasing too much when the person lies down.

- **Maintaining blood pressure:** Standing up slowly may help prevent blood pressure from decreasing too much or too fast when a person stands, as may wearing an abdominal binder or compression stockings. These garments help maintain blood pressure by promoting blood flow from the legs to the heart and, thus, prevent too much blood from staying (pooling) in the legs.
- **Non-drug treatments:** In addition to the above suggested measures including "head-up tilt" (elevating the head of the whole bed by about 10 degrees), ingesting salt tablets or increasing salt in the diet, generous intake of fluids, and pressure (elastic) stockings, and abdominal binders, the following non-drug treatments are also recommended. Avoidance of triggers of low blood pressure, such as hot weather, alcohol, and dehydration are crucial. Moving and transferring from sitting to standing slowly to decrease risk of falls and limiting the effect of postural hypotension. Instruction in ankle pumping helps to return blood in the legs to the systemic circulation.

- **Body fluids production**
  - **Decreasing production of body fluids:** If sweating is reduced or absent, people should avoid warm environments to avoid overheating the body. Good dental care and regular check-ups are essential for people with dry mouth. Artificial tears (eye drops containing substances that resemble real tears) applied every few hours may relieve dry eyes.
  - **Urinary retention:** If needed, people can learn to insert a catheter (a thin rubber tube) into the bladder themselves. They insert it several times a day. It is inserted through the urethra, allowing urine in the bladder to drain out. People remove the catheter after the bladder is empty. This measure helps prevent the bladder from stretching and urinary tract infections from developing. Washing the hands, cleansing the area around the urethra, and using a sterile or clean catheter also help prevent infections. Inserting a catheter becomes more difficult as coordination deteriorates.
  - **Urinary incontinence:** Certain drugs (see section below) may be used to relax the muscles of an overactive bladder. If incontinence persists, using a catheter inserted into the bladder may help. Certain drugs (see section below) may stimulate contractions of the bladder and, thus, help the bladder empty.

- **Constipation**
  - A high-fiber diet and stool softeners are recommended. If constipation persists, enemas may be necessary.

- **Erectile dysfunction**
  - Usually, treatment consists of drugs (see section below).

## Symptoms management

Currently, no specific treatment can reverse or halt the progression of the disease, but symptoms can be managed.

- **Orthostatic hypotension:** It is associated with reduced physical activity, and the consequent de-conditioning and problems associated with it. Management will include:
  - Management of postural hypotension.
  - Management of constipation, urinary incontinence, and falls.
  - Physical activity, especially in water, to prevent physical de-conditioning.
  - Speech therapy, which may be required to help with speech and swallowing.
- **Movement disorder:** Usually treated with drugs, but their effectiveness may be limited.
- **Functional capacity:** Recombinant erythropoietin (see section below) has been shown to correct anemia and improve standing blood pressure.

## Pharmacological therapy

Patients require pharmacological therapy because the disorder is progressive and fatal. The therapy targets PD, parkinsonism and autonomic failure. The extrapyramidal and cerebellar aspects of the disease are debilitating and difficult to treat. The drug Tiluzole is ineffective in treating MSA or PSP.

- **Autonomic failure:**
  - **Increasing blood pressure:** Fludrocortisone (taken by mouth) helps the body retain salt and water and, thus, may increase blood pressure as needed when a person stands. Other drugs, such as Midodrine or Droxidopa, taken by mouth, may also help.
  - **Orthostatic hypotension:** Treatment includes intravascular volume expansion with salt and water supplementation and sometimes Fludrocortisone (0.1 to 0.4 mg, orally, once a day) or alpha-adrenoreceptor stimulation with Midodrine (10 mg, orally, 3 times a day) may help. However, Midodrine also increases peripheral vascular resistance and supine blood pressure (BP), which may be problematic. Alternatively, Droxidopa may be used; its action is similar to that of Midodrine, but duration of action is longer.

- **Urinary retention**: Bethanechol (10-50 mg, orally, 3 or 4 times a day) is used to stimulate contractions of the bladder and, thus, help the bladder empty.
- **Urinary incontinence:** Certain drugs such as Oxybutynin chloride (5 mg, orally, 3 times a day), Mirabegron (25-50 mg, once a day), Tamsulosin (0.4-0.8 mg, once a day), or Tolterodine (2 mg, taken by mouth, 2 times a day), may be used to relax the muscles of an overactive bladder. Tamsulosin may be effective for urinary urgency. Unlike Tamsulosin, the beta-3 adrenergic agonist Mirabegron does not worsen orthostatic hypotension.
- **Erectile dysfunction:** Sildenafil, Tadalafil (2.5-5 mg, daily), Vardenafil, or Avanafil, taken orally, as needed, can be used.
- **Functional capacity:** Recombinant erythropoietin increases the functional capacity of patients, particularly if there is associated mild anemia, which is common. It has been shown to correct anemia and improve standing blood pressure.

- M**ovement disorders:** Usually treated with Levodopa, dopaminergic agonists, anticholinergic agents, or Amantadine, but effectiveness may be limited.
- **PD:** Drugs used to treat PD, such as Levodopa plus Carbidopa (taken by mouth) may be tried, but this combination usually has little effect or is effective for only a few years.
- **Parkinsonism:** Levodopa (L-Dopa) improves parkinsonian symptoms in a small percentage of MSA patients. Levodopa/Carbidopa (25-100 mg, taken orally at bedtime) may be tried to relieve rigidity and other parkinsonian symptoms, but this combination is usually ineffective or provides modest benefit. Other agents that are much less often used include NSAIDs (non-steroidal anti-inflammatory drugs), antihistamines, somatostatin analogues, caffeine, and Yohimbine. (Note: A recent trial reported that only 1.5% of MSA patients experienced any improvement at all when taking Levodopa, their improvement was less than 50%, and even that improvement was a transient effect lasting less than one year. Poor response to L-Dopa has been suggested as a possible element in the differential diagnosis of MSA from PD.)
- **Postural hypotension:** It often responds to Fludrocortisone, a synthetic mineralocorticoid. Another common drug treatment is the alpha-agonist Midodrine.

## Supervision

Ongoing care from a neurologist specializing in movement disorders is recommended because the complex symptoms of MSA are often not familiar to less-specialized neurologists. Hospice/homecare services can be very useful as disability progresses.

## Rehabilitation

Management by rehabilitation professionals including physiatrists, physiotherapists, occupational therapists, speech therapists, and others for difficulties with walking/ movement, daily tasks, and speech problems is essential.

Physiotherapists can help to maintain the patient's mobility and will help to prevent contractures. Instructing patients in gait training will help to improve their mobility and decrease their risk of falls. A physiotherapist may also prescribe mobility aids such as a cane or a walker to increase the patient's safety.

Physical and occupational therapists can teach people ways to compensate when walking, doing daily activities, and speaking become difficult. Social workers can help people find support groups and, when symptoms become disabling, home health care or hospice services.

Speech therapists may assist in assessing, treating, and supporting speech (dysarthria) and swallowing difficulties (dysphagia). Speech changes mean that alternative communication may be needed, for example, communication aids or word charts.

Early intervention of swallowing difficulties is particularly useful to allow for discussion around tube feeding further in the disease progression. At some point in the progression of the disease, fluid and food modification may be implemented.

## Supportive care

As the disease progresses, people may need a breathing tube and/or a feeding tube (usually surgically inserted), or both.

Clinicians should advise patients to prepare advance directives soon after MSA is diagnosed.

Facts sheets for most MSA drugs are provided in Sidebar 11.1. These drugs include: Amantadine HCl, Avanafil, Betanechol HCl, Carbidopa, Droxidopa, Fludrocortisone, Levodopa, Midodrine HCl, Mirabegron, Oxybutynin HCl, Rinuzole, Sildenafil, Tdalafil, Tamsulosin, Tolteradine tartrate, and Vardenafil HCl.

## Take-away points

- At present, no available treatment can cure MSA. However, a combination of simple measures and drugs may help relieve symptoms. For parkinsonism, continuing to do as many daily activities as possible, including regular stretching and exercise. For orthostatic hypotension, stabilizing the sudden changes in blood pressure. For body fluids, decreasing their production, taking measures against urinary retention or incontinence. For constipation, change diet or/and use over-the-counter (OTC) products. For erectile dysfunction, treatment consists of a variety of drugs.

- Whilst no specific treatment can reverse or halt the progression of the disease, symptoms can be managed for orthostatic hypotension, postural hypotension management, constipation, urinary incontinence, and falls, Remain physically active, and seek speech therapy. For movement disorder, treat with drugs but their effectiveness may be limited. For functional capacity, recombinant erythropoietin has been shown to correct anemia and improve standing blood pressure.
- Pharmacological therapy is required because the disorder is progressive and fatal. It targets Parkinson's Disease, parkinsonism and autonomic failure. The extrapyramidal and cerebellar aspects of the disease are debilitating and difficult to treat. Several medications are available for Parkinson's, parkinsonism, movement disorders, postural hypotension, and autonomic failure.
- Most of the available drugs have been indicated, including detailed Fact Sheets.
- Supervision and ongoing care is required from a neurologist specializing in movement disorders.
- Management by rehabilitation professionals including physiatrists, physiotherapists, occupational therapists, speech therapists, and others for difficulties with walking/ movement, daily tasks, and speech problems is essential.
- Supportive care is needed as the disease progresses.

## Sidebar 11.1 - MSA drugs Facts Sheets

### Amantadine HCl

Amantadine is used to treat Parkinson's disease, as well as side effects caused by drugs (such as drug-induced extrapyramidal symptoms), chemicals, and other medical conditions. In these cases, this medication may help to improve the range of motion and ability to exercise. It works by restoring the balance of natural chemicals (neurotransmitters) in the brain. This medication is an antiviral, not a vaccine.

#### Uses

This medication works best when the amount of medicine in the body is kept at a constant level. In PD, the effects of the medication may not be noticed for several weeks. It may not work as well after it has been taken for several months.

#### Side Effects

Blurred vision, nausea, stomach upset, drowsiness, dizziness, headache, dry mouth, constipation, nervousness, or trouble sleeping may occur.

Many people using this medication do not have serious side effects. Such effects include: Seizures, falling asleep during usual daily activities (talking on the phone, driving, sleep may rarely occur without any feelings of drowsiness beforehand), purplish-red blotchy spots on the skin, swelling of the ankles/feet, difficulty urinating, vision changes, shortness of breath, mental/mood changes (depression, suicidal thoughts/attempts), muscle stiffness, uncontrolled muscle movements, unusual sweating, fast heartbeat, unexplained fever, unusual strong urges (increased gambling, increased sexual urges). The risk of the sleep effect is increased by using alcohol or other medications that can make one drowsy. A very serious allergic reaction to this drug is rare, including: rash, itching/swelling (especially of the face/tongue/throat), severe dizziness, trouble breathing.

Older adults may be at a greater risk for side effects while taking this drug.

During pregnancy, this medication should be used only when clearly needed as it passes into breast milk and may have undesirable effects on a nursing infant.

### Precautions

One should not overdo physical activity as one's condition improves because this may increase the risk of falls.

### Drug interactions

Drug interactions may change how medications work or increase the risk for serious side effects. Amantadine may interfere with the effect of certain vaccines, such as flu vaccine inhaled through the nose.

## Avanafil

Avanafil is used to treat male sexual function problems (impotence or erectile dysfunction-ED). In combination with sexual stimulation, Avanafil works by increasing blood flow to the penis to help a man get and keep an erection. This drug does not protect against sexually transmitted diseases (such as HIV, hepatitis B, gonorrhea, syphilis).

### Uses

This medication is available in different doses. The dosage is based on the medical condition, response to treatment, and other medications one may be taking.

### Side effects

This drug may cause dizziness or vision changes, which may be exacerbated by alcohol or marijuana (cannabis). Rarely, a sudden decrease or loss of hearing, sometimes with ringing in the ears and dizziness, or/and a painful or prolonged erection lasting 4 or more hours, may occur,. A very serious allergic reaction is rare, including: rash, itching/swelling (especially of the face/tongue/throat), severe dizziness, trouble breathing.

### Precautions

Use of this medication depends on existing medical conditions, especially heart problems (such as heart attack or life-threatening irregular heartbeat in the past 6 months, chest pain/angina, heart failure), stroke in the past 6 months, kidney disease (dialysis), liver disease, high or low blood pressure, dehydration, penis conditions (such as angulation, fibrosis/scarring, Peyronie's disease - PD), history of painful/prolonged erection (priapism), conditions that may increase the risk of priapism (such as sickle cell anemia, leukemia, multiple myeloma), eye problems (such as retinitis pigmentosa, sudden decreased vision, NAION), bleeding disorders, active stomach ulcers.

### Drug interactions

Drug interactions may change how medications work or increase the risk for serious side effects.

A product that may interact with this drug is Riociguat.

Avanafil should not be used with any of the following: certain drugs used to treat chest pain/angina (nitrates such as Nitroglycerin, Isosorbide), recreational drugs called "poppers" containing amyl or butyl nitrite. Avanafil can cause a serious drop in blood pressure when used with nitrates, which can lead to dizziness, fainting, and rarely heart attack or stroke.

If also taking an alpha blocker medication (such as Doxazosin, Tamsulosin) to treat an enlarged prostate/BPH or hypertension, blood pressure may get too low, leading to dizziness or fainting.

Other medications can affect the removal of Avanafil, including: Azole antifungals (such as Itraconazole, Ketoconazole), Cobicistat, macrolide antibiotics (such as Clarithromycin, Erythromycin), HIV protease inhibitors (such as Indinavir, Ritonavir), hepatitis C virus protease inhibitors (such as Boceprevir, Relaprevir), Nefazodone, Ribociclib, Rifampin, among others.

## Bethanechol chloride

Bethanechol is used to treat certain bladder problems such as the inability to urinate or empty the bladder completely. It helps the bladder muscle to squeeze better, thereby improving the ability to urinate.

### Uses

This medication is available in different doses. The dosage is based on the medical condition, response to treatment, and other medications one may be taking.

### Side effects

Dizziness, lightheadedness, nausea, vomiting, abdominal cramps/pain, diarrhea, increased saliva/urination, sweating, flushing, watery eyes, or headache may occur. Serious allergic reactions to this drug are rare, including: rash, itching/swelling (especially of the face/tongue/throat), severe dizziness, trouble breathing.

### Precautions

This product may contain inactive ingredients, which can cause allergic reactions or other problems. It should not be taken if there has been a recent stomach/intestinal/bladder surgery, stomach/intestinal problems (such as ulcers, blockage, spasms), peritonitis, blockage of the bladder, a certain nerve problem (vagotonia), overactive thyroid (hyperthyroidism), lung disease (such as asthma, chronic obstructive pulmonary disease-COPD), heart problems (such as coronary artery disease, slow heartbeat), seizures, Parkinson's disease, blood pressure problems. Alcohol or marijuana (cannabis) can cause dizziness.

### Drug interactions

This medication may interfere with certain laboratory tests (including amylase/lipase levels), possibly causing false test results.

## Carbidopa

Cabidopa is used in combination with Levodopa to treat symptoms of Parkinson's disease or Parkinson-like symptoms (such as shakiness, stiffness, difficulty moving). If used alone, Carbidopa has no effect on Parkinson's symptoms. Levodopa changes into dopamine in the brain, helping to control movement. Carbidopa prevents the breakdown of Levodopa in the bloodstream so more Levodopa can enter the brain. Carbidopa can also reduce some of Levodopa's side effects such as nausea and vomiting.

### Uses

The dosage is based on medical condition and response to treatment. Since this medication is always taken with a Levodopa-containing product, it is best to avoid a high-protein diet (it decreases the amount of Levodopa that the body takes in) during treatment. It should be separated by as many hours as possible from any iron supplements or products containing iron (such as multivitamins with minerals) one may take. Iron can reduce the amount of Levodopa absorbed by the body.

### Side effects

This drug may cause dizziness and drowsiness, which may be exacerbated by alcohol or marijuana (cannabis). During pregnancy, this medication should be used only when clearly needed.

### Precautions

Some patients may experience a "wearing-off" (worsening of symptoms) before the next dose is due. An "on-off" effect might also occur, in which sudden short periods of stiffness occur.

### Drug interactions

Drug interactions may change how your medications work or increase your risk for serious side effects.

Some products that may interact with this drug (or Levodopa) include: Antipsychotic drugs (such as Chlorpromazine, Haloperidol, Thioridazine), certain drugs used to treat high blood pressure (such as Methyldopa, Tetrabenazine). Taking MAO inhibitors with this medication (along with a Levodopa-containing product) may cause a serious (possibly fatal) drug interaction. Avoid taking MAO inhibitors (Isocarboxazid, Linezolid, Metaxalone, Methylene blue, Moclobemide, Phenelzine, Procarbazine, Tranylcypromine). Most MAO inhibitors should also not be taken for two weeks before treatment with this medication. However, certain MAO inhibitors (Rasagiline, Safinamide, Selegiline) may be used with careful monitoring.

This medication (or Levodopa) may interfere with certain laboratory tests (including urine catecholamine/glucose/ketone tests), possibly causing false test results.

## Droxidopa

Droxidopa is used to treat symptoms of low blood pressure when standing such as dizziness, lightheadedness, or the "feeling that you are about to black out", caused by a certain medical condition (neurogenic orthostatic hypotension-NOH). It is thought to work by making the blood vessels become more narrow, which increases blood pressure.

### Uses

The dosage is based on the medical condition and response to treatment. Since it is unknown if this medication will work longer than 2 weeks, it should be continued only if symptoms continue to get better during treatment.

### Side effects

Headache, nausea, or dizziness may occur. This medication can increase blood pressure, especially when lying down (supine hypertension). It may rarely cause very serious symptoms that are like a condition called neuroleptic malignant syndrome (NMS). A very serious allergic reaction to this drug is rare including: rash, itching/swelling (especially of the face/tongue/throat), severe dizziness, trouble breathing.

### Precautions

This product may contain inactive ingredients, which can cause allergic reactions or other problems. It may cause dizziness or increase blood pressure. During pregnancy, this medication should be used only when clearly needed. It is unknown if this medication passes into breast milk

## Fludrocortisone

Fludrocortisone is a man-made form of a natural substance (glucocorticoid) made by the body. It is used along with other medications (such as Hydrocortisone) to treat low glucocorticoid levels caused by disease of the adrenal gland (such as Addison's disease, adrenocortical insufficiency, salt-losing adrenogenital syndrome). Glucocorticoids are needed in many ways for the body to function well. They are important for salt and water balance and keeping blood pressure normal. They are also needed to break down carbohydrates in the diet. Fludrocortisone makes the body hold on to salt (sodium) and get rid of other salts (such as calcium, potassium).

### Uses

The dosage is based on the medical condition and response to therapy. Some conditions may become worse when the drug is suddenly stopped.

### Side effects

Stomach upset, headache, and menstrual changes (such as delayed/irregular/absent periods) may occur. Serious side effects include: Change in skin appearance (such as color changes, thinning, fatty areas), easy bleeding/bruising, dizziness, slow wound healing, signs of infection (such as sore throat that does not go away, fever, skin sores), bone/joint/muscle pain, puffy face, swelling of the hands/feet, severe tiredness, increased thirst/urination, unusual weight gain, muscle weakness, eye problems (such as pain, redness, vision changes), severe/continuous headaches, fast/pounding/irregular heartbeat, mental/mood changes (such as agitation, depression, mood swings), seizure, symptoms of stomach/intestinal bleeding (such as stomach/abdominal pain, black/tarry stools, vomit that looks like coffee grounds).

A very serious allergic reaction to this drug is rare including: rash, itching/swelling (especially of the face/tongue/throat), severe dizziness, trouble breathing.

### Precautions

This product may contain inactive ingredients, which can cause allergic reactions or other problems depending on medical history, especially of: bleeding problems, blood clots, brittle bones (osteoporosis), diabetes, eye problems (such as cataracts, glaucoma, infection of the eye), heart problems (such as congestive heart failure), high blood pressure, infections (such as candidiasis, valley fever, herpes, tuberculosis), kidney disease, liver disease (such as cirrhosis), mental/mood disorders (such as anxiety, depression, psychosis), low blood minerals (such as calcium, potassium), stomach/ intestinal problems (such as diverticulitis, peptic ulcer disease, ulcerative colitis), seizures, thyroid problems.

This medication may mask signs of infection or put at greater risk of developing very serious infections (such as sore throat that doesn't go away/fever/cough, pain while urinating, skin sores) that occur during treatment.

Do not have immunizations/vaccinations and avoid contact with people who have recently received oral polio vaccine or flu vaccine inhaled through the nose. Avoid exposure to chickenpox or measles infection.

Using corticosteroid medications for a long time can make it more difficult for the body to respond to physical stress.

This medication may slow down a child's growth if used for a long time. Older adults may be more sensitive to the side effects of this drug, especially water retention, bone loss/ pain, stomach/intestinal bleeding, and mental/mood changes (such as confusion).

During pregnancy, this medication should be used only when clearly needed. Infants born to mothers who have been using this medication for an extended time may have low levels of corticosteroid hormone. This medication passes into breast milk and may have undesirable effects on a nursing infant.

### Drug interactions

Some products that may interact with this drug are: Aldesleukin, Digoxin, drugs that can cause bleeding/bruising (including antiplatelet drugs such as Clopidogrel, "blood thinners" such as Dabigatran/warfarin, NSAIDs such as Aspirin/Celecoxib/Ibuprofen), hormones (such as androgens, birth control pills, estrogens), immunosuppressants (such as Cyclosporine), Mifepristone, vaccines, drugs affecting liver enzymes that remove Fludrocortisone from the body (including Rifamycins such as Rifampin/Rifabutin, certain anti-seizure medicines such as barbiturates/Phenytoin).

This medication may interfere with certain laboratory tests, possibly causing false results.

## Levodopa (see Carbidopa}

## Midodrine HCl

Midodrine is used for certain patients who have symptoms of orthostatic hypotension. It is known as a sympathomimetic (alpha receptor agonist) that acts on the blood vessels to raise blood pressure.

### Uses

Dosage is based on your medical condition and response to treatment

### Side effects

Skin tingling, chills, "goose bumps," stomach pain, or urinary problems (strong/frequent urge to urinate, frequent urination, trouble urinating) may occur. Less common side effects include: dry mouth, dizziness, drowsiness, trouble sleeping, or leg cramps.

This medication can cause the blood pressure to increase, especially when lying down (supine hypertension)., and rarely cause dizziness, drowsiness, or vision blur.

Serious side effects may include: Slow heartbeat, unusual feeling in the chest, fainting, pressure/fullness in the head, confusion, anxiety, weakness, vision problems.

A very serious allergic reaction to this drug is rare.

### Precautions

This product may contain inactive ingredients, which can cause allergic reactions or other problems.

It is unknown if this medication passes into breast milk.

### Drug interactions

Drug interactions may change how medications work or increase the risk for serious side effects. Some products have ingredients that could raise the blood pressure. products, diet aids, or NSAIDs such as ibuprofen/naproxen).

## Mirabegron

Mirabegron is used to treat certain bladder problems (overactive bladder, neurogenic detrusor overactivity). Overactive bladder is a problem with how the bladder stores urine. Neurogenic detrusor overactivity is a bladder control condition caused by brain, spinal cord, or nerve problems. Symptoms of these conditions may include frequent urination, strong sudden urges to urinate that are hard to control, or involuntary loss of urine (incontinence). Mirabegron works by relaxing a certain bladder muscle (detrusor), which helps the bladder hold more urine and lessens symptoms of overactive bladder and neurogenic detrusor overactivity.

### Uses

The dosage is based on medical condition and response to treatment. Children's dose is also based on weight.

## Side effects

Nausea, dizziness, fast heartbeat, runny/stuffy nose, or headache may occur. This medication may raise the blood pressure. Many people using this medication do not have serious side effects.

A very serious allergic reaction to this drug is rare, including: rash, itching/swelling (especially of the face/tongue/throat), severe dizziness, trouble breathing.

## Precautions

This product may contain inactive ingredients, which can cause allergic reactions or other problems. It may cause dizziness, which alcohol or marijuana (cannabis) can worsen.

During pregnancy, this medication should be used only when clearly needed. It is unknown if it passes into breast milk.

## Drug interactions

This medication can slow down the removal of other medications from the body, which may affect how it works. Examples of affected drugs include Flecainide, Propafenone, Thioridazine, among others.

# Oxybutinin chloride

Oxybutynin belongs to a class of drugs known as antispasmodics. The manufacturer does not recommend using this medication in children younger than 5 years of age.

## Uses

Oxybutynin is used to treat certain bladder and urinary conditions (such as overactive bladder). It relaxes the muscles in the bladder to help decrease problems of urgency and frequent urination. The dosage is based on the medical condition and response to therapy.

## Side effects

Dry mouth, dizziness, drowsiness, blurred vision, dry eyes, nausea, vomiting, upset stomach, stomach pain, constipation, diarrhea, headache, unusual taste in mouth, dry/flushed skin, and weakness, dizziness, drowsiness or blurred vision may occur.

This drug may increase the risk for heatstroke because it causes decreased sweating.

Serious side effects may include: Decreased sexual activity, difficulty urinating, fast/pounding heartbeat, signs of kidney infection (such as burning/painful/frequent urination, lower back pain, fever), mental/mood changes (such as confusion, hallucinations), swelling of arms/legs/ankles/feet, vision problems (including eye pain), seizures, stomach/intestinal blockage (such as nausea/vomiting that doesn't stop, prolonged constipation).

A very serious allergic reaction to this drug is rare including: rash, itching/swelling (especially of the face/tongue/throat), severe dizziness, trouble breathing.

### Precautions

This product may contain inactive ingredients, which can cause allergic reactions or other problems.

During pregnancy, this medication should be used only when clearly needed. It is unknown if it passes into breast milk.

### Interactions

Drug interactions may change how medications work or increase the risk for serious side effects.

Some products that may interact with this drug include: Pramlintide, drugs that can irritate the esophagus/stomach (such as potassium tablets/capsules, oral bisphosphonates including Alendronate, etidronate).

## Riluzole

Riluzole is used to treat a certain type of nerve disease called amyotrophic lateral sclerosis (ALS, also commonly called Lou Gehrig's disease). It helps to slow down the worsening of this disease and prolong survival.

### Side effects

Drowsiness, nausea, vomiting, or numbness/tingling around the mouth may occur.

Many people using this medication do not have serious side effects, including: fast heartbeat, signs of liver disease (nausea/vomiting that does not stop, loss of appetite, stomach/abdominal pain, yellowing eyes/skin, dark urine), signs of infection (such as sore throat that doesn't go away, fever), signs of lung problems (such as shortness of breath, cough).

This product may contain inactive ingredients, which can cause allergic reactions or other problems. However, a very serious allergic reaction to this drug is rare.

### Precautions

This drug may cause dizziness or drowsiness, which may be exacerbated by alcohol or marijuana (cannabis). Liquid products may contain sugar and/or aspartame, which is not advised when having diabetes, phenylketonuria (PKU), or any other condition that requires to limit/avoid these substances in the diet. Ask your doctor or pharmacist about using this product safely.

During pregnancy, this medication should be used only when clearly needed. It is unknown if this drug passes into breast milk. Consult your doctor before breast-feeding.

**Drug interactions**

Drug interactions may change how medications work or increase the risk for serious side effects.

## Sildenafil

Sildenafil is used to treat high blood pressure in the lungs (pulmonary hypertension). It works by relaxing and widening the blood vessels in the lungs, which allows the blood to flow more easily. Decreasing high blood pressure in the lungs allows the heart and lungs to work better and improves the ability to exercise. This medication is not recommended for use in children.

**Uses**

Use as directed.

**Side effects**

Dizziness, lightheadedness, headache, flushing, stomach upset, nosebleeds, trouble sleeping, or swollen hands/ankles/feet (edema) may occur. Vision changes such as increased sensitivity to light, blurred vision, or trouble telling blue and green colors apart may also occur.

Many people using this medication do not have serious side effects. Rarely, sudden decreased vision, including permanent blindness, in one or both eyes (NAION) may occur. Rarely, a sudden decrease or loss of hearing, sometimes with ringing in the ears and dizziness, may occur.

Rarely, males may have a painful or prolonged erection lasting 4 or more hours (priapism).

A very serious allergic reaction to this drug is rare.

**Precautions**

This product may contain inactive ingredients, which can cause allergic reactions or other problems, including:.dizziness or vision problems.

During pregnancy, Sildenafil should be used only when clearly needed.

### Drug interactions

Drug interactions may change how medications work or increase the risk for serious side effects. Some products that may interact with this drug are: Riociguat, Vericiguat.

Sildenafil should not be used with any drugs used to treat chest pain/angina (nitrates such as Nitroglycerin, Isosorbide), recreational drugs called "poppers" containing amyl nitrate, amyl nitrite, or butyl nitrite, alpha blocker medication (such as Doxazosin, Tamsulosin), to treat an enlarged prostate/BPH or high blood pressure.

Other medications can affect the removal of sildenafil from the body, including: azole antifungals (such as Itraconazole, Ketoconazole), Cobicistat, macrolide antibiotics (such as Clarithromycin, Erythromycin), Mifepristone, HIV protease inhibitors (such as Saquinavir), Rifampin, Ritonavir, among others.

## Tadalafil

Tadalafil is thought to work by relaxing the smooth muscle in the prostate and bladder. This drug does not protect against sexually transmitted diseases (such as HIV, hepatitis B, gonorrhea, syphilis).

### Uses

Tadalafil is used to treat male sexual function problems (impotence or erectile dysfunction-ED). In combination with sexual stimulation, It works by increasing blood flow to the penis to help a man get and keep an erection. It is also used to treat the symptoms of an enlarged prostate (benign prostatic hyperplasia-BPH). It helps to relieve symptoms of BPH such as difficulty in beginning the flow of urine, weak stream, and the need to urinate frequently or urgently.

The dosage is based on the medical condition, response to treatment, and other medications. It may also be taken with Finasteride to treat symptoms of BPH. To treat erectile dysfunction-ED, there are 2 ways that Tadalafil may be prescribed either at least 30 minutes before sexual activity or taking it regularly, once a day every day.

### Side effects

Headache, stomach upset, back pain, muscle pain, stuffy nose, flushing, or dizziness may occur. Many people using this medication do not have serious side effects.

Rarely, sudden decreased vision, including permanent blindness, in one or both eyes (NAION) may occur. There is a slightly greater chance of developing NAION if one has heart disease, diabetes, high cholesterol, certain other eye problems ("crowded disk"), high blood pressure, if aged over 50, or if smoking.

Rarely, a sudden decrease or loss of hearing, sometimes with ringing in the ears and dizziness, may occur.

A very serious allergic reaction to this drug is rare.

Tadalafil can cause a serious drop in blood pressure when used with nitrates, which can lead to dizziness, fainting, and rarely heart attack or stroke.

### Precautions

This product may contain inactive ingredients, which can cause allergic reactions or other problems. This drug may cause dizziness.

This brand of the drug is not usually used in women. During pregnancy, Tadalafil should be used only when clearly needed.

### Drug interactions

Drug interactions may change how medications work or increase the risk for serious side effects.

Do not use any of the following with tadalafil or within 48 hours of the last dose of Tadalafil: certain drugs used to treat chest pain/angina (nitrates such as Nitroglycerin, Isosorbide), or recreational drugs called "poppers" containing amyl or butyl nitrite.

If also taking an alpha blocker medication (such as Doxazosin, Tamsulosin) to treat an enlarged prostate/BPH or high blood pressure, the blood pressure may get too low, which can lead to dizziness or fainting.

Other medications can affect the removal of tadalafil from the body, including: Azole antifungals (such as Itraconazole, Ketoconazole), macrolide antibiotics (such as Clarithromycin, Erythromycin), HIV protease inhibitors (such as Fosamprenavir, ritonavir), hepatitis C virus protease inhibitors (such as Boceprevir, Telaprevir), rifampin, among others.

Do not take this medication with any other product that contains tadalafil or other similar medications used to treat erectile dysfunction-ED or pulmonary hypertension (such as Sildenafil, Vardenafil).

## Tamsulosin

Tamsulosin belongs to a class of drugs known as alpha blockers. It should not be used to treat high blood pressure.

### Uses

Tamsulosin is used by men to treat the symptoms of an enlarged prostate (benign prostatic hyperplasia-BPH). It does not shrink the prostate, but it works by relaxing the muscles in the prostate and the bladder. This helps to relieve symptoms of BPH such as difficulty in beginning the flow of urine, weak stream, and the need to urinate often or urgently (including during the middle of the night). It may cause a sudden drop in your blood pressure, which could lead to dizziness or fainting.

It may take up to 4 weeks before symptoms improve.

### Side effects

Dizziness, lightheadedness drowsiness, runny/stuffy nose, or ejaculation problems may occur. Many people using this medication do not have serious side effects.

Rarely, males may have a painful or prolonged erection lasting 4 or more hours.

A very serious allergic reaction to this drug is rare.

### Precautions

This drug may contain inactive ingredients, which can cause allergic reactions or other problems. It my cause dizziness or drowsiness, which are enhanced by alcohol or marijuana (cannabis).

Older adults may be more sensitive to the side effects of this drug, especially dizziness and low blood pressure when getting up from a sitting or lying position. These side effects can increase the risk of falling.

During pregnancy, this medication should be used only when clearly needed. It is unknown if this medication passes into breast milk.

### Drug interactions

Drug interactions may change how medications work or increase the risk for serious side effects. Some products that may interact with this drug include: other alpha blocker drugs (such as Prazosin, Terazosin).

If also taking a drug to treat erectile dysfunction-ED or pulmonary hypertension (such as Sildenafil, Tadalafil), blood pressure may get too low, which can lead to dizziness or fainting. Your doctor may need to adjust your medications to minimize this risk.

Other medications can affect the removal of Tamsulosin from the body, which may affect how it works, including: Azole antifungals (such as Itraconazole, Ketoconazole),

Clarithromycin, Cobicistat, HIV protease inhibitors (such as Lopinavir), Mifepristone, Tibociclib, Ritonavir, among others.

## Tolterodine tartrate

This medication belongs to the class of drugs known as antispasmodics.

This medication is used to treat an overactive bladder. By relaxing the muscles in the bladder, it improves the ability to control urination. It helps to reduce leaking of urine, feelings of needing to urinate right away, and frequent trips to the bathroom.

### Uses

The dosage is based on medical condition (especially kidney and liver disease), response to treatment, and other medications one may be taking.

### Side effects

Dry mouth, dry eyes, headache, constipation, stomach upset/pain, dizziness, drowsiness, tiredness, or blurred vision may occur. Many people using this medication do not have serious side effects including: vision changes, severe stomach/abdominal pain, trouble urinating, or signs of kidney infection (such as burning/painful urination, lower back pain, fever).

Very serious side effects include: fast/slow/irregular heartbeat, severe dizziness, fainting.

A very serious allergic reaction to this drug is rare. However, get medical help right away if you notice any symptoms of a serious allergic reaction, including: rash, itching/swelling (especially of the face/tongue/throat), severe dizziness, trouble breathing is rare.

### Precautions

This product may contain inactive ingredients, which can cause allergic reactions or other problems. It may cause a condition that affects the heart rhythm (QT prolongation) although QT prolongation can rarely cause serious (rarely fatal) fast/irregular heartbeat and other symptoms (such as severe dizziness, fainting) that need immediate medical attention.

The risk of QT prolongation may be increased for certain medical conditions such as taking other drugs that may cause QT prolongation and for the following conditions: certain heart problems (heart failure, slow heartbeat, QT prolongation in the EKG), and family history of certain heart problems (QT prolongation in the EKG, sudden cardiac death).

Low levels of potassium or magnesium in the blood may also increase the risk of QT prolongation. This risk may increase if certain drugs are used (such as diuretics/"water pills") or if for some conditions (severe sweating, diarrhea, or vomiting).

Older adults may be more sensitive to the side effects of this drug, especially QT prolongation, drowsiness, confusion, constipation, or trouble urinating. Drowsiness and confusion can increase the risk of falling.

This drug may cause dizziness or drowsiness or vision blurring, which are exacerbated by alcohol or marijuana (cannabis). It may also make one sweat less, making that person more likely to get heat stroke.

During pregnancy, this medication should be used only when clearly needed.

**Drug interactions**

Drug interactions may change how medications work or increase the risk for serious side effects. Some products that may interact with this drug include: Anticholinergic drugs (such as Atropine, Scopolamine), other antispasmodic drugs (such as Dicyclomine, Propantheline), certain anti-Parkinson's drugs (such asTrihexyphenidyl), Belladonna alkaloids, Mifepristone, Potassium tablets/capsules, Pramlintide.

Many drugs besides Tolterodine may affect the heart rhythm (QT prolongation), including Amiodarone, Dofetilide, Pimozide, Procainamide, Quinidine, Sotalol, Macrolide antibiotics (such as Erythromycin), among others.

## Vardenafil HCl

Vardenafil is used to treat male sexual function problems (impotence or erectile dysfunction-ED). In combination with sexual stimulation, It works by increasing blood flow to the penis to help a man get and keep an erection. This drug does not protect against sexually transmitted diseases (such as HIV, hepatitis B, gonorrhea, syphilis).

**Uses**

The dosage is based on medical condition, response to treatment, and other medications one may be taking.

**Side effects**

Headache flushing, stuffy/runny nose, or dizziness may occur. Vision changes such as increased sensitivity to light, blurred vision, or trouble telling blue and green colors apart may also occur. Grapefruit can increase the chance of side effects with this medicine. Many people using this medication do not have serious side effects.

Rarely, sudden decreased vision, including permanent blindness, in one or both eyes (NAION) may occur. The chance of developing NAION is greater if one has heart disease, diabetes, high cholesterol, certain other eye problems ("crowded disk"), high blood pressure, being over 50, or smoking. Rarely, a sudden decrease or loss of hearing, sometimes with ringing in the ears and dizziness, may occur.

A very serious allergic reaction to this drug. including: rash, itching/swelling (especially of the face/tongue/throat), severe dizziness, trouble breathing is rare

## Precautions

This product may contain inactive ingredients, which can cause allergic reactions or other problems. It may cause dizziness or vision changes, which are exacerbated by alcohol or marijuana (cannabis). It is unlikely to be used during pregnancy or breast-feeding.

## Drug interactions

Drug interactions may change how medications work or increase the risk for serious side effects. Some products that may interact with this drug are: Riociguat and Vericiguat.

Vardenafil can cause a serious drop in blood pressure when used with nitrates, which can lead to dizziness, fainting, and rarely heart attack or stroke. It should not be used with any of the following: certain drugs used to treat chest pain/angina (Nitrates such as Nitroglycerin, Isosorbide), recreational drugs called "poppers" containing amyl or butyl nitrite; and alpha blocker s (such as Doxazosin), Ramsulosin) to treat an enlarged prostate/BPH or high blood pressure,.

Other medications can affect the removal of Vardenafil from the body, which may affect how Vardenafil works. Examples include Azole antifungals (such as iIraconazole, Ketoconazole), Macrolide antibiotics (such as larithromycin, Erythromycin), HIV protease inhibitors (such as Indinavir), Titonavir, among others.

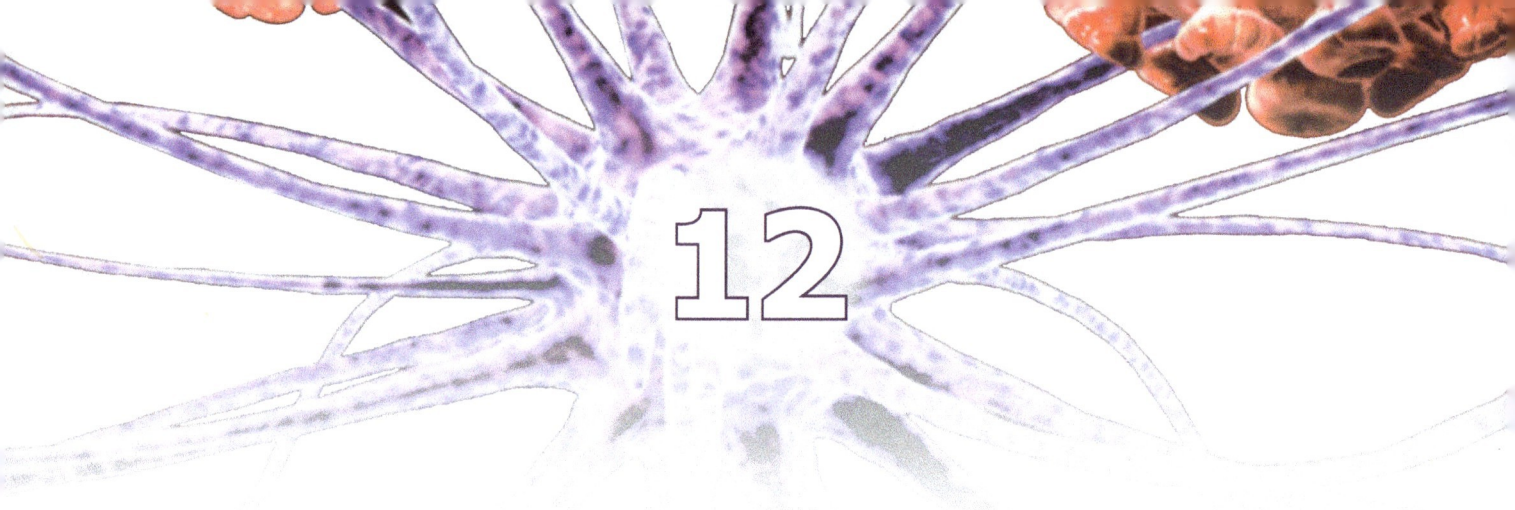


# Treatment portfolio: I. Pharmacological

The disease etiology not being fully understood, there are currently no treatments to delay or arrest the progressive neurodegeneration of MSA, and there is no cure. The condition progresses gradually and eventually leads to death. However, there are alleviating treatments to help people cope with the symptoms of MSA. They include lifestyle changes and medications, which were discussed at great length in Chapter 11.

Management options remain very limited and novel treatment options are continuously being investigated. This chapter is dedicated to pharmacological treatments and the following three chapters (Chapters 13-15) will dwell on other treatment options.

## Why are treatments a priority for people living with a rare disease?

Once a child or adult is diagnosed with a rare disease, their next logical step is to search for a treatment.

Treatments provide relief to people living with a rare disease and their families. A treatment can slow down the progression of a disease, treat the symptoms or cure the disease. They ease the reality of living with a rare disease every day.

For people living with a rare disease, there are various forms of treatments, including assistive technologies, digital devices, medical devices, orphan medicines, pediatric medicines, physiotherapy, radiotherapy, and surgery.

A significant part of treatments experienced by patients has also not yet been approved for the treatment of their disease. Many patients reported that they have experienced treatments that were indicated to treat or cure a different disease than theirs through off-label use.

# Treating MSA

**The following are the treatments usually prescribed for the conditions indicated:**

## Bladder control problems

Bladder control problems are treated according to the nature of the problem. Anticholinergic drugs, such as Oxybutynin or Tolteridine, may help reduce the sudden urge to urinate.

## Dystonia

Fixed abnormal muscle postures (dystonia) may be controlled with injections of botulinum toxin.

## Mobility issues

Physical therapy helps maintain mobility, reduce contractures (chronic shortening of muscles or tendons around joints, which prevents the joints from moving freely), and decrease muscle spasms and abnormal posture.

## Motor function

For some individuals, those in the variation MSA-P, the Parkinson's drug Levodopa may improve motor function, but the benefit may not continue as the disease progresses.

## Orthostatic hypotension

The fainting and lightheadedness from orthostatic hypotension may be treated with interventions such as wearing compression stockings, adding extra salt and/or water to the diet, and avoiding heavy meals. The drugs Fludrocortisone and Midodrine are usually prescribed.

In the U.S., the Food and Drug Administration (FDA) has approved the medication Droxidopa for the treatment of orthostatic hypotension seen in MSA. Dihydroxyphenylserine helps replace chemical signals called neurotransmitters which are decreased in the autonomic nervous system in MSA. Some medications used to treat orthostatic hypotension can be associated with high blood pressure when lying down, so affected individuals may be advised to sleep with the head of the bed tilted up.

## Sleep problems

Sleep problems such as rapid eye movement/sleep behavior disorder (REM/SBD) can be treated with medicines including Clonazepam, Melatonin, or some antidepressants.

### Swallowing difficulties

Some individuals with MSA may have significant difficulties with swallowing and may need a feeding tube or nutritional support. Speech therapy may be helpful in identifying strategies to address swallowing difficulties.

## Complications

The progression of MSA varies, but the condition does not go into remission. As the disorder progresses, daily activities become more difficult.

Possible complications include:

### Motor complications

They are usually related to the use of anti-parkinsonian medication, and include:

- Deteriorating function.
- Dyskinesia.
- Falls and resulting injuries caused by poor balance or fainting.
- Freezing of gait.
- Loss of ability to care for oneself in day-to-day activities.
- Loss of drug effect.
- Motor fluctuations.
- Progressive immobility that can lead to secondary problems such as a breakdown of skin.

### Non-motor complications

- Cognitive impairment.
- Dementia.
- Impulse control disorders.
- Mental health conditions:
    1. Anxiety.

2. Apathy.
3. Depression.
4. Psychotic symptoms (delusions and hallucinations).

## Autonomic dysfunctions

- Bladder issues.
- Breathing problems during sleep.
- Constipation.
- Dysphagia.
- Excessive salivation and sweating.
- Increased difficulty swallowing.
- Orthostatic hypotension.
- Sexual problems.
- Vocal cord paralysis, which makes speech and breathing difficult.
- Weight loss,

## Other complications

- Aspiration pneumonia.
- Nausea and vomiting.
- Pain.
- Pressure sores.
- Sleep disturbance and daytime sleepiness.

Sidebar 12.1-3 respectively address the subjects of pharmacovigilance, orphan medicines, and compassionate use.

## Take-away points

- Because of our incomplete understanding of the disease, there are currently no treatments to delay or arrest the progressive neurodegeneration of MSA, and there is no cure. The condition progresses gradually and eventually leads to death.
- There are alleviating symptomatic treatments that include lifestyle changes and medications.
- Management options are very limited and are offered for issues of motor function, orthostatic hypotension, mobility issues, dystonia, bladder control problems, sleep problems, and swallowing difficulties.
- The progression of MSA varies and the condition does not go into remission. As the disorder progresses, daily activities become more difficult.
- Possible complications are of the following nature: motor, non-motor, autonomic dysfunctions, and others.
- No neuroprotective treatment is available. However, potential drug candidates have been considered, including: Growth hormone therapy, Minocycline, Rasagiline, Rifampicin, and Mesenchymal stem cell therapy.
- Management options remain very limited and novel treatment options are continuously being investigated.

### Sidebar 12.1 - Pharmacovigilance

Even though medicines go through rigorous toxicity testing prior to becoming available on the market, there can be unplanned adverse or side effects once they are used by patients.

**Pharmacovigilance** is the science and activities relating to the detection and reporting of side effects of a medicine, together with measures to minimize these risks.

Individuals may be treated with one or several medicines. Their experience with taking these medicines is precious when shared with other patients by reporting them to authorities. This increases the knowledge we have on these medicines, such as how different people react to the same product.

Patients are not just passively taking the treatments that doctors prescribe: they have an active role to play to generate more knowledge about these products. They are vigilant when taking a new medicine, want to be informed of its properties, its effects (both positive and negative), and want this experience to be collected. The below information sets out how one can report adverse events and side effects of a medicine.

## What is a side effect? What is an adverse drug reaction?

A totally safe and still fully effective medicine does not exist. Even penicillin, which has saved millions of lives can cause severe allergies, which can be deadly.

All drugs have an effect on the body: Part of the effect is desired (to prevent, treat or cure a given disease, or ameliorate its symptoms), but part of the effects may be undesired (adverse events). A medicine is authorized to be used in humans when experts estimate that the desired effects on the disease outweigh the undesired effects on the body.

When one does not feel well right after taking a medicine, it may or may not be caused by the medicine. When the undesired effect occurs, it is named an "Adverse Effect", or "Undesired Effect". Sometimes, it is called a "Side Effect", "Adverse Event", or "Undesired Event", or the term "Suspected Adverse Reaction". It is only when it is certain that the undesirable effect is due to the medicine that the term "Adverse Drug Reaction" applies. Literally, this means healthcare professionals have established that the undesired effect is a direct reaction to the drug.

When experts decide to authorize a medicine, they still wish to learn more about the effect of the medicine as more patients start taking it. When more patients than expected report the same undesired events, and it can be proven that the medicine is the cause, then the experts may revise their decision, adopt measures to diminish the risks when possible, or ultimately decide to withdraw the drug from the market if the effect is severe.

It cannot be guaranteed that all risks are known at the time a medicine first enters the market. It is likely that some risks will only become known after a medicine receives market approval.

For these reasons, rather than talking about the "safety profile" of a medicine, it is more accurate to use the term "toxicity profile" as all drugs come with some degree of risks.

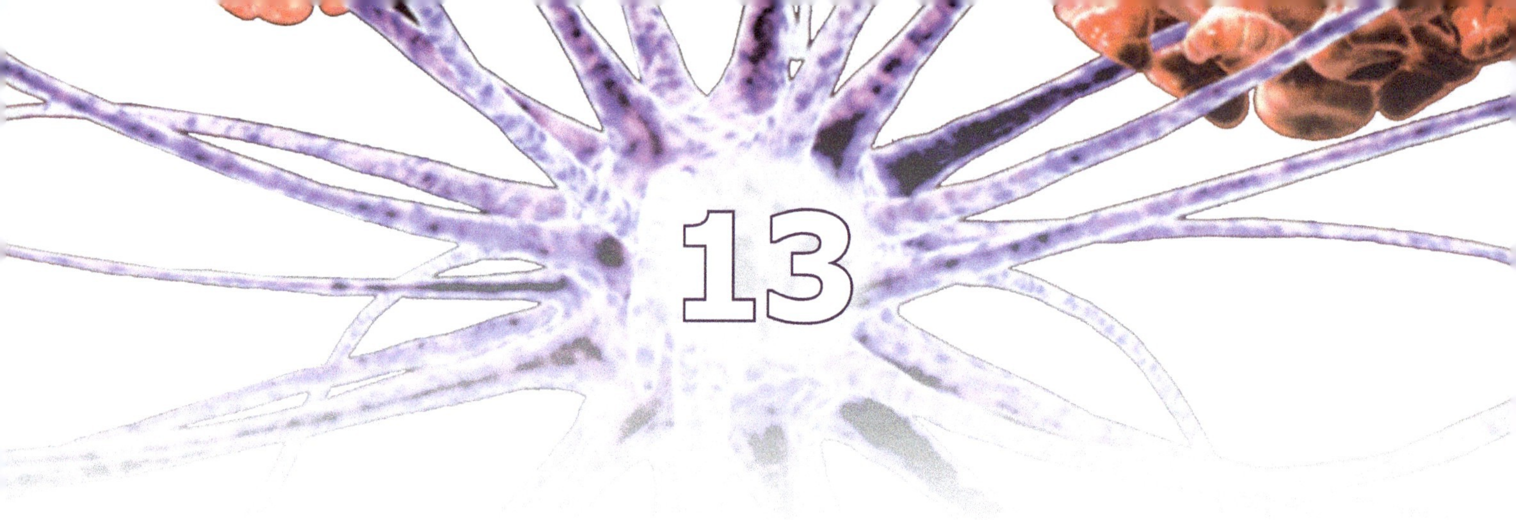


# Treatment portfolio: II. Orphan, repurposed, off-label, and compassionate use medicines

This chapter is devoted to orphan, repurposed, off-label, and compassionate use medicines for rare diseases. While it merely describes the European situation, similar descriptions apply to other countries and are not discussed here.

## Orphan medicines

### Definition

Orphan medicines are intended for the diagnosis, prevention or treatment of rare diseases. They may also be pediatric medicines for the treatment of rare diseases in children, or advanced therapies. These medicines were called "orphan" because under normal market conditions (i.e. in the absence of an orphan regulation), the pharmaceutical industry has little interest in developing and marketing products intended for only a small number of patients, when the high cost of bringing a medicinal product to market may not be recovered by the expected sales of the product.

In Europe, the EU Orphan Medicinal Products Regulation (2000) brought into place a range of incentives aimed at encouraging the development of medicines for rare diseases. Since 1999, there have been over 2000 orphan designations and around 200 orphan medicines authorized for market.

## Advanced therapy medicinal products (ATMP)

ATMPs are medicines for human use that are based on genes, tissues or cells. They are highly relevant for the treatment of rare diseases as they might, for example, target the genetic cause of a rare disease. Research to develop ATMPs for rare diseases creates a pool of knowledge that can be highly valuable for the development of medicinal products for more common diseases.

## Other treatment forms available for rare diseases

Assistive technologies and digital devices, medical devices, physiotherapy, radiotherapy, and surgery may also be used in the treatment of rare diseases.

## Development and authorization of orphan medicines

### At the European level

In Europe, the sponsor (public or private) developing an orphan medicine can apply to the European Medicines Agency (EMA) for orphan designation. After full review, the EMA's Committee for Orphan Medicinal Products (COMP) issues an opinion recommending whether the orphan designation should be granted and the European Commission (EC) makes the final decision.

Once designation is granted and the development has progressed, the sponsor must submit an application for marketing authorization to the EMA for assessment through the centralized procedure. The benefit-risk ratio of the medicine (i.e. the balance between the efficacy and the safety of the medicine) is assessed by EMA's Committee for Medicinal Products for Human Use (CHMP). The EMA's CHMP makes a recommendation on whether or not a medicine should be authorized for use in humans (i.e. whether a market authorization should be granted). Of note, designated orphan medicines are eligible for conditional marketing authorization.

In parallel, the COMP reviews the criteria for orphan designation in order to assess whether the orphan status still holds. Then, the EC takes the final decision on whether to authorize the medicine based on that recommendation and whether to maintain this orphan status or not. (Note: The EMA has an interactive tool setting out the development and authorization of medicines for human use.)

### At the country level

Once a medicine is authorized at the EU level, the process moves to the national level. The national competent authorities for pricing and reimbursement decide whether the medicine can be provided and how. In many cases, a health technology assessment (HTA) body assesses whether the medicine is health and cost effective in comparison to existing medicines available in that country and provides a recommendation on whether that medicine should be reimbursed by the national healthcare system. The ultimate goal is to have authorized medicines available, affordable, and accessible for rare disease patients.

## Protocol assistance

The EMA can provide medicine developers with advice on the most appropriate way to design and conduct a clinical development in order to generate robust evidence on a medicine's benefits and risks. It provides scientific advice to support the timely and sound development of high-quality, effective, and safe medicines for the benefit of patients. Protocol assistance is a form of scientific advice for orphan medicines.

## List of orphan medicines authorized at the EU level

A list of the latest marketing authorizations and orphan medicinal products designations is available. One can also view the list of Community Register of orphan medicinal products.

In addition to orphan medicines (i.e. authorized medicines with an orphan status), some medicines are authorized at the EU level with an indication for a rare disease but without an orphan status (consult the Orphanet Report Series). In addition, some medicines (without an orphan status) are used to treat rare diseases patients and are authorized at the national level.

Once a medicine is authorized at the EU level, the next step is for the national authorities to negotiate a price for the medicine and decide if it will be reimbursed through the national healthcare system. Unfortunately, this decision is not always immediately positive. They may decide the price is too high, negotiations with the company may break down, or they may assess that the effectiveness of the medicine and its added value in comparison to an existing medicine available in that country is not high enough.

## Development and authorization of orphan medicines

### Accessing treatment in another country through cross-border healthcare

EU citizens have the right to access healthcare in any EU country and to be reimbursed for care abroad by their home country.

The conditions under which a patient may travel to another EU country to receive medical care and reimbursement are set out in the following agreements:

1. Directive 2011/24/EU on patients' rights in cross-border healthcare.
2. Regulation (EC) No 883/2004 of the European Parliament.
3. Council of 29 April 2004 on the coordination of social security systems.

The Directive covers healthcare costs as well as the prescription and delivery of medications and medical devices. However, it is not yet fully applied by Member States and the process to access the right to cross border care may not result in a suitable outcome.

### Safety

Pharmacovigilance is the science and activities related to the detection and reporting of side effects of a medicine, together with measures to minimize these risks (see Sidebar 12.1).

## Repurposed medicines

A repurposed medicine is a medicine already approved for human use in a certain indication and for which researchers or clinicians identify new disease(s) that the medicine could treat (i.e. a new indication). Because the medicine is already in use, some data are already available, especially regarding the safety profile of the medicine. Additional data have to be collected through a clinical study to confirm the efficacy of the medicine in the new patient population. However, the repurposing approach brings advantages for a rare disease as it saves money and time as a new compound does not have to be found and developed from scratch.

## Off-label use of a treatment

When doctors prescribe a medicine for a use different from what is authorized on the label, this is called "off label" use, for example, when the drug is prescribed for a different disease or when the dosage differs from the one stated on the label. Patients with rare diseases and their families are often familiar with this practice, or may not even realize that they are taking products that are prescribed "off-label".

## Compassionate use medicines

### What is a compassionate use program (CUP)?

A medicinal product given on a compassionate basis is first and foremost a treatment. It is a medicinal product not yet fully evaluated but prescribed to treat people with no other therapeutic options.

Running a Compassionate Use Program (CUP) consists of making a medicinal product available for compassionate reasons to a group of patients (or sometimes individual patients on a case-by-case basis) with a chronically or seriously debilitating disease or whose disease is considered to be life-threatening, and who cannot be treated satisfactorily by an authorized medicinal product.

- The demand is made by the doctor to the pharmaceutical company that is developing the product, and to national authorities who need to accept the compassionate use.
- In Europe, the legislation (for medicines authorized via the centralized procedure) states that the medicinal product concerned must either be the subject of an application for a marketing authorization or must be undergoing clinical trials. In

other terms, it is not requested that the medicine in question be already authorized somewhere in the world. If the product has been or is currently being tested in a clinical trial for the disease under consideration, the patient's doctor can request a compassionate use authorization.

- Most EU Member States have a special scheme to dispense a medicine on a compassionate basis. Many other European and North American countries have similar processes. These processes are more or less complex and time consuming.

## What a compassionate use program is not

- ***A CUP is not an experiment or a clinical trial:*** It is intended to treat the person. By definition, a compassionate use is a treatment, yet not fully evaluated, for patients who do not have other options. Other circumstances when a medicine is given should *not* be confused with compassionate use.
- ***Neither a clinical trial nor an experiment:*** in no case can the medicinal product given on a compassionate use be a placebo, nor a treatment or combination of treatments that the patient has had before, lacking efficacy or poorly tolerated. Even though it is not completely certain whether the treatment the patient receives on a compassionate use basis is useful, if there is no other option and there is the slightest chance that the product will be effective, the patient should benefit from it.
- ***A substitute for product development:*** *A* CUP cannot replace clinical trials. Again, it is not an experiment. It cannot conclude whether the product is safe and effective on a group of patients. A CUP can be organized in parallel to clinical trials, but it can only be authorized if clinical trials are already in progress, and recruitment in a CUP should not be an obstacle for the recruitment of patients in clinical trials (for example, if patients prefer to receive the medicine on a compassionate basis and not take the risk of receiving a placebo as might be the case in a clinical trial).
- ***An off-label use:*** A medicine used off-label is, by definition, a medicine used in a different way than the authorized one. For example, a medicine can be given for a different disease, or at a different dose than indicated on the label. Thus, off-label use only applies to medicines that are already authorized. Compassionate use only applies to medicines that are not yet authorized for any condition.
- ***A financial aid program or a humanitarian program:*** Financial aid programs (also called humanitarian programs) are for medicines that are authorized and placed on the market, but at a cost that the patient cannot afford (for example, medicines that are not 100% reimbursed or covered by the health care system). In some cases, the marketing authorization holder creates a financial assistance program for patients who do not have enough revenue. This is not compassionate use; it is a marketing tool to open access to a larger group of patients.
- ***A way to place a product on the market prior to marketing authorization:*** Some companies can be tempted to provide a medicine they develop to a large group of patients, prior to its authorization. This is to make sure the medicine is

already largely used, at an early stage, to "capture" a large market share and make it more complex for competitor products to make their own market share. This is why a CUP needs to be properly authorized and monitored by national competent authorities. A CUP cannot be used for investigational purposes or commercial pre-authorization activities. Promotion of the medicinal product in question, or the CUP itself, is not permitted.

- ***A "favor" or a "gift" to clinicians who achieve their objectives in recruiting for clinical trials:*** Completing enrollment of patients in a clinical trial is a key factor of success for a clinical trial and, thus, for the product development and evaluation. Clinicians who are also investigators of clinical trials are precious to the trial sponsor, e.g. a pharmaceutical company, as they can ask their own patients to participate in a clinical trial. In a very competitive world, a company can be tempted to gain the favors of clinicians by offering them access to the medicine on a compassionate basis if they manage to enroll high numbers of patients. This practice is not official but does exist, and is not recommended as it creates inequity in accessing the medicine on a compassionate basis.

## Can anyone access medicines on a compassionate basis?

Before a medicine is authorized and placed on the market, it must be duly evaluated to learn more about its efficacy and safety. The first priority is to conduct clinical trials that will respond to these questions. Only patients who cannot be part of a clinical trial are eligible for a compassionate use.

- Under compassionate use, the treatment that is given to the patient is a medicine, not a placebo. The patient receiving it is expected to benefit from it. In a clinical trial, the medicinal product is tested against a comparative treatment which may be a placebo. People enrolled in clinical trials correspond to specific biomedical criteria, and people who should not be enrolled in a clinical trial are also defined (so-called exclusion criteria). A common example involves patients who are too severely ill, with multi-organ impairment, or severe liver or renal deficiency. They are usually excluded from clinical trials. However, they can receive the treatment on a compassionate basis. This ensures the optimum care for the more severely ill. They cannot take the risk of receiving a placebo or a treatment that would not help them. Even though it has not been determined whether the treatment patients receive on a compassionate use basis is useful, if there is the slightest chance the treatment may work, patients should benefit from it.
- When authorizing a compassionate use, regulators can do so on a named-patient basis (the doctor makes a request for a given patient), or for a group of patients (a so-called cohort). On a named-patient basis, authorization will be on a case-by-case basis. For a cohort compassionate use, regulators will define the patient population eligible for the program. For example, in a disease for which only two medicines exist, regulators may decide the CUP is only open for patients who have

already been treated with both medicines with no response, or who cannot tolerate either product.

### Are there unlimited supplies of a medicine that can be used on a compassionate use?

A company developing a new product first produces necessary quantities of the product for its clinical trials (a few hundred to a few thousands of patients, pilot production). When the product is authorized, the company needs to manufacture enough product to satisfy the demand in a larger population (commercial batches). Between these two stages, the size of a CUP may vary.

The manufacturing capacities for a medicinal product also vary with time. When the product is first tested in the laboratory or in animals, only small quantities are needed (usually a few grams to a few kilograms).

When the product is then tested in humans, the first clinical trials are limited in size (typically, a few dozens to a few hundred patients). Thus, quantities of product are still limited. When early results are obtained, the company analyzes them and may decide the chances that the medicinal product is safe and effective are high; therefore it elects to launch larger confirmatory trials and prepare to submit a marketing authorization application. This is called the *Go/No go decision*. At this point, the company needs to produce larger quantities of the medicine, as confirmatory clinical trials may enroll thousands of patients.

As a consequence, there is a phase where larger quantities of a product become available. Before this, the company may be very limited if the demand for compassionate use is high. After this, production can increase and when authorities grant authorization for a compassionate use, the company should be able to satisfy the demand. But, there is a period beginning with the Go/No go decision where it is not certain all demands can be satisfied, as it takes time to build a manufacturing site and to validate the production quality.

## Accessing unauthorized medicines

### Through a compassionate use program

A compassionate use program (CUP) consists of making a medicinal product available for compassionate reasons to a group of patients (or sometimes individual patients on a case-by-case basis) with a chronically or seriously debilitating disease or whose disease is considered to be life-threatening, and who cannot be treated satisfactorily by an authorized medicinal product.

### Other mechanisms to bring rare disease medicines to patients more quickly

The EMA has put in place such mechanisms. These voluntary schemes are based on enhanced interaction and early dialogue with developers of promising medicines to optimize development plans and speed up evaluation so these medicines can reach patients earlier.

The EC has also proposed a Regulation to make European cooperation on health technology assessment permanent, stable, and sustainable. Pooling expertise together aims to support the decision-making on added value, pricing, and reimbursement of health technologies across European countries, both for those who already have high capacity in assessing the value of new technologies and for those who have none.

## Patient engagement in the development of medicines for rare diseases

It is vital that patients be engaged in the development of treatments for rare diseases. By providing feedback on their real-life needs throughout the life-cycle development of medicines, they can play a role in ensuring the end-product truly serves its purpose and to improve their health outputs and quality of life.

### Tools available to facilitate the engagement of patients

The PARADIGM partnership has developed a series of tools that all stakeholders involved in the development of medicines – including patient organizations – can use to facilitate patient engagement.

## Take-away points

- Orphan medicines are intended for the diagnosis, prevention or treatment of rare diseases. They may also be pediatric medicines for the treatment of rare diseases in children, or advanced therapies. They are thus called because they are of insufficient commercial interest to the pharmaceutical industry.
- Advanced therapy medicinal products are medicines for human use that are based on genes, tissues or cells. They are highly relevant for the treatment of rare diseases.
- Assistive technologies and digital devices, medical devices, physiotherapy, radiotherapy, and surgery may also be used in the treatment of rare diseases.
- In Europe, the process of developing an orphan medicine is regulated from the application stage to the development stage to the follow-up as to their efficacy and safety. Once a medicine is authorized at the European level, the process moves to the national level.
- A list of the latest marketing authorizations and orphan medicinal products designations is available.

- Under certain conditions, European citizens have the right to access healthcare in any European Union country and to be reimbursed for care abroad by their home country.
- A repurposed medicine is a medicine already approved for human use in a certain indication and for which researchers or clinicians identify new disease(s) that the medicine could treat. A new compound does not have to be found and developed from scratch.
- Off-label use is the use of a drug prescribed for a different disease or when the dosage differs from the one stated on its label.
- A compassionate use is the use of a medicinal product available for compassionate reasons to patients with a chronically, seriously debilitating, or life-threatening disease and who cannot be treated satisfactorily by an authorized medicinal product.
- It is vital that patients be engaged in the development of treatments for rare diseases. They can play a role in ensuring the end-product truly serves its purpose and to improve their health outputs and quality of life. Tools are available to facilitate the engagement of patients.
- Health technology assessment is the assessment of whether a medicine is effective/ cost effective in comparison to existing medicines available. The ultimate goal is to have authorized medicines available, affordable, and accessible for rare disease patient. The assessment consists of examining the long-term effects of any existing or new health care technology, including drugs, medical devices, procedures and organizational systems used in health care. It also evaluates the medical, social, ethical, and economic implications of these interventions. The goal is to support health care decisions and to serve policy making through objective information.

## Sidebar 13.1 - Health technology assessment (HTA)

HTA is a multi-disciplinary field and a process performed by competent authorities or sometimes academics to inform health policies. It consists of examining the long-term effects of any existing or new health care technology, including drugs, medical devices, procedures, and organizational systems used in health care. The goal is to support health care decisions and to serve policy making through objective information.

HTA plays an important role in determining pricing negotiations, reimbursement decisions, and the organization of the health systems (including for orphan medicinal products and rare diseases). It also evaluates the medical, social, ethical, and economic implications of these interventions.

HTA is mainly performed at the national level to inform governments' policies. Since 1988 European Countries have tried to cooperate on HTA to make it more evidence-based, timely, and transparent. The EC has been funding several projects of voluntary cooperation among national competent authorities. Today, the EC has proposed a Regulation to make European cooperation on HTA permanent and beneficial for all EU countries.

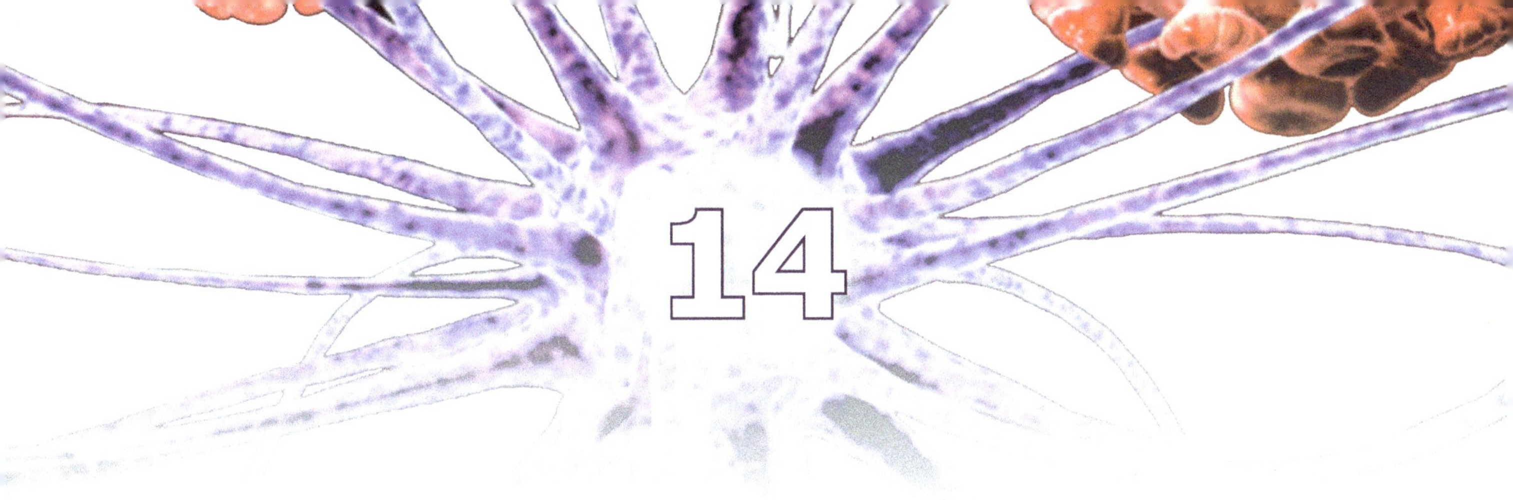

# 14

# Treatment portfolio: III. Clinical trials

Clinical trials are prospective biomedical or biobehavioral research studies on human participants designed to answer specific questions about biomedical or biobehavioral interventions, including new treatments (such as novel vaccines, drugs, dietary choices, dietary supplements, and medical devices) and known interventions that warrant further study and comparison. They generate data on dosage, safety, and efficacy and look at new ways to prevent, detect, or treat diseases. Treatments might be new drugs or new combinations of drugs, new surgical procedures or devices, or new ways to use existing treatments. They can also look at other aspects of care such as improving the quality of life for people with chronic illnesses. Their overriding goal is to determine if a new test or treatment works and is safe.

Sidebar 14.1 provides the main particulars of clinical trials. The following sections will present those trials that are currently recruiting participants and might be of interest to MSA patients, their families, and carers.

## Questions usually asked by potential MSA participants

### Can an MSA patient participate in a clinical trial?

Yes, and it is encouraged for those eligible participants. The best way to find out about drug trials and to express interest in participating in one of them is to be referred by one's own neuroradiologist or physician. That healthcare professional will be able to identify possible suitable trials for the existing medical condition, make a referral, and facilitate the enrollment process, as appropriate.

### Is the list of clinical trials available?

It can be found on line: www.clinicaltrials.gov. This site lists all registered trials across the world and their status (recruiting, not recruiting, completed, or suspended). The latest information on current drugs in the pipeline and clinical trials is posted at: hps://defeatmsa.org/msa-research/pipelines/ But, always stay in touch with these pages for updates.

### Does it cost anything to participate in a clinical trial?

Participation is usually free.

## Currently recruiting clinical trials

The number of clinical trials that are currently recruiting may vary depending on the particular date at which the website clinicaltrials.gov is searched. At the date of the preparation of this chapter, there were 58 such trials. For the reader's convenience, only the first 44 of them are provided below. These have been classified as:"Clinical" [C], "Drug-related" [D], "Gene therapy" [G], Immunotherapy" [I], "Rehabilitation [R], "Stem cell therapy" [S], and "Therapy" [T]. They are further specified below:

[C]: Trial numbers: 1, 4, 10, 12, 14, 20, 24, 25, 28, 30, 34, 35, 36, 39, 40, 41, 42, 43, and 44: 19 trials.
[D]: 3, 7, 8, 11, 19, 26, and 38: 7 trials.
[G]: 5: 1 trial.
[I]: 23: 1 trial.
[R]: 15: 1 trial.
[S]: 9, 16, 17, and 18: 4 trials.
[T]: 2, 6, 13, 21, 22, 27, 29, 31, 32, 33, and 37: 11 trials.

Useful information can be obtained on these and other trials (those completed, not recruiting, etc.).

- **Synaptic Loss in Multiple System Atrophy**
  University of Exeter, England.

It is known from pathological studies that the synapses are affected in MSA, but is not known how, to what extent, and how early. An imaging tool called Positron Emission Tomography (PET) will study the integrity of the synapses by the use of a dedicated tracer 11C]UCB-J. The results are anticipated to help in understanding better the mechanisms underlying this disease and open new avenues for its treatment.

- **Quality of Life of Caregivers and Patients Suffering From Multiple System Atrophy**
  University Hospital, Bordeaux, France.

As in other neurodegenerative diseases, many MSA patients require caregivers for assistance with daily living. Caregiving can also be extremely stressful, and many caregivers experience declines in mental health. All of these repercussions contribute to the deterioration of the caregiver's quality of life and they can have an impact on the patient, in particular, on the patient's survival. Improving quality of life is a major element and identifying effective targeted interventions would bring immediate and direct benefit to patients and their families. A multimodal intervention proposed by the NYU Caregiver Counseling and Support Intervention (NYUCI) could contribute to improve disease management and better coping with daily living difficulties.

- **Study of ATH434 in Participants With Multiple System Atrophy**
  Alterity Therapeutics, Australia.

This study will assess the safety and efficacy of the drug ATH434 in participants with MSA.

- **Insulin Resistance in Multiple System Atrophy**
  University Hospital, Bordeaux, France.

*Post-mortem* findings suggest insulin resistance, i.e. reduced insulin signaling, in the brains of MSA patients. The aim of this study is to complete the target validation of insulin resistance for future treatment trials.

- **GDNF Gene Therapy for Multiple System Atrophy**
  Brain Neurotherapy Bio, Inc., USA.

This Phase 1 investigation will evaluate the safety and potential clinical effect of AAV2-GDNF delivered to the putamen in subjects with either a possible or probable diagnosis of MSA.

- **Spinal Cord Stimulation for Multiple System Atrophy**
  Ruijin Hospital, China.

Spinal cord stimulation (SCS) is a mature technique in the treatment of chronic pain. It is generally accepted by patients because of its non-destructive and reversible nature, few complications, no side effects, and avoidance of unnecessary surgical procedures. This study proposes an innovative treatment protocol for MSA with SCS in C2-4 segment to evaluate the improvement of dysarthria, dysphagia, urinary retention, and orthostatic hypotension in MSA patients before and after SCS treatment, and shed new light on the treatment for MSA.

- **A Study of TAK-341 in Treatment of MSA**
  Takeda, Japan and Astra Zeneca, Britain-Sweden.

This study will investigate how TAK-341 works after 52 weeks in participants with MSA as measured by the Unified Multiple System Atrophy Rating Scale Part I (UMSARS). It will be conducted in North America, Europe, and Asia.

- **Trial to Evaluate the Efficacy and Safety of KM-819 Treatment to Slow the Progression of MSA**
  South Korea and Parexel, USA.

This trial will evaluate the efficacy and safety of the drug KM819.

- **Randomized Double-Blind Placebo-Controlled Adaptive Design Trial Of Intrathecally Administered Autologous Mesenchymal Stem Cells In MSA**
  Mayo Clinic, USA.

This study will assess optimal dosing frequency, effectiveness, and safety of adipose-derived autologous mesenchymal stem cells delivered into the spinal fluid of patients with MSA.

- **Multiple System Atrophy Multidisciplinary Clinic**

  University of Texas Southwestern Medical Center, USA.

This study will examine the disease burden of MSA and the impact of multidisciplinary care on quality of life and caregiver burden.

- **Study to Evaluate the Safety, Tolerability, and Pharmacokinetics of ION464 Administered to Adults With MSA**

  Ionic Pharmaceuticals, Inc., USA.

This study will evaluate the safety and tolerability of multiple doses of ION464 administered via intrathecal (IT) injection (Part 1) and to evaluate the long-term safety and tolerability of ION464 (Part 2) in participants with MSA. It will also evaluate the pharmacodynamic (PD) effect of ION464 on the level of a potential biomarker of target engagement (Parts 1 and 2) and to evaluate the pharmacokinetic (PK) profile of ION464 in serum (Part 1).

- **TRACK-MSA: A Longitudinal Study to Define Outcome Measures in MSA**

  NYU Langone Health, USA.

This is an observational, non-interventional, and longitudinal natural history study to define changes in clinical, neurological, blood, CSF, and neuroimaging biomarkers in patients with MSA.

- **DBS and SCS Therapy Improve Motor Function in MSA With Predominant Parkinsonism**

  Zhangyuqing, Xuanwu Hospital, Beijing, China.

The parkinsonian type of MSA (MSA-P) does not respond to the established treatment for Parkinson's disease (deep brain stimulation at the sub-thalamic nucleus or globus pallidus internal). The improvement in motor function is short-lasting and rapidly followed by the early appearance of freezing of gait (FOG) and postural instability, and often leads to significant disability and loss of quality of life. This study will investigate the safety and therapeutic outcome of SCS for FOG and the effectiveness of DBS combined with SCS for symptomatic treatment of MSA-P.

- **Observational Study in MSA**

  H. Lundbeck A/S, Denmark.

Talisman, a global clinical study (20058N) in MSA patients will be conducted in two regions (China and the European Union [EU]).

- **Comprehensive Swallowing Rehabilitation in Patients With MSA**

  Seoul National University Hospital, South Korea.

Although the symptoms of dysphagia in the two subtypes of MSA - the parkinsonian variant and the cerebellar variant - are different, there is no significant difference in the latency to onset of tube feeding. Therefore, effective intervention is needed to improve the safety and efficiency of swallowing regardless of the subtypes of MSA. This study will assess a comprehensive swallowing therapy focused on functional muscle training, compensatory swallowing maneuvers, and thermal-tactile stimulation and investigate its effects. in patients with MSA.

- **Potential Use of Autologous and Allogeneic Mesenchymal Stem Cells (MSC) in Patients With MSA**

  Indonesia University, Indonesia..

Clinical improvement with MSCs will be evaluated for three treatment groups in six different time frames.

- **Study to Evaluate Investigational Allogeneic Cell Therapy Product hOMSC300 for Treatment of Early- to Moderate Stage MSA**

  Cytora, Ltd., England.

Purpose of this phase 1/2a study is to assess the safety and efficacy of intrathecal administration of allogeneic human oral mucosa stem cells in patients suffering from early to moderate stage MSA.

- **Pre-Gene Therapy Study in Parkinson's Disease and MSA**

  Asklepios Biopharmaceutical, Inc., USA.

The objective of this study is to describe disease progression in study participants diagnosed with early Parkinson's Disease or MSA (P) up to 18 months as delineated by clinical and biochemical parameters.

- **Phase 3 Efficacy and Durability of Ampreloxetine for the Treatment of Symptomatic nOH in Participants With MSA**

  Theravance Biopharma, USA.

This Phase 3 study will evaluate the efficacy and durability of Ampreloxetine in participants with MSA and symptomatic nOH after 20 weeks of treatment. It will include 4 periods: Screening, open label, randomized withdrawal, and long-term treatment extension.

- **Progressive Supranuclear Palsy (PSP), Cortico-Basal Degeneration (CBD), and MSA Longitudinal Study**

  University College, London, England.

This longitudinal will collect standardized clinical data over time.

- **MotIoN aDaptive Deep Brain Stimulation for MSA (MINDS)**

  University of Oxford, England.

In MSA patients undergoing therapeutic DBS, the effects on autonomic parameters such as blood pressure and bladder symptoms has been shown to be improved. This study uses a novel technique of adaptive DBS in order to provide stimulation dependent on patient physiological or positional factors. The aim is to make stimulation more responsive and patient-specific.

- **Systematic Assessment of Laryngopharyngeal Function in Patients With MSA, PD, and 4repeat Tauopathies (FEEMSA)**

  Kliniken Beelitz GmbH, Germany.

This is a non-interventional observational study designed to systematically record the results of routine laryngeal examinations and specific characteristics of dysphagia in patients with MSA, PD, PSP, and related repeat tauopathies.

- **UB-312 in Patients With Synucleinopathies**

  NYU Langone Health, USA.

This is a Phase 1b study to determine the safety, tolerability, and immunogenicity of UB-312 in participants with MSA, and in participants with Parkinson's disease (PD). UB-312 is a UBITh®-enhanced synthetic peptide-based vaccine and may provide an active immunotherapy option for treating synucleinopathies including the most prevalent form, PD; and the most rapidly progressive form, MSA.

- **Pain and Autonomic Symptoms in Parkinson's Disease and Atypical Parkinsonisms**

  I, Italy.

The goal of this observational study is to learn about the impact of the different types of pain and of the domains involved in the autonomic disorders of inpatients and outpatients diagnosed with PD and MSA. The main aims are to evaluate the prevalence of pain, the effect of rehabilitation on pain and autonomic symptoms, and the prevalence of autonomic symptoms.

- **The Effect of Gluten-free Diet on Parkinsonism (GFREEPARK)**

  General University Hospital, Prague, Czechoslovakia.

Recent data suggest that the brain-gut axis, chronic intestinal inflammation, and microbiome may contribute to the pathogenesis of neurodegenerative diseases with alpha-synucleinopathy (PD and MSA). Environmental factors e.g. diets, microbiome, metabolites, and immune mechanisms may play important role in pathogenesis of these diseases. This project will address effects of an anti-inflammatory gluten-free diet (GFD) on motor and non-motor symptoms as well as its effects on immune and metabolomic characteristics. The anti-inflammatory gluten-free diet and its related mechanisms represent a novel, promising, and relatively straightforward approach in a search to improve symptoms of PD as well as MSA or even in their prevention.

- **Proof of Mechanism Study to Evaluate Binding of Alpha-synuclein**

  Invicro, USA.

The overall goal of this protocol is to evaluate [18F]UCB-2897 as an α-synuclein targeted radiopharmaceutical, its safety and tolerability of microdose, and its pharmacokinetics/metabolism.

- **Treatment of Transcranial Alternating Current Stimulation (tACS) on Cerebellar Ataxia**

  First Affiliated Hospital of Fujian Medical University, China.

Transcranial alternating current stimulation (tACS) is a relatively recent method that non-invasively modulates brain oscillations, and can effectively stimulate deep brain regions, affect brain rhythm, increase neural plasticity, change neurotransmitter levels, and improve brain function. It is a comfortable, safe, effective, non-invasive, and easy-to-operate method, which means it has development potential in relevant medical fields. It has been approved by the FDA for clinically treating neuropsychiatric diseases.

- **Clinical Laboratory Evaluation of Chronic Autonomic Failure**

  National Institute of Neurological Disorders and Stroke (NINDS), USA.

Researchers want to improve the tests used to diagnose autonomic failure and orthostatic hypotension.

- **Evaluation of the Efficacy of a Two-week EMST on Dysphagia in Parkinsonian Patients (EMST-PS)**

  Kliniken Beelitz GmbH, Germany.

This is an interventional therapy study designed to evaluate the efficacy of a two-week intervention, i.e. training with a specialized exhalation training device (called expiratory muscle strength training; EMST150 or EMST75; Aspire Products, Gainesville, FL) on swallowing function in patients with neurodegenerative Parkinsonian disorders.

- **Facilitating Diagnostics and Prognostics of Parkinsonian Syndromes Using Neuroimaging**

  University of Texas Southwestern Medical Center, USA.

The goals of this study are to identify biomarkers using neuroimaging that are associated with progression rate using statistical methods and biomarkers that are associated with the differential diagnosis of Parkinson's disease and atypical parkinsonism.

**Mobility in Atypical Parkinsonism: a Trial of Physiotherapy (Mobility-APP)**

Universitätsklinik für Neurologie, Innsbruck, Austria.

Patients with atypical parkinsonism often show gait and mobility impairment manifesting in early disease stages. In order to maintain mobility and physical autonomy as long as possible for these patients, this study will examine the effect of two types of physiotherapy in patients with MSA, PSP, and idiopathic PD.

- **Abdominal Binders to Treat Orthostatic Hypotension in Parkinsonian Syndromes (ABOH-PS)**

  Universitätsklinik für Neurologie, Innsbruck, Austria.

The purpose of this clinical trial is to determine whether the use of an elastic abdominal binder is effective in the non-pharmacological management of symptomatic, neurogenic orthostatic hypotension (OH) in individuals suffering from PD or MSA-P.

- **Automated Abdominal Binder for Orthostatic Hypotension**

  Vanderbilt University Medical Center, USA.

The automated inflatable abdominal binder is an investigational device for the treatment of orthostatic hypotension in patients with autonomic failure. The purpose of this study is to determine the safety and effectiveness of this device in improving orthostatic tolerance.

- **Biomarkers in Parkinsonian Syndromes (BIOPARK)**

  University Hospital, Bordeaux, France.

PD, MSA, and PSP are neurodegenerative disorders. PD and MSA are alpha-synucleinopathies characterized by the abnormal accumulation of alpha-synuclein, while tau protein accumulates in PSP. The development of biological markers for the diagnosis and prognosis in these three disorders remains an unmet need. Such biological markers are crucial for future disease-modification and neuroprotection trials. The main objective is to compare oligomeric alpha-synuclein cerebrospinal fluid levels between PD, MSA, and PSP patients.

- **Unstructured Eye Tracking as a Diagnostic and Prognostic Biomarker in Parkinsonian Disorders**

  Conor Pearson and Queen's University, Ireland.

No accurate tests currently exist to diagnose PD and the conditions which mimic it (atypical parkinsonism) at a very early stage. Similarly there are no accurate ways to track how these diseases progress in a very precise manner. Recording eye movements and pupil changes may be a very sensitive way of doing this and may contain important information about a patient's diagnosis and their cognitive and motor function.

- **Neurodegenerative Diseases Registry (NDD Registry)**

  Vincent Mok, Chinese University of Hong Kong

With the increase in life expectancy of our population due to advancement of medical diagnosis and treatments, the incidence of age-dependent neurodegenerative diseases increased, including Alzheimer's disease (AD), parkinsonian syndromes (PS), small vessel disease (SVD) and motor neuron disease (MND). In spite of the progress of knowing the pathogenesis of various neurodegenerative diseases at molecular and genetic level, they are still very incompletely understood and often cause diagnostic and therapeutic challenges to physicians. Due to the overlapping presentation and similar brain pathology, especially in the early stage of the diseases, it is difficult to differentiate idiopathic Parkinson's disease (iPD) from atypical parkinsonian syndromes, such as MSA and PSP. Similarly, distinguishing AD from other dementia syndromes including frontotemporal dementia (FTD), dementia with Lewy Bodies (DLB), corticobasal degeneration (CBD) and vascular dementia can be difficult. It is necessary to develop accurate and comprehensive diagnostic tests to properly prognosticate the diseases, start treatments in early stage of the diseases, and maximize the accuracy of drug trials for more effective preventive and therapeutic measures for these neurodegenerative diseases. Therefore, the registry aims to generate a large database of cognitive, behavioral, lifestyle, and psychological information of the subjects who suffered from neurodegenerative diseases, as well as to examine the genetic basis of neurodegenerative diseases to help decode their pathogenic mechanisms. The registry may provide important information to understand symptom development of the neurodegenerative diseases, which may help physicians to diagnose the diseases more accurately and provide better treatment plans.

- **Overnight Trials With Heat Stress in Autonomic Failure Patients With Supine Hypertension**

  Vanderbilt University Medical Center, USA

Patients with autonomic failure are characterized by disabling orthostatic hypotension (low blood pressure on standing), and at least half of them also have high blood pressure while lying down (supine hypertension). Exposure to heat, such as in hot environments, often worsens their orthostatic hypotension. The causes of this are not fully understood. The purpose of this study is to evaluate whether applying local heat over the abdomen of patients with autonomic failure and supine hypertension during the night would decrease their nocturnal high blood pressure while lying down. This will help us better understand the mechanisms underlying this phenomenon, and may be of use in the treatment of supine hypertension.

- **Hemodynamic Mechanisms of Abdominal Compression in the Treatment of Orthostatic Hypotension in Autonomic Failure**

  Vanderbilt University Medical Center, USA.

Compression garments have been shown to be effective in the treatment of orthostatic hypotension in autonomic failure patients. The purpose of this study is to determine the hemodynamic mechanisms by which abdominal compression (up to 40 mm Hg) improve the standing blood pressure and orthostatic tolerance in these patients, and to compare them with those of the standard of care Midodrine.

- **[18F]F-DOPA Imaging in Patients With Autonomic Failure**

  Daniel Claassan, Vanderbilt University Medical Center, USA.

Alpha-synucleinopathies refer to age-related neurodegenerative and dementing disorders, characterized by the accumulation of alpha-synuclein in neurons and/or glia. The anatomical location of alpha-synuclein inclusions (Lewy Bodies) and the pattern of progressive neuronal death (e.g. caudal to rostral brainstem) give rise to distinct neurological phenotypes, including Parkinson's disease (PD), Multiple System Atrophy (MSA), Dementia with Lewy Bodies (DLB). Common to these disorders are the involvement of the central and peripheral autonomic nervous system, where Pure Autonomic Failure (PAF) is thought (a) to be restricted to the peripheral autonomic system, (b) a clinical risk factor for the development of a central synucleinopathy, and (c) an ideal model to assess biomarkers that predict phenoconversion to PD, MSA, or DLB. Such biomarkers would aid in clinical trial inclusion criteria to ensure assessments of disease-modifying strategies to delay or halt the neurodegenerative process. One of these biomarkers may be related to the neurotransmitter dopamine agonist (DA) and related changes in the substantia nigra (SN) and brainstem. [18F]F-DOPA is a radiolabeled substrate for aromatic amino acid decarboxylase (AADC), an enzyme involved in the production of dopamine. Use of this radiolabeled substrate in positron emission tomography (PET) may provide insight to changes in monoamine production and how they relate to specific phenoconversions in PAF patients. Overall, this study aims to identify changes in dopamine production in key regions including the SN, locus coeruleus, and brainstem to distinguish between patients with PD, MSA, and DLB, which may provide vital information to predict conversion from peripheral to central nervous system disease.

- **Longitudinal Tracking of Patients Diagnosed With Neurodegenerative Movement Disorders**

  Brigham and Women's Hospital, USA.

The purpose of this protocol is to create an active natural history cohort of patients with degenerative movement disorders, tracked in a clinical setting with clinical rating scales and neuroimaging. The overarching rationale is that neurodegenerative diseases may be heterogeneous, complex disorders. A new way of performing clinical trials in these patients may be in order and this protocol aims to build a longitudinally tracked clinical trial-ready cohort of patients.

- **Accelerometer for Quantification of Neurogenic Orthostatic Hypotension Symptoms**

  Vanderbilt Univrsity Medical Center, USA.

This study aims to find a more objective and accurate way to assess the efficacy of the treatment for neurogenic orthostatic hypotension. An activity monitor will be used to determine the amount of time patients spend in the upright position (standing and walking; upright time) during a given time period compared to regular medicines (Midodrine or Atomoxetine).

- **Effect of Midodrine vs Abdominal Compression on Cardiovascular Risk Markers in Autonomic Failure Patients**

  Vanderbilt Univrsity Medical Center, USA.

The purpose of this study is to learn more about the effects of abdominal compression and the medication Midodrine, two interventions used for the treatment of orthostatic hypotension (low blood pressure on standing), on hemodynamic markers of cardiovascular risk.

- **Effects of Midodrine and Droxidopa on Splanchnic Capacitance in Autonomic Failure**

  Vanderbilt Univrsity Medical Center, USA.

The purpose of this study is to learn more about the effects of Midodrine and Droxidopa, two medications used for the treatment of orthostatic hypotension (low blood pressure on standing), on the veins of the abdomen of patients with autonomic failure.

- **Cerebro Spinal Fluid Collection (CSF) (Analzheimer)**

  University Hospital, Strasbourg, France.

Cognitive neurodegenerative diseases are a major public health issue. At present, the diagnosis of certainty is still based on anatomopathological analyses. Even if the diagnostic tools available to clinicians have made it possible to improve probabilistic diagnosis during the patient's lifetime, there are still too many diagnostic errors and sub-diagnosis in this field. The arrival of biomarkers has made it possible to reduce these diagnostic errors, which were of the order of 25% to 30%, a high error rate is due to different parameters. These diseases are numerous and often present common symptoms due to the fact that common brain structures are affected. These diseases evolve progressively over several years. When the symptoms are discrete, their early diagnosis, makes them even more difficult to diagnose at this stage. In addition, co-morbidities are common in the elderly, further complicating the diagnosis of these diseases. At present, the only cerebrospinal fluid (CSF) biomarkers that are routinely used for the biological diagnosis of neurodegenerative cognitive pathologies are those specific to Alzheimer's disease: Aβ42, Aβ40, Tau-total and Phospho-Tau. These biomarkers represent an almost indispensable tool in the diagnosis of dementia. It is therefore important to determine whether Alzheimer's biomarkers can be disrupted in other neurodegenerative cognitive pathologies, but also to find biomarkers specific to these different pathologies by facilitating the implementation of clinical studies which will thus make it possible to improve their diagnosis.

## Take-away points

1. Clinical trials are prospective biomedical or biobehavioral research studies on human participants designed to answer specific questions about biomedical or biobehavioral interventions, including new treatments and known interventions that warrant further study.
2. Treatments might be new drugs or new combinations of drugs, new surgical procedures or devices, or new ways to use existing treatments. They can also look at other aspects of care, such as improving the quality of life for people with chronic illnesses.
3. The overriding goal of clinical trials is to determine if a new test or treatment is safe and effective.
4. Participation in clinical trials is encouraged for eligible participants. An updated list of clinical trials is available on-line and it usually costs nothing to participate.

### Sidebar 14.1 – A brief primer on clinical trials

Clinical trials (CT) are prospective biomedical or biobehavioral research studies on human participants designed to answer specific questions about biomedical or biobehavioral interventions, including new treatments (such as novel vaccines, drugs, dietary choices, dietary supplements, and medical devices) and known interventions that warrant further study and comparison. They are part of clinical research at the heart of all medical advances. They look at new ways to prevent, detect, or treat diseases by new drugs or new combinations of drugs, new surgical procedures or devices, or new ways to use existing treatments. They can also look at other aspects of care, such as improving the quality of life for people with chronic illnesses Their goal is to determine if a new test or treatment is safe and effective.. Some CT involve healthy subjects with no pre-existing medical conditions, others pertain to people with specific health conditions who are willing to try an experimental treatment. Pilot experiments are conducted to gain insights for design of the CT to follow.

Except for small, single-location trials, the design and objectives are specified in a document called a clinical trial protocol (CTP). This is the trial's "operating manual" to ensure that all researchers perform the trial in the same way, on similar subjects, and that the data is comparable across all subjects. As a trial is designed to test hypotheses and rigorously monitor and assess outcomes, it can be seen as an application of the scientific method, specifically the experimental step.

CT generate data on dosage, safety, and efficacy. They are conducted only after they have received regulatory approval (health authority and ethics committee approval), which vet the risk/benefit ratio of the trial and allow or deny it.

Depending on product type and development stage, investigators initially enroll volunteers or patients into small pilot studies, and subsequently conduct progressively larger-scale comparative studies.

CT can vary in size and cost, and can involve a single research center or multiple centers, in one or in multiple countries. The clinical study design aims to ensure the scientific validity and reproducibility of the results. Costs for clinical trials can range into the billions of dollars per approved drug. The sponsor may be a governmental organization or a pharmaceutical, biotechnology, or medical device company. Certain functions necessary to the trial, such as monitoring and laboratory work, may be managed by an outsourced partner, such as a contract research organization (CRO) or a central laboratory. Only 10% of all drugs started in human clinical trials become approved drugs.

## Overall goals

There are two goals to testing medical treatments: to learn whether they work well enough, called "efficacy" or "effectiveness"; and to learn whether they are safe enough, called "safety". Neither is an absolute criterion and both safety and efficacy are evaluated relative to how the treatment is intended to be used, what other treatments are available, and the severity of the disease or condition. The benefits must outweigh the risks.

The sponsor designs the trial in coordination with a panel of expert clinical investigators who also consider what alternative or existing treatments exist to compare to the new drug and what type(s) of patients might benefit.

## Categories of trials

There are three trial categories:

### Drugs

They are the most common to evaluate new pharmaceutical products, biologics, diagnostic assays, psychological therapies, or other interventions.

### Devices

Similarly to drugs, manufacturers of medical devices may compare a new device to an established therapy, or may compare similar devices to each other. They are required for pre-market approval.

## Procedures

Similarly to drugs, medical or surgical procedures may be subjected to clinical trials, They compare different surgical approaches in treatment.

# Types of trials

CT are classified by the research objective(s) or purpose(s) of the investigators:

**By research objectives**

This will depend on the kind of study. Thus, in an:

- **Observational study:** The investigators observe the subjects and measure their outcomes. They do not actively manage the study.
- **Interventional study:** The investigators give the research subjects an experimental drug, use of a medical device, a surgical procedure, diagnostic or other intervention to compare the treated subjects with those receiving no treatment or the standard treatment. Then, the researchers assess how the subjects' health changes.

## By research purposes

There are ten such types:

- **Prevention trials:** They look for ways to prevent disease in people who have never had the disease or to prevent a disease from returning. These approaches may include drugs, vitamins or other micronutrients, vaccines, or lifestyle changes.
- **Screening trials:** They test for ways to identify certain diseases or health conditions.
- **Diagnostic trials:** They are conducted to find better tests or procedures for diagnosing a particular disease or condition.
- **Treatment trials:** They test experimental drugs, new combinations of drugs, or new approaches to surgery or radiation therapy.
- **Quality of life trials or supportive care trials:** They evaluate how to improve comfort and quality of care for people with a chronic illness.
- **Genetic trials:** They are conducted to assess the prediction accuracy of genetic disorders making a person more or less likely to develop a disease.
- **Epidemiological trials:** They have the goal of identifying the general causes, patterns or control of diseases in large numbers of people.
- **Compassionate use trials** or **expanded access trials:** They provide partially tested, unapproved therapeutics to a small number of patients who have no other realistic options. Usually, this involves a disease for which no effective therapy has

been approved, or a patient who has already failed all standard treatments and whose health is too compromised to qualify for participation in randomized clinical trials. Usually in the U.S., case-by-case approval must be granted by both the FDA and the pharmaceutical company for such exceptions.

- **Fixed trials:** They consider existing data only during the trial's design, do not modify the trial after it begins, and do not assess the results until the study is completed.
- **Adaptive trials:** They use existing data to design the trial, and then use interim results to modify the trial as it proceeds. Modifications include dosage, sample size, drug undergoing trial, patient selection criteria and "cocktail" mix.

## Trial phases

CT are conducted typically in four phases (Phases I to IV), with each phase using different numbers of subjects and having a different purpose to construct focus on identifying a specific effect. However, for new drugs, there are five phases (Phases 0 and I to IV), each phase being treated as a separate CT.

Table 14.1 recapitulates the aims of these phases:

**Table 14.1 – Phases of clinical trials**

| Phase | Aim | Notes |
|---|---|---|
| **0** | **Pharmacodynamics** (what the drug does to the body) and **pharmacokinetics** (what the body does to the drug) in humans | o Optional<br>o Sub-therapeutic doses<br>o Small number of subjects (10-15) for preliminary data<br>o Trial documents the absorption, distribution, metabolization, and clearance (excretion) of the drug, and the drug's interactions within the body, to confirm that these appear to be as expected |
| **I** | **Safety** | o Small number of subjects (20-30)<br>o Determine safe dosage ranges<br>o Identify side effects |
| **II** | **Iia. Dosing**<br>**Iib. Efficacy** | o IIa: Dosing requirements<br>o Iib: Efficacy to establish therapeutic dose range |
| **III** | **Confirmation of safety and efficacy** | o Large group of subjects (1,000-3,000)<br>o Monitor side effects<br>o Compare to commonly-used treatments |
| **IV** | **Post-marketing safety** | o Delineate benefits, risks, optimal use<br>o Ongoing during the drug's lifetime of active medical use |

*Reference: Wikipedia*

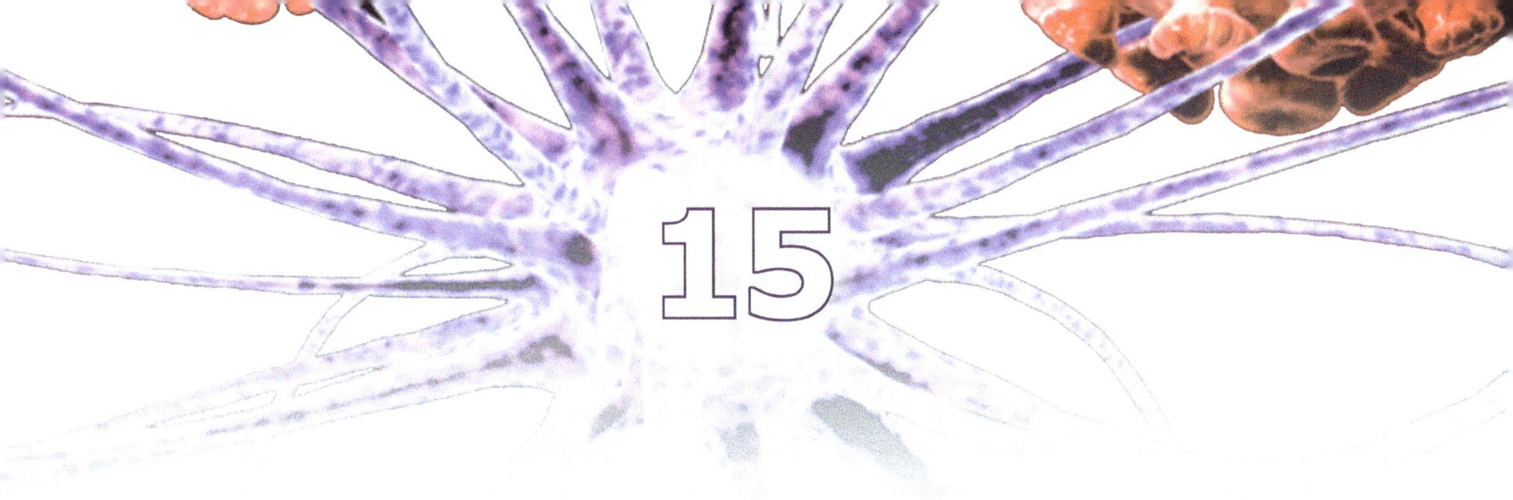

# 15

# Treatment of MSA: IV. Experimental disease-modifying therapies

The treatment approaches discussed in this chapter are based on our current understanding of the pathogenesis of MSA and the results of preclinical and clinical therapeutic studies conducted over the last two decades. They point to putative targets for disease modification, including the leading disease-modifying drugs/therapies (DMD/T): Targeting alpha-synuclein (α-syn) pathology, modulating neuroinflammation, and enhancing neuroprotection.

While the pathogenic mechanisms underlying MSA remain inconclusive, the evidence collected from *post-mortem* studies and preclinical models classifies MSA as a **primary oligodendrogliopathy**, included in the category of **alpha-synucleinopathies** together with PD and dementia with Lewy Bodies (DLB) (Spillantini and Goedert 2000). The presence of α-syn aggregates in the cytoplasm of oligodendrocytes defines MSA as a unique alpha-synucleinopathy. By contrast, in PD and DLB, α-syn pathology occurs mostly in the cytoplasm of neurons (Trojanowski and Revesz 2007; Goedert *et al.,* 2017). These observations result in several questions that we cannot completely answer so far. For instance, what is the source of α-syn within oligodendrocytes? Are the α-syn inclusions a disease trigger or an epiphenomenon? Where should we focus when defining therapeutic targets in MSA?

## Targeting alpha-synuclein pathology

α-syn is an intrinsically disordered protein widely distributed in the central nervous system (CNS), more precisely in the pre-synaptic terminals of neurons, with a suggested physiological role in synaptic homeostasis, vesicle recycling, and synaptic neurotransmission (Maroteaux *et al.,* 1988; Jakes *et al.,* 1994; Iwai *et al.,* 1995). Under pathological conditions, such as α-syn mutations, multiplications, and post-translational modifications or stress-induced changes in the cellular environment, α-syn becomes highly prone to aggregate into pathological oligomeric and large fibrillary structures such as GCIs and Lewy Bodies (LBs) (Spillantini *et al.*, 1998; Anderson *et al.*, 2006; Auluck *et al.*, 2010; Wales *et al.*, 2013). To date, the process of α-syn accumulation and aggregation is considered one of the main pathological events underlying α-synucleinopathies, leading to neuronal dysfunction, neuroinflammation, and neurodegeneration (Mahul-Mellier *et al.*, 2020). Specifically, pathological forms of α-syn seem to interact with cellular components and pathways affecting the cellular homeostasis. Recently, it was observed that in the process of α-syn aggregation, the formation of different fibrillary strains can arise in MSA as compared to PD or DLB (Schweighauser *et al.*, 2020; Shahnawaz *et al.*, 2020).

## Enhancing the degradation of α-syn

- **Inducing α-syn degradation by stimulating macroautophagy:** Initial studies ere conducted using Rapamycin, Lithium, and Nilotinib. Lithium was discarded due to severe adverse effects and Nilotinib did not show neuroprotective effects. A phase II, double-blind clinical trial with Sirolimus (Rapamycin) in MSA patients has been completed (NCT03589976), but no results have been published yet.
- **Promoting α-syn degradation by microglial cells:** It increases the extracellular a-Syn clearance.
    1. **Up-regulating toll-like receptor 4 (TLR4) in microglia:** TLR4 plays an important role in the microglial α-syn clearance (Stefanova *et al.*, 2011); Fellner *et al.,* 2013). It was tested experimentally using monophosphoryl lipid A (MPLA), a TLR4 selective agonist and vaccine component with lower pro-inflammatory toxicity. It showed that the administration of MPLA led to a significant motor improvement, preservation of nigral dopaminergic neurons, and decreased levels of GCIs (Venezia *et al.*, 2017).
    2. **Disrupting the oligomerization process of α-syn:** The small molecule ATH434 (formerly, PTB434) is a moderate iron chelator shown to reduce α-syn accumulation by redistributing labile iron in the brain. It preserves dopaminergic neurons, lowers ferric iron in the brain, and reduces α-syn oligomerization, resulting in improvement of the motor deficits (Heras-Garvin *et al.*, 2021; Stamler *et al.,* 2019, 2020). In the preclinical stage, two more therapeutic candidates are being evaluated: the molecular tweezer CLR01 and the caspase-1 inhibitor VX-765. CLR01.
    3. **Using antisense oligonucleotides (ASOs):** It suppresses the production of α-syn, and therefore, reduces its intracellular toxic accumulation.

In summary, the prevention of α-syn aggregation as well as the enhancement of its degradation constitute promising therapeutic strategies for disease modification in MSA. Since it became widely accepted that α-syn accumulation, spreading, and aggregation constitute major driving forces leading to neurodegeneration, a majority of the developed therapeutic approaches has been focused on enhancing α-syn degradation and preventing or disrupting its aggregation (Brundin *et al.*, 2017). A considerable amount of preclinical evidence supports targeting α-syn pathology for disease modification in MSA as well as in other α-synucleinopathies. Successful clinical trials with α-syn targeting in MSA that prove efficacy of the approach in patients are currently awaited.

## Targeting microglia activation and neuroinflammation

Neuroinflammation is a crucial part of the neuropathological process in MSA and other α-synucleinopathies. It is mediated by the activation of quiescent microglia cells that respond to neuronal damage and pathological α-syn by secreting pro- and anti-inflammatory cytokines, chemokines, and reactive oxygen species (ROS). Whether such inflammatory responses are directly associated with the pathogenesis of the disease, or they represent a downstream effect triggered by the pathological accumulation of α-syn, is still under debate. Although still not well understood, the processes of microglial activation and neuroinflammation have been getting increased attention and exploited for disease-modifying therapies in MSA.

According to PET and neuropathological studies in MSA brains, the process of microglial activation and neuroinflammation can be already detected at early-disease stages. Such observations raise the possibility that reduction of microglial pro-inflammatory activity and anti-inflammatory strategies may represent a promising approach for disease modification in MSA.

## Targeting cellular dysfunction and loss (neuroprotection)

The selective striatonigral degeneration observed in MSA-P patients can lead to the dysfunction of corticostriatal glutamatergic, as well as striatal GABAergic projections. The impairment of such projections can result in neurotoxicity and add to the neurodegenerative cascade. On the other hand, the accumulation of α-syn aggregates within oligodendrocytes leads to the dysfunction of these cells, hampering the neurotrophic support by brain-derived neurotrophic factor (BDNF) and glial-derived neurotropic factor (GDNF) and resulting in neuronal death (Ubhi *et al.*, 2010).

- **Improving impaired growth factors:** Insulin/insulin-like growth factor-1 (IGF-1) signaling and insulin resistance in MSA patients, as well as increased IGF-1 brain levels in MSA mice have been reported (Ubhi *et al.*, 2010; Numao *et al.*, 2014; Bassil *et al.*, 2017). Insulin and IGF-1 appear to be involved in several cellular processes including the synthesis of the myelin sheaths and oligodendrocyte maturation as well as neuronal homeostasis, thereafter their deficits lead to neurotoxicity and consequent neurodegeneration. This strategy aims to prevent oligodendroglial dysfunction and provides neuroprotection of the affected neuronal populations.
- **Use of small molecules:** Rasagiline appears to induce neuroprotection and ameliorate motor deficits but in very high doses, which may not be appropriate in humans due to the associated side effects. Exendin-4 (Exenatide), an anti-diabetic drug presents neuroprotective effects. At present, a phase II clinical trial assesses

its efficacy in disease progression of MSA patients. Other preclinical studies provided rationale for MSA therapy with Sodium phenylbutyrate, an unspecific histone deacetylase inhibitor, and Benztropine, an anti-cholinergic drug (Ettle *et al.,* 2016). Despite the promising preclinical data, both Sodium phenylbiturate and Benzotropine have not yet progressed to clinical trials. In the former case, because of the expected side effects of the drug. In the latter case because, among other reasons, the contribution of the demyelination in early stages of the disease and its causative role for the neurodegeneration has remained uncertain.

- **Supplementation of the co-enzyme Q10** (reduced form Ubiquinol): It is linked to the contribution of mutations in the COQ2 gene in rare familial MSA cases. It has been proposed as an individualized therapeutic approach for patients carrying the mutation/polymorphisms. At a high yet tolerable dose, it improves mitochondrial oxidative metabolism. Currently, a phase II clinical trial with high-dose coenzyme Q10 is underway in Japanese MSA patients.

To summarize, the preclinical evidence supports a number of approaches for the therapy of MSA, which still await confirmation in a clinical setting.

## Major obstacles and open questions

Despite the existence of prominent therapeutic strategies supported by extensive preclinical testing and target validation, a serious gap remains in their translation into successful clinical trials in MSA patients. The major difficulties are linked to the following intertwined factors:

- **Absence of useful biomarkers** (early in the disease and as the disease progresses)**.**
- **Challenge in making an early diagnosis.**
- **Discrepancies in the design of preclinical and clinical studies.**
- **Failure of treatment outcome measurements in clinical trials.**
- **Limited knowledge about the root cause of the disease.**
- **Failure in defining the best therapeutic target(s) for disease modification.**

In summary, progress will be contingent upon resolving the above factors. Additionally, since MSA is a multifactorial disease, multi-target individualized therapies might be necessary to unravel the root cause of MSA and arrive at a cure. In the meantime, tentative and limited symptomatic therapies might continue to be prescribed.

### Take-away points

- Current treatment approaches point to putative targets for disease modification: Alpha-synuclein pathology, neuroinflammation modulation, and neuroprotection enhancement..

- While the pathogenic mechanisms underlying MSA remain elusive, the evidence collected from post-mortem studies and preclinical models classifies MSA as a primary oligodendrogliopathy included in the category of alpha-synucleinopathies.
- In MSA, t\he presence of α-syn aggregates is in the cytoplasm together with the formation of different fibrillary strains. By contrast, in Parkinson's disease and dementia with Lewy bodies, the aggregates occur in the cytoplasm of neurons without fibrillary strains.
- To date, the process of α-syn accumulation and aggregation is considered one of the main underlying pathological events leading to neuronal dysfunction, neuroinflammation, and neurodegeneration.
- The majority of the developed therapeutic approaches has been focused on enhancing α-syn degradation and preventing or disrupting its aggregation.
- Enhancing the degradation of α-syn includes: Inducing α-syn degradation by stimulating macroautophagy; promoting α-syn degradation by microglial cells; up-regulating toll-like receptor 4 (TLR4) in microglia; disrupting of the oligomerization process of α-syn; or/and using antisense oligonucleotides.
- When targeting microglia activation and neuroinflammation, it is not known whether such inflammatory responses are directly associated with the pathogenesis of the disease or represent a downstream effect triggered by the pathological accumulation of α-syn.
- Reduction of microglial pro-inflammatory activity and anti-inflammatory strategies may possibly represent a promising approach for disease modification in MSA.
- Targeting cellular dysfunction and loss (neuroprotection) involves improving impaired growth factors, using small molecules, or supplementing the co-enzyme Q10
- The preclinical evidence supports a number of approaches for the therapy of MSA, which still await confirmation in a clinical setting.
- Despite the existence of prominent therapeutic strategies, major obstacles and open questions remain including the absence of useful biomarkers (whether early in the disease or as the disease progresses), the challenge in making an early diagnosis, the discrepancies in the design of preclinical and clinical studies, the failure of treatment outcome measurements in clinical trials, the limited knowledge about the root cause of the disease, and the failure in defining the best therapeutic target(s) for disease modification.

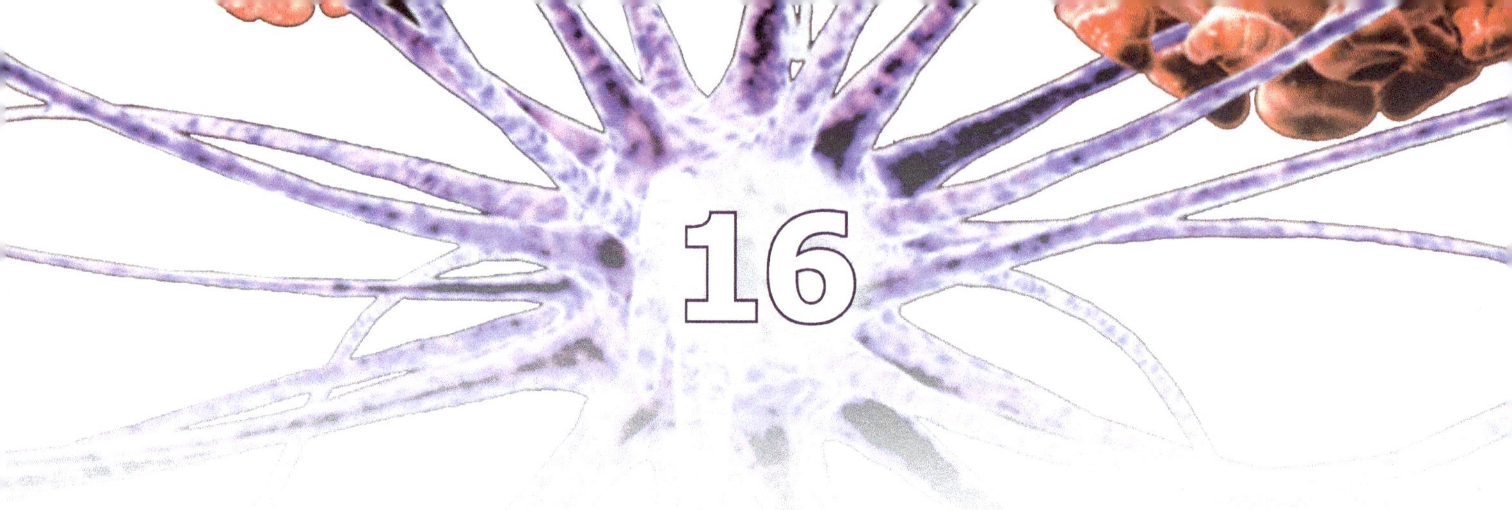


# Treatment portfolio: V. Future therapeutic options

Future therapeutic options will be considered in the following sections, including growth hormone therapy, immunotherapy, gene therapy, and mesenchymal stem cell therapy.

## Growth hormone therapy (GHT)

Experimentally, GHT appears to slow the progression of the disease but not significantly.

### Minocycline

Mynocycline is a tetracycline with neuroprotective efficacy in transgenic MSA mice, which has shown some promise in the early stages of the disease in laboratory studies.

### Rasagiline

Rasagiline is a monoamine-oxidase-B inhibitor which appears to have disease-modifying effects and is soon expected to enter phase 3 trials.

### Rifampicin

Rifampicin has been shown to have the property of preventing α-synuclein aggregation and so is also being considered as a therapeutic candidate.

## Immunotherapy

Immunotherapy or biological therapy is "*the treatment of disease by activating or suppressing the immune system*". Immunotherapies designed to elicit or amplify an immune response are classified as activation immunotherapies, while immunotherapies that reduce or suppress are classified as suppression immunotherapies. Immunotherapy is under preliminary research for its potential to treat MSA.

### Principle and use

The principle of immunotherapy (passive or active) is based on the specific binding of the antigen α-syn and its respective antibody, followed by clearance of the complexes (Mandler *et al.,* 2015; El-Agnaf *et al.,* 2017).

The use of immunotherapy for the treatment of neurodegenerative disorders consists in the development of anti-α-Syn immunotherapies to enhance the degradation and clearance of α-syn.

## Activation immunotherapy

Activation immunotherapy employs the following antibodies:

### Affitope®

Activation immunization for targeting the α-syn pathology has been carried out with short synthetic peptide fragments (AFFITOPEs®), mimicking parts of the native sequence and structure of the human α-Syn protein.

An 'epitope', also known as 'antigenic determinant', is the part of an antigen that is recognized by the immune system, specifically by antibodies, B-cells, or T-cells. The part of an antibody that binds to the epitope is called a 'paratope'. Although epitopes are usually non-self proteins, sequences derived from the host that can be recognized (as in the case of autoimmune diseases) are also epitopes.

The immunogenic peptide, i.e., AFFITOPE, operates a B-cell epitope and is responsible for the specificity of the immune response. Initial studies in PD, DLB, and MSA mouse models demonstrated the efficacy of the AFFITOPE® PD01 and PD03. It triggered specific antibody generation with CNS penetration and lowered α-Syn aggregates and oligomers, leading to neuroprotection and improvement of locomotor behavior in PD and MSA mice, respectively (Mandler *et al.,* 2014, 2015; Lemos *et al.,* 2020).

### PD01 and PD03

The first phase I clinical trial with PD patients using PD01 suggested good immunogenicity, safety, and tolerability (Volc *et al.,* 2020).

In 2020, a clinical trial with PD01 and PD03 in MSA patients showed that both AFFITOPEs® presented immunogenicity and good tolerability. However, the authors noticed that the antibody levels in the plasma were higher in individuals receiving PD01 than in patients receiving PD03 (Meissner *et al.,* 2020). In contrast, substantial levels of PD03-induced antibodies were reported in PD patients (Poewe *et al.,* 2021). These differences in plasma antibody levels between PD and MSA patients receiving PD03 immunotherapy and the evidence of different α-Syn strains in PD and MSA (Schweighauser *et al.,* 2020; Shahnawaz *et al.,* 2020), led the researchers to speculate that vaccines may have different binding of the antibodies to disease-specific α-syn conformations. These differences may result in the observed difference in plasma antibody levels reported in the clinical trials in PD and MSA. In support of this hypothesis, PD03 immunotherapy in MSA mice showed high binding of IgGs in the brain, suggesting that the PD03-induced antibodies entered the brain and accumulated at the sites of α-Syn pathology.

## Anle138b

Anle138b is a small molecule that modulates the oligomerization of α-syn. It can be delivered orally and crosses the blood–brain barrier (BBB). If the MSA mice received in parallel to PD03 also Anle138b, the IgG binding in the brain was significantly decreased (Heras-Garvin *et al.,* 2019; Lemos *et al.,* 2020). This phenomenon was accompanied by an increase in the measured plasma antibodies to α-syn in the mice receiving combined therapy. These observations support the hypothesis that the plasma levels of anti-α-syn antibodies may reflect not simply the immunogenicity of the used vaccine, but also the level of selective binding to a specific α-syn conformation.

The use of small molecules such as Anle138b has shown promising results in preventing α-syn accumulation or disrupting the formation of toxic oligomeric species. Preclinical studies with Anle138b in a MSA mouse model suggested neuroprotection associated with decreased α-syn oligomerization, lower microglial activation, resulting in motor improvement. Recently, a phase I clinical trial with Anle138b in healthy patients was successfully completed (NCT04208152) and confirmed its safety. A follow-up phase II study in MSA patients is currently in preparation.

Taken together, the clinical and preclinical evidence reinforce the relevance of disease-specific α-syn strains for the efficacy of active immunotherapy in α-synucleinopathies.

## Suppression immunotherapy

Approaches of suppression immunotherapy target α-syn pathology using antibodies targeting different α-syn species have been extensively tested pre-clinically in PD models (Zella *et al.,* 2019). Several clinical trials testing passive immunization in PD have been launched. First preclinical data supporting the efficacy of passive immunization approach in MSA were also reported and the clinical application in MSA is currently discussed (Kallab *et al.,* 2018).

## AAV2-GDNF

Currently, a phase I clinical trial with AAV2-GDNF gene therapy in MSA patients is in progress (NCT04680065).

## Gene therapy

Gene therapy is the insertion of genes into an individual's cells and tissues to treat hereditary diseases where deleterious mutant alleles can be replaced with functional ones. The genes are usually placed within a non-pathogenic virus, which serves as the vector to penetrate the cells. It can also be used to correct non-genetic deficiencies such as the loss of dopamine in MSA, to modify the function of a group of cells (e.g. convert an excitatory structure to one that is inhibitory) or to provide a source of growth factors.

Fewer than 10% of rare diseases have FDA-approved treatments. About 80% of rare diseases are caused by known alterations in a single gene. This common feature makes these diseases potential candidates for gene therapy, which entails replacing or correcting a defective gene. Developing gene therapies for rare diseases, however, is complex, time consuming, and expensive. The gene therapy development process is hampered by a lack of access to proprietary tools and methods, a dearth of standards, and a one-disease-at-a-time approach. As of December 2021, only two rare diseases have an FDA-approved gene therapy.

## Mesenchymal stem cell therapy (MSC)

Cell therapies have been of interest in MSA for a long time. Initial efforts in toxin SND models have aimed at restoration of the dopaminergic response (Stefanova *et al.,* 2005). MSCs applied intravenously were found to delay the progression of neurological deficits in patients with MSA-cerebellar type. They may also suppress the exacerbated neuroinflammatory cellular environment by producing anti-inflammatory cytokines and neurotrophic factors and exert neuroprotection in a transgenic MSA mouse model (Stemberger *et al.,* 2011).

The treatment with autologous MSCs has been attempted in MSA patients indicating some positive trends (Lee *et al.,* 2008, 2012; Singer *et al.,* 2019). However, due to some insufficiencies in the designs of these clinical trials, further studies are required and currently performed (e.g., NCT02795052, NCT02315027, NCT04876326, NCT04495582) to better evaluate the therapeutic potential of MSCs in MSA patients (Table 16.1).

In summary, many alternative approaches to improve the cellular function and induce neuroprotection in MSA have been proposed, expanding from drug repurposing to gene and cell therapies. No reliable approach has been identified yet, despite the extensive preclinical evidence. However, many clinical trials are still underway as listed.

**Table 16.1 - FDA-approved therapies and corresponding drugs**

| Type of therapy | Drugs |
|---|---|
| **Anti-inflammatory therapies** | o Intravenous immunoglobulins (IVIg)<br>o Lenalidomide<br>o Rituximab |
| **Alpha-synuclein targeted therapies** | o Affitopac (R) PD01A<br>o Belmacasan (VX-766)<br>o FTY220 (Fingolimod)<br>o Kalliterein-6<br>o Lu AF82422 (alpha-synuclein mAD)<br>o MPLA<br>o NBMI<br>o Sirolinus<br>o Synuclean-D<br>o TAK-34 |
| **Neuroprotective therapies** | o BNN-20<br>o Exonatide<br>o Gene therapy (AAV 2-GDNF)<br>o Inosine 5 – Monophosphate<br>o Intranasal insulin (INI)<br>o Stearoyl-coA desaterase inhibition<br>o Stem cells<br>o Ubiquinofi<br>o Verdiperstat (BHV-3241) |
| **Diagnosis & Biomarkers** | o Alpha-synuclein<br>o Alzheimer's disease biomarkers<br>o Brain network activation<br>o DaTscanTM Iofluopane (12) injection/ SPECT imaging<br>o Digital speech analysis (Bvoice 4P D-MSA)<br>o (18-F)F-Dopa imaging<br>o Gait analysis<br>o Magnetic Resonance Imaging (MRI)<br>o Morphomer TM library PET tracer specific for alpha-synuclein<br>o Transcranial magnetic stimulation (TMS)<br>o Web-based automated imaging |

| | |
|---|---|
| **Symptomatic treatments** | o Abdominal binder<br>o Ampreloxetine/TD-9855<br>o Atomoxetine<br>o Botilunum A toxin<br>o Continuous positive airway pressure (CPAP)<br>o Deep brain stimulation (DBS)<br>o Droxidopa<br>o Expiratory muscle strength training (EMST)<br>o Fipamezole (JP-1730)<br>o Midodrine<br>o Midodrine + Droxidopa<br>o Nebivolol<br>o NDMA modulator<br>o Repetitive transcranial magnetic stimulation (rTMS)<br>o Riluzole<br>o Safinamide<br>o Zoledronic acid |

*Source: (U.S.) FDA*

## Take-away points

- The principle of immunotherapy (passive or active) is based on the specific binding of the antigen α-syn and its respective antibody, followed by clearance of the complexes. Its use for the treatment of neurodegenerative disorders consists in the development of anti-α-syn immunotherapies to enhance the degradation and clearance of α-syn.
- Active immunotherapy employs the following antibodies: Affitope® PD01 and PD03. A 2020 clinical trial with PD01 and PD03 in MSA patients led to the speculation that vaccines may have different binding of the antibodies to disease-specific α-syn conformations, suggesting that the PD03-induced antibodies entered the brain and accumulated at the sites of α-syn pathology.
- The use of other small molecules such as Anle138b has shown promising results in preventing α-syn accumulation or disrupting the formation of toxic oligomeric species.
- Approaches of passive immunization to target α-syn pathology using antibodies targeting different α-syn species have been extensively tested pre-clinically in Parkinson's disease models. Passive immunization approach in MSA have been reported.
- Gene therapy is the insertion of genes into an individual's cells and tissues to treat hereditary diseases where deleterious mutant alleles can be replaced with functional ones. The genes are usually placed within a non-pathogenic virus, which serves as the vector to penetrate the cells.

- Gene therapy can also be used to correct non-genetic deficiencies such as the loss of dopamine in MSA, to modify the function of a group of cells, or to provide a source of growth factors.
- Cell therapies have been of interest in MSA for a long time. Mesenchymal stem cells applied intravenously were found to suppress the exacerbated neuroinflammatory cellular environment by producing anti-inflammatory cytokines and neurotrophic factors and exert neuroprotection.
- The treatment with autologous mesenchymal stem cells has been attempted in MSA patients indicating some positive trends. However, due to some insufficiencies in the designs of these clinical trials, further studies are required and are currently being performed.
- Many alternative approaches to improve the cellular function and induce neuroprotection in MSA have been proposed, expanding from drug repurposing to gene and cell therapies. Unfortunately, no reliable approach has been identified yet, despite the extensive preclinical evidence.

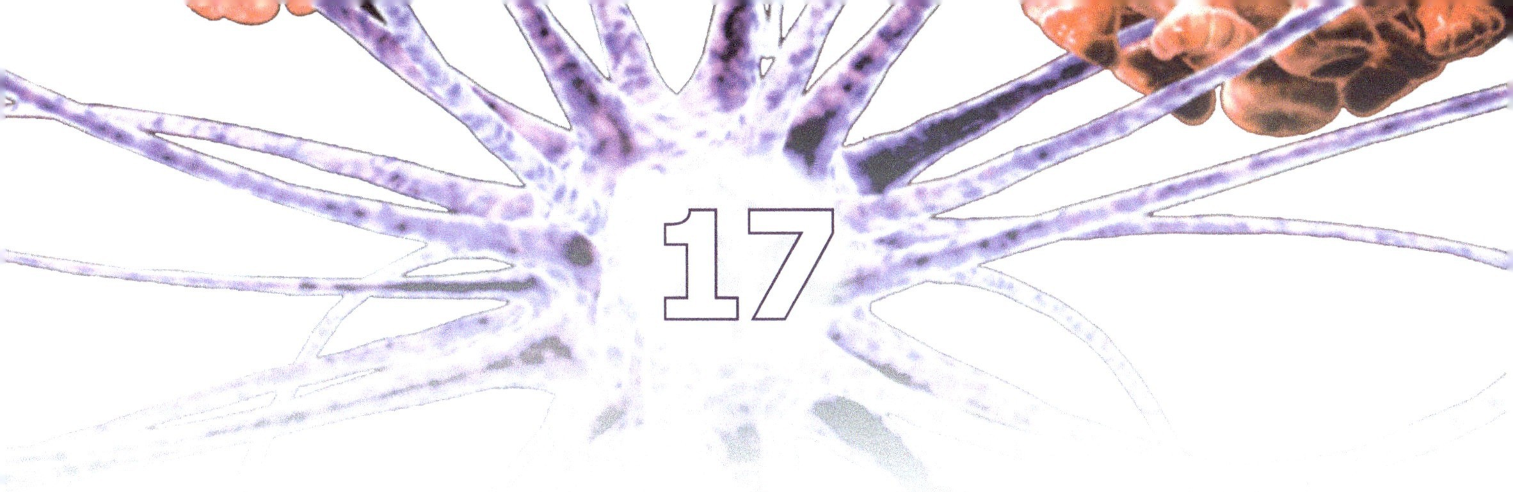

# 17

# Prognosis and future outlook

MSA is rapidly progressive and is associated with wheelchair dependence, unintelligible speech, intermittent urinary catheterization, disabling orthostatic hypotension, and cognitive impairment (executive dysfunction). Disease progression is assessed using the unified MSA rating scale (UMSARS), which rates activities of daily life, autonomic and motor impairment, as well as overall disability. Prognosis is poor with a median survival of 6-9 years.

For those individuals in the MSA-P category, it may be of interest to know the prognosis in Parkinson's disease (PD). As is well known, PD is, by contrast, typically slowly progressive, but the rate of progression is variable. The mortality rate for elderly people aged 70-89 years with PD is 2-5 times higher than for age-matched controls in some studies. The risk of dementia is about 2-6 times higher in people with PD than in healthy controls.

## Prognosis

The disease progresses without remission at a variable rate. Those who present at an older age, those with parkinsonian features, and those with severe autonomic dysfunction have a poorer prognosis. By contrast, those with predominantly cerebellar features (MSA-C) and those who display autonomic dysfunction later have a better prognosis.

People who have MSA will usually develop movement-related symptoms first. This condition gets progressively worse over time. About half of people with this condition need help walking within this time frame. That usually means walking with a cane, walker or another type of assistive device. About 60% of people with MSA need to use a wheelchair about five years after the onset of MSA. Within six to eight years, at least half of those with this condition are bedridden.

As the disease worsens, many people need additional procedures or interventions to maintain or modify body processes and avoid dangerous complications. Some of these interventions include:

- **Tracheotomy** (a surgical operation of opening into the trachea): To preserve breathing ability.
- **Tube feeding** (enteral nutrition).
- **In-dwelling catheters.**
- **Urostomy** (the establishment of an artificial cutaneous opening into the urethra)**:** For urinary incontinence.
- **Colostomy** (the establishment of an artificial cutaneous opening into the colon): For fecal incontinence.

## Future outlook

The outlook for MSA is poor. The symptoms of this condition get progressively worse and always disrupt body function, leading to deadly complications. It is a permanent condition that lasts the rest of a person's life. It is also a grave disease with a rapid progression of clinical symptoms. The mean life expectancy following the onset of symptoms is about 6 – 10 years and approximately seven yers after diagnosis. In less severe cases, people can survive up to 15 years.

In very severe cases, survival time may be much lower. These cases usually involve the following features and characteristics:

- **Older age at time of diagnosis.**
- **Autonomic symptoms** that reach severe levels before motor symptoms begin.
- **Movement symptoms** that cause repeated falls.

One review found prognostic indicators that showed a shorter survival for older age at onset, early bladder catheterization, and early generalized autonomic failure. Approximately 60% of patients require a wheelchair within five years of onset of the motor symptoms, and few patients survive beyond 12 years.

## Causes of death

The most common causes of death are:

- **Sudden death** (usually at night, because of disruptions in how the brain controls breathing while sleeping).
- **Death caused by infections**, which include:
  1. **Urinary catheterization infections:** They lead to sepsis or the presence of various pus-forming and other organisms, or their toxins, in the blood or tissues.
  2. **Feeding tube infections.**
  3. **Bronchopneumonia:** An acute inflammation of the walls of the smaller tubes, with irregular areas of consolidation due to the spread of the inflammation

into peribronchiolar alveoli and the alveolar ducts, It may become confluent or may be hemorrhagic. Complications include: necrosis and abscess formation.
4. **Pulmonary embolus:** A blood clot in the lungs.
5. **Cachexia** (also known as "wasting syndrome")**:** A general lack of nutrition and wasting occurring in the course of the disease

## Take-away points

- The mortality rate for elderly people with Parkinson's disease (PD) and aged 70-89 years is 2-5 times higher than for age-matched controls in some studies. The risk of dementia is about 2-6 times higher in people with PD than in healthy controls.
- MSA progresses without remission at a variable rate. Older people with parkinsonian features, (MSA-P) and those with severe autonomic dysfunction have a poorer prognosis. By contrast, those with predominantly cerebellar features (MSA-C) and those who display autonomic dysfunction later have a better prognosis.
- People who have MSA will usually develop movement-related symptoms first, a condition that gets progressively worse over time.
- As the disease worsens, many people need additional procedures or interventions to maintain or modify body processes and avoid dangerous complications. Some of these interventions include: Tracheotomy, tube feeding, in-dwelling catheters, urostomy, and colostomy.
- The outlook for MSA is poor. The symptoms get progressively worse and always disrupt body function, leading to deadly complications.
- The mean life expectancy following the onset of symptoms is about 6 – 10 years and approximately seven years after diagnosis. In less severe cases, people can survive up to 15 years. In very severe cases, survival time may be much lower.
- The most common causes of death are: Sudden death and death caused by infections, which include: Urinary catheterization infections, feeding tube infections, bronchopneumonia, pulmonary embolus, and cachexia:

# D. LIVING WITH THE DISEASE

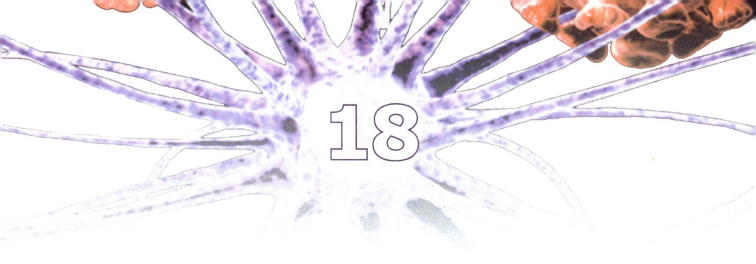

18

# Living with MSA

As with common diseases, the personal and economic burdens of rare diseases are immense. People who live with rare diseases often struggle for years before they receive an accurate diagnosis, with some remaining undiagnosed for a decade or longer. The diagnostic odyssey includes countless doctor visits, unnecessary tests and procedures, and wrong diagnoses. For people in rural and low-income communities, lack of access to care is an additional barrier to an accurate diagnosis. And a diagnosis often does not lead to better health—only about 5% of rare diseases have FDA-approved treatments.

Most rare diseases have no cure, so living with a rare disease is an ongoing learning experience for patients and families. Collections of stories and videos from people who have generously shared their experiences of living with a rare disease can be found in the websites of the several advocating and supporting organizations (see Chapter 19). MSA patients are generally encouraged to share their own experiences.

One of the first places many newly diagnosed rare disease patients and their families turn to is the NORD Rare Diseases Database to locate their particular disease of concern. NORD can provide valuable assistance in navigating its database. It also offers patient assistance programs and help with access care.

## Patient Assistance Programs

The following patient assistance programs are offered to help individuals living with rare diseases:

1. Obtain medication.
2. Receive financial help with insurance premiums and co-pays.
3. Get diagnostic testing assistance.
4. Receive travel assistance for clinical trials or consultation with disease specialists.
5. Provide caregiver respite.
6. Offer support during emergencies.

7. Gain knowledge about rare diseases.
8. Connect with other patient assistance programs.

## Help with financial assistance

Collectively, the personal burdens of those with rare diseases impose a significant economic cost on their respective nation. In the U.S., for example, the health care expenses for people with rare diseases are 3-5 times greater than those without rare diseases. Further, the total direct medical costs for those with rare diseases is approximately $400 billion annually. Including indirect and non-medical costs, this latter figure resulting in a higher total economic burden of nearly $1 trillion annually. Financial assistance programs, such as RareCare are therefore quite welcome.

The RareCare program helps patients obtain life-saving or life-sustaining medication, which they could not otherwise afford. The program also provides financial assistance with insurance premiums and co-pays, diagnostic testing assistance, and travel assistance for clinical trials or consultation with disease specialists.

## Help with caregiver aid

Caring for a loved one demands significant amounts of time, attention, patience, and dedication. The Respite Program provides financial assistance to enable caregivers a break away from caregiving.

## Help with emergency relief

NORD has teamed up with the MedicAlert Foundation to provide protection to rare disease patients in emergency situations. The program provides eligible individuals with a MedicAlert product and three years of membership.

## Help with educational support

The Rare Disease Educational Support Program reimburses registration costs for rare disease-specific educational offerings such as workshops, nutrition classes, and conferences as well as limited financial assistance for travel and lodging costs.

## End-of-life issues

Because the disorder is progressive and ultimately fatal, people should prepare advance directives soon after the disorder is diagnosed. These directives should indicate what kind of medical care people want at the end of their life.

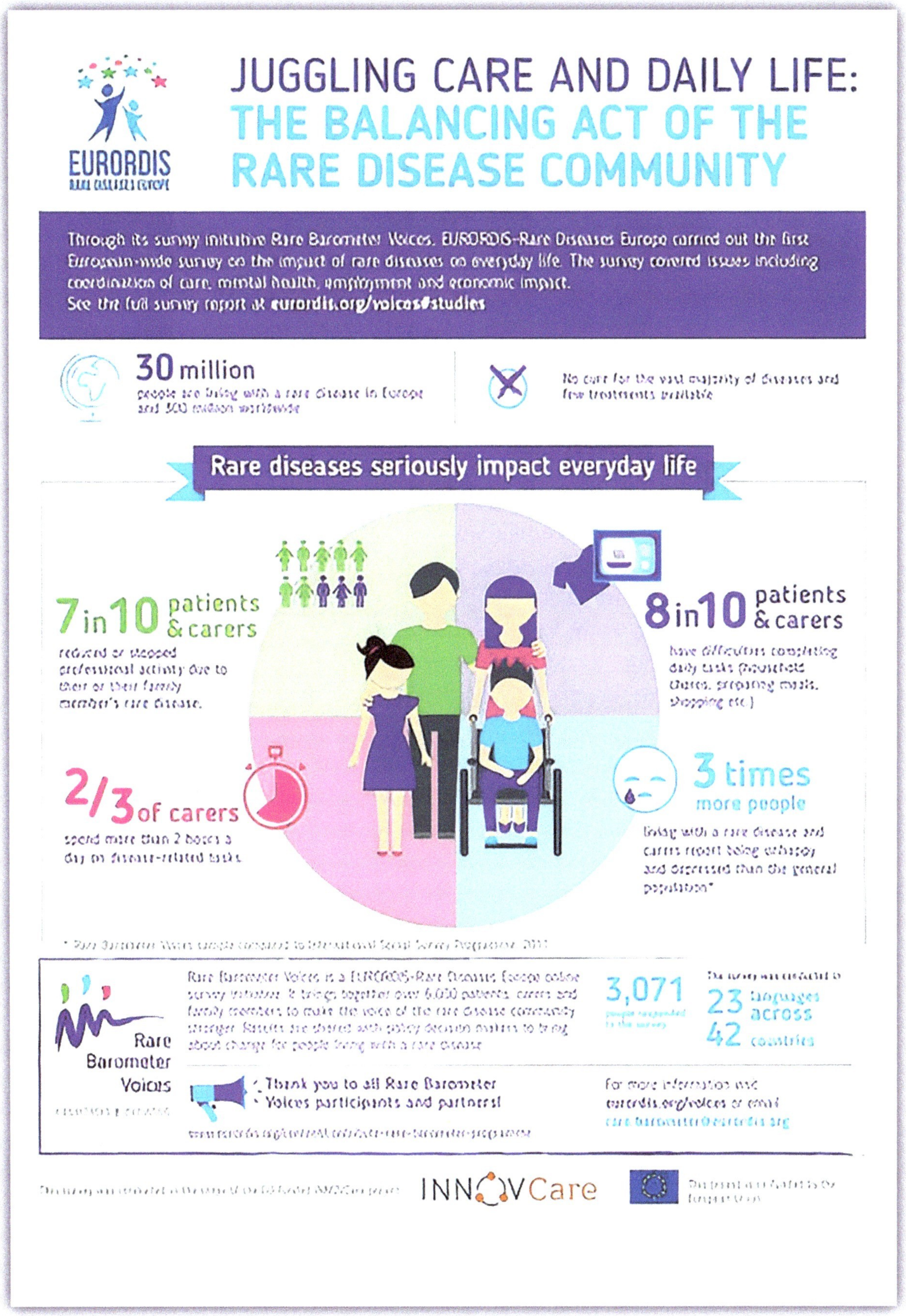
EURORDIS
JUGGLING CARE AND DAILY LIFE:
THE BALANCING ACT OF THE RARE DISEASE COMMUNITY
Through its survey initiative Rare Barometer Voices, EURORDIS-Rare Diseases Europe carried out the first European-wide survey on the impact of rare diseases on everyday life. The survey covered issues including coordination of care, mental health, employment and economic impact.
See the full survey report at eurordis.org/voices#studies
30 million
people are living with a rare disease in Europe and 300 million worldwide
No cure for the vast majority of diseases and few treatments available
Rare diseases seriously impact everyday life
7 in 10 patients & carers
reduced or stopped professional activity due to their or their family member's rare disease.
8 in 10 patients & carers
have difficulties completing daily tasks (household chores, preparing meals, shopping etc.)
2/3 of carers
spend more than 2 hours a day on disease-related tasks.
3 times more people
living with a rare disease and carers report being unhappy and depressed than the general population*
Rare Barometer Voices
3,071
23 languages across
42 countries
Thank you to all Rare Barometer Voices participants and partners!
For more information visit eurordis.org/voices or email
INNOVCare

Figure 18.1 is an infographic from the European Organization of Rare Disorders (EURORDIS). It shows the results of a survey it conducted and titled 'Juggling care and daily life: The balancing act of the rare disease community'. It was conducted via Rare Barometer Voices (Rare Barometer is a EURORDIS global survey initiative, available is 23 languages, which aims to make the voice of rare disease patients stronger) and, in the scope of the EU-funded INNOVCare project, focused on promoting person-centered care for rare diseases. 'Rare Barometer' is a EURORDIS global survey initiative, available is 23 languages. It aims to make the voice of rare disease patients stronger. INNOVCare gives a voice to the social and everyday needs of people living with a rare disease and addresses the need for coordination between service providers in European Union Member States.

## Take-away points

- As with common diseases, the personal and economic burdens of rare diseases are immense.
- Most rare diseases have no cure, so living with a rare disease is an ongoing learning experience for patients and families.
- One of the first places many newly diagnosed rare disease patients and their families turn to is the NORD Rare Diseases Database to locate their particular disease of concern. NORD can provide valuable assistance in navigating its database.
- NORD also offers patient assistance programs and help with: Access care, caregiver aid, help with emergency relief, help with educational support, and help with end-of-life issues.
- Because the disorder is progressive and ultimately fatal, people should prepare advance directives soon after the disorder is diagnosed.

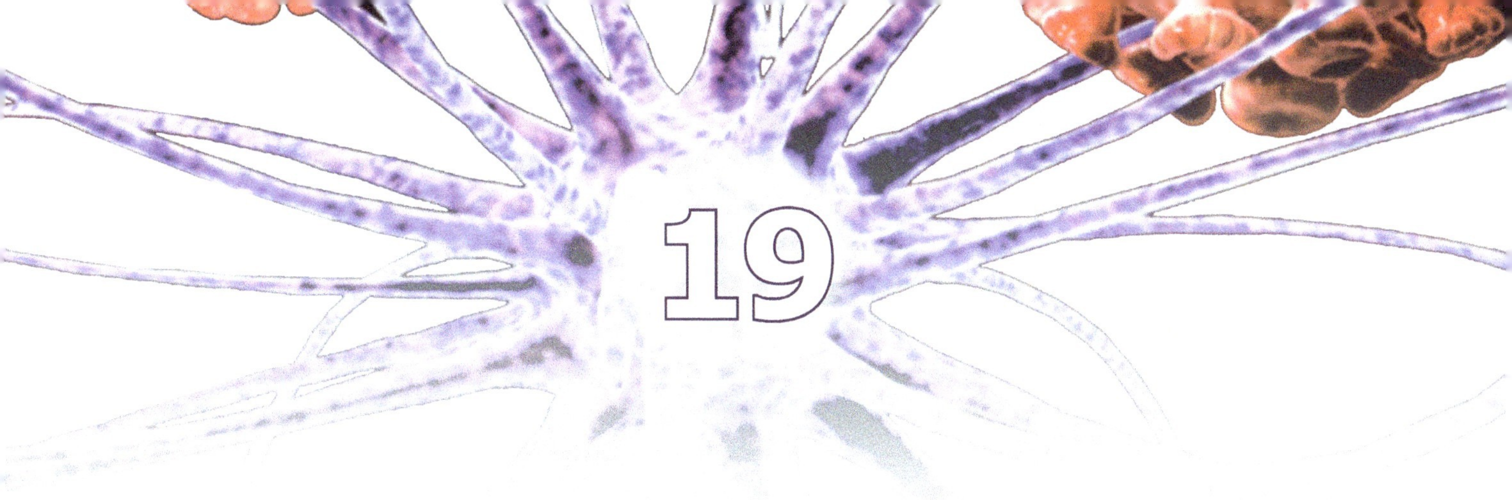

# 19

# What can you do about MSA? Resources and support

## How can a patient organization be helpful?

Patient advocacy and support organizations offer many valuable services and often drive the research and development of treatments for their disease(s). Because these organizations include the life experiences of many different people who have a specific disease, they may best understand the resources needed by those in their community. Although missions of organizations may differ, services may include, but are not limited to:

- Ways to connect to others and share personal stories.
- Easy-to-read information.
- Latest treatment and research information.
- Lists of specialists or specialty centers.
- Financial aid and travel resources.

### What do disease-specific organizations do?

Some organizations build a community of patients and families impacted by a specific disease or group of related diseases. These organizations usually have more disease-specific information and services, including helping new members find others who have the same disease.

### What do organizations that focus on a medical condition do?

These organizations usually have information and services focused more on the medical condition(s), but may also have information about associated diseases.

### What do umbrella organizations do?

Rare disease umbrella organizations focus on improving the lives of all those impacted by rare diseases through education and advocacy efforts. They provide a range of services for patients, families, and disease-specific organizations.

## Where can I find more information about multiple system atrophy?

Information may be available from the following organizations and resources, and others:

**Worldwide Education and Awareness for Movement Disorders**
www.movementdisorders.org/MDS.htm

**International Parkinson & Movement Disorder Society (IP&MDS)**
555 East Wells Street, Suite 1100
Milwaukee, WI 53202-3823 USA
Tel: +1 (414) 276-2145
Fax: +1 (414) 276-3349
E-mail: info@movementdisorders.org

The IP&MDS is a professional society of clinicians, scientists, and other healthcare professionals who are interested in some of the most challenging diseases to diagnose and treat: movement disorders, including Parkinson's disease, related neurodegenerative and neurodevelopmental disorders, hyperkinetic movement disorders, and abnormalities in muscle tone and motor control. It operates exclusively for scientific, scholarly, and educational purposes.

**International Society for Autonomic Neuroscience (ISAN)**
www.autonomicneuroscience.info

The ISAN is a scientific society of researchers studying the autonomic nervous system. The society organizes scientific meetings, publishes a scientific journal, and supports students through awards and travel grants.

**Progressive Supranuclear Palsy Support Group – Australia (via Fight Parkinson's)**
fightparkinsons.org.au/atypical-parkinsonspsp-australia.org.au

**Defeat Multiple System Atrophy Australia**
MSAdownunder.org.au

**European Organization of Rare Disorders (EURORDIS)**
EURORDIS-Rare Diseases Europe,
Plateforme Maladies Rares,
96, rue Didot,

75014 Paris,
France
Tel: +33 1 56 53 52 10

EURORDIS-Rare Diseases Europe
Fondation Universitaire,
Rue d'Egmont 11,
1000 Brussels,
Belgium
Tel: +32 2 882 77 2

EURORDIS-Rare Diseases Europe,
Recinte Modernista Sant Pau,
Pabellón de Santa Apolonia,
Calle Sant Antoni Mª Claret 167,
08025 Barcelona,
Spain

EURORDIS-Rare Diseases Europe is a unique, non-profit alliance of over 1000 rare disease patient organizations from 74 countries that work together to improve the lives of over 300 million people living with a rare disease globally.

By connecting patient, families, and patient groups as well as by bringing together all stakeholders and mobilizing the rare disease community, EURORDIS strengthens the patient voice and shapes research, policies, and patient services.

Through interactions with policy makers, companies, regulators and payers, EURORDIS advocates for better access to rare disease treatments and also improved engagement of patients in the R&D process for rare disease treatments.

Its advocacy and the positions it takes on important topics around rare disease treatments are bolstered by the views and experience of its member patient organizations, who collectively represent the 30 million people living with a rare disease in Europe. It collects their input through consultations (often held through webinars and events) or through Rare Barometer surveys, as can be seen in the results of their 2019 treatments survey.

EURORDIS has proposed a four-pillar approach to tackling the challenges that prevent patients' access to medicines, including the ambition to have 3 to 5 times more new rare disease therapies approved per year, 3 to 5 times cheaper than today by 2025.

In cooperation with its member patient organizations and on behalf of the wider rare disease community, EURORDIS advocates for better access to treatments at several stages.

**It improves access to gene and cell therapies, repurposing of treatments, and safety of treatments.**

**Its 'Resource Centers' are a one-stop shop service specifically designed for people living with a rare disease. A European network of resource centers for rare diseases is under creation.**

**Its 'RareResourceNet' is a European Network of Resource Centers for Rare Diseases, which aims at accelerating the development and the implementation of holistic high quality care pathways.**

**It also offers Case Management Services in which a case manager coordinates the services for the user, especially for users facing complex and long-term needs.**

**(U.K.) Multiple System Atrophy Trust**
msatrust.org.uk

**(U.S.) Food & Drug Administration (FDA)**
10903 New Hampshire Ave
Silver Springs, MD 20993-0002
Tel: +1 888-463-6332 (+1 888-INFO-FDA)
www.fda.gov

**Center for Drug Evaluation and Research (CDER)**
Division of Drug Information
10001 New Hampshire Avenue
Hillandale Building, 4th Floor
Silver Spring, MD 20993
Tel: +1 301-796-3400

The Food and Drug Administration (FDA) is responsible for protecting the public health by ensuring the safety, efficacy, and security of human and veterinary drugs, biological products, and medical devices; and by ensuring the safety of the nation's food supply, cosmetics, and products that emit radiation.

FDA is also responsible for advancing the public health by helping to speed innovations that make medical products more effective, safer, and more affordable and by helping the public get the accurate, science-based information they need to use medical products and foods to maintain and improve their health.

**(U.S.) National Institutes of Health (NIH)**
9000 Rockville Pike, Bethesda, Maryland 20892
301-496-4000
www.nih.gov; medlineplus.gov/ency/article/000757.htm

The National Institutes of Health (NIH), Department of Health and Human Services, is one of the world's foremost medical research centers and the Federal focal point for health research. It is the steward of medical and behavioral research for the Nation. Its mission is to seek fundamental knowledge about the nature and behavior of living systems and the application of that knowledge to enhance health, lengthen life, and reduce illness and disability. In the pursuit of its goals, the NIH provides leadership and direction to programs designed to improve the health of the Nation by conducting and supporting research in:

- The causes, diagnosis, prevention, and cure of human diseases.
- The processes of human growth and development.
- The biological effects of environmental contaminants.
- The understanding of mental, addictive and physical disorders.
- Directing programs for the collection, dissemination, and exchange of information in medicine and health.

*Of its 27 member Institutes and Centers, those of most direct relevance to MSA are the:*

- **National Center for Translational Research (NCTR).**
- **National Center for Advancing Translational Sciences (NCATS).**
- **National Institute of General Medical Sciences (NIGMS).**
- **National Institute of Mental Health (NIMH).**
- **National Institute of Neurological Diseases and Stroke (NINDS):** The mission is to seek fundamental knowledge about the brain and nervous system and to use that knowledge to reduce the burden of neurological disease.
- www.ninds.nih.gov/health-information/disorders/multiple-system-atrophy
- **National Library of Medicine (NLM).**

In particular, NCATS works with patients, advocates, clinicians, and researchers to meet the public health challenge of rare diseases. Driving those conversations are three overarching goals to help people living with rare diseases get the high-quality care they need, faster:

- **Shorten the duration of the diagnostic odyssey by more than half: From the current average of 7 years.**
- **Develop treatments for more than one rare disease at a time: Approximately, 80%–85% of rare diseases are genetic.**
- **Make it easier and more efficient for scientists to discover and develop treatments for rare diseases**.

The NIH **MSA Coalition Center** provides support, education, research, advocacy.

**American Academy of Neurology (AAN)**
201 Chicago Avenue
Minneapolis, MN 55415
Tel: +1 800-8791960
or +1 612-928-6000 (International)
Fax: (612) 454-2746
E-mail: info@aan.com

The AAN aims to promote the highest quality patient-centered neurologic care. Among others, its goals are to:

- Demonstrate and assert the value of neurology and brain health to policymakers, patients, the public, and other major stakeholders.
- Grow the neurology workforce and innovate care delivery to meet the future needs for patient care.
- Ensure the health of the global neurology community.
- Expand and support neuroscience research.
- Create novel ways to educate and assist members in providing high-value, team-based, and patient-centered clinical care.

**Autonomic Disorders Consortium (ADC)**
(also known as the Autonomic Rare Disorders Clinical Research Consortium)
Tel: +1 888-205-2311
E-mail: GARDinfo@nih.gov (GARD=Genetic and Rare Diseases Information Center)

ADC helps the public find reliable information about rare and genetic diseases.

ADC investigators and associated patient advocacy groups aim to find better ways to identify rare autonomic diseases, elucidate fundamental mechanisms of their pathogenesis, and discover therapeutic strategies to treatment. They are dedicated to finding new therapies to treat and cure rare diseases including including, in particular, Lewy Body Disease, Multiple System Atrophy, parkinsonism with autonomic failure, and others.

**Multiple System Atrophy Coalition (MSAC)**
1660 International Drive
Suite 600
McLean, VA USA 22102
Tel: +1 866-737-5999 (support hot line)
**E-mail:** info@multiplesystematrophy.org

MSAC aims to improve the quality of life for the MSA community by expanding access to care and support while advancing research toward treatment and a cure. It is devoted to improving quality of life and building hope for people affected by multiple system atrophy through:

- Providing patients and care partners with trusted and compassionate emotional **support.**
- **Educating** patients, care partners, and healthcare professionals with credible, critically important, and relevant information.
- Building a sense of **community** by connecting and unifying people affected by MSA.
- Funding patient-centric collaborative **research** aimed at alleviating symptoms, slowing disease progression, and discovering a cure.
- Playing a leading role in raising awareness and **advocating** for those impacted by the disease.

The MSAC offers print, DVD, online, and downloadable resources for patients, caregivers and families.

Current MSAC partners include but are not limited to the following MSA and related disease charity organizations:

USA:

- MSA NJ (Howell, NJ).
- Move Over MSA (Boise, ID).
- Blandford-Rees Foundation (Richmond, VA),
- CureMSA (Fremont, CA).
- CurePSP (New York, NY).
- Michael J Fox Foundation (New York, NY).

UK:

- MSA Trust (London, UK).

BELGIUM:

- MSA Belgium (Borsbeek, Belgium).

FRANCE:

- ARAMISE (Orleans, France).

National Organization for Rare Disorders (NORD)
1900 Crown Colony Drive
Suite 310
Quincy, MA 02169
Tel: +1 617-249-7300

55 Kenosia Avenue
Danbury, CT 06810
Tel: +1 203-263-9938
Fax: +1 203-263-9938

1779 Massachusetts Avenue
Suite 500
Washington, DC 20036
Tel: +1 202-588-5700

**NORD aims to improve the health and well-being of people with rare diseases by driving advances in care, research, and policy. It strives for:**

- A national awareness and recognition of the challenges faced by people living with rare diseases and the associated costs to society.
- A nation where people with rare diseases can secure access to care that extends and improves their lives.
- A social, political, and financial culture of innovation that supports both the basic and translational research necessary to create tests and therapies for all rare disorders.
- A regulatory environment that encourages development and timely approval of safe and effective treatments for patients with rare diseases.

**New York University Langone Health**
info@nyulangone.org
Tel: + 1 212-263-7225.

**Clinical Trials**
www.clinicaltrials.gov

**Cure PSP**
1216 Broadway
2nd Floor
New York, NY 10001
Tel: +1 800-457-4777 or 410-785-7004
Hope Line: 800-457-4777
Fax: 410-785-7009
E-mail: info@curepsp.org

CurePSP is dedicated to the awareness, care, and cure for MSA and two other neurodegenerative diseases: progressive supranuclear palsy (PSP) and corticobasal degeneration (CBD). As a catalyst for new treatments and a cure, it establishes important partnerships and funds critical research. Through its advocacy and support efforts, it enhances education, care delivery, and quality of life for people living with MSA, PSP, CBD and their families.

It boasts centers of care – a network of specialized medical centers across the U.S. and Canada dedicated to the comprehensive care of MSA; locally-organized support groups; quality of life respite programs; peer support network; and bereavement support to families as they navigate the complexity of the grief journey.

Further, it offers printed resources including: a catalog of educational materials (Answers booklets, Care Partner Guidebook, and Medical Alert Wallet Cards); community educational events, including: biannual Family Conferences and regular Ask the Expert and Community Conversation webinars for individuals and families to gather useful information for their care journey.

Still further, it provides an educational support series that offers information and connection for people who are newly diagnosed.

Lastly, it advocates and actively implements new and expanded programs aimed at increasing awareness of MSA and advocates for legislation that would result in improved quality of care and life for people with MSA.

**Defeat MSA Alliance**
29924 Jefferson Avenue
Saint Clair Shores
Michigan 48082, USA
Tel: +1 855- 542-5672 (855 KICK-MSA)
Facebook: https://www.facebook.com/DefeatMSA/
Twitter: @DefeatMSA
Instagram: defeatmsa

Realizing that much of the current attention is focused on more widely known diseases, and that MSA is often overlooked, it aspires to balance efforts to support patients, educate medical professionals, raise public awareness, nurture promising research, and advocate for the MSA community.

**EveryLife Foundation for Rare Diseases**
1012 14th Street, NW
Suite 500
Washington, DC 20005
Tel: +1 202-697-RARE(7273)

It aims to empower the rare disease patient community to advocate for impactful, science-driven legislation and policy that advances the equitable development of, and access to, lifesaving diagnoses, treatments, and cures.

**The MSA Coalition (USA)**
multiplesystematrophy.org

**Closed Facebook Support Group**
facebook.com/groups/MSAOZNZ/

## Additional support

Social workers and occupational therapists can also help with coping with disability through the provision of equipment and home adaptations, services for caregivers and access to healthcare services, both for the person with MSA as well as family caregivers.

## Take-away points

- Patient advocacy and support organizations offer many valuable services and often drive the research and development of treatments for their disease(s). Because these organizations include the life experiences of many different people who have a specific disease, they may best understand the resources needed by those in their community.
- Some organizations build a community of patients and families impacted by a specific disease or group of related diseases. These organizations usually have more disease-specific information and services, including helping new members find others who have the same disease.

- Some organizations build a community of patients and families impacted by a medical condition, like MSA or related conditions, heart problems that may also be a symptom in other diseases, etc. These organizations usually have information and services focused more on the medical condition(s), but may also have information about associated diseases.

- Detailed information about supporting and advocating organizations is provided for worldwide, international, national, and private organizations.

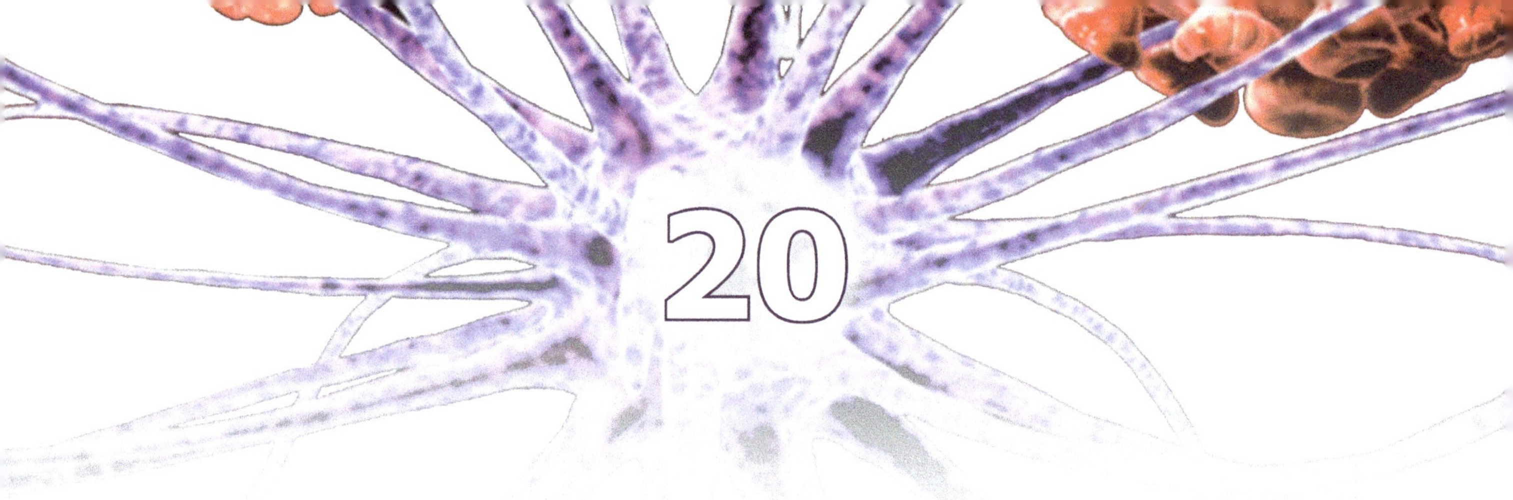


# Frequently asked questions

It is important for the MSA patient to have concerns addressed and questions answered. Below are some of the frequently asked questions by people who are afflicted by MSA, and others. Many of these have been gleaned across the literature. They may not represent the totality of frequently asked questions.

## About the MSA disease

### What is MSA?

Multiple system atrophy (MSA) is a degenerative brain disease, meaning it causes parts of your brain to deteriorate. This disrupts how you move around and your body's automatic processes like breathing, digestion, and blood pressure. The disease is usually fatal within 10 years, but may have a shorter or longer life expectancy depending on severity.

### Is MSA contagious?

MSA is not contagious, and you cannot spread it to, or catch it from, others.

### Who does MSA affect?

MSA affects adults over age 30. The symptoms are most likely to start between ages 50 and 59. The condition does not affect people differently depending on sex.

### How common is MSA?

MSA is a rare condition. Experts estimate an average of 0.6 to 0.7 new cases per 100,000 people yearly. The estimated number of total cases is between 3.4 and 4.9 per 100,000 people.

### Who is more likely to get MSA?

MSA is a rare disease, affecting potentially 15,000 to 50,000 Americans, including men and women of all racial groups. The cause of MSA is unknown. The vast majority of cases are sporadic, meaning they occur at random.

A distinguishing feature of MSA is the accumulation of the protein alpha-synuclein in glia, the cells that support nerve cells in the brain. The deposits of alpha-synuclein particularly occur in oligodendroglia, a type of cell that makes myelin (a coating on nerve cells that allows them to conduct electrical signals rapidly). This protein also accumulates in Parkinson's disease, but in nerve cells. Because they both have a buildup of alpha-synuclein in cells, MSA and Parkinson's disease are sometimes referred to as synucleinopathies. A possible risk factor for the disease is variations in the synuclein gene SCNA, which provides instructions for the production of alpha-synuclein.

## About learning from others who have MSA

### Are there others in the community who have MSA?

MSA is an individual disease. While one cannot compare oneself with others in terms of the type of disease, the course of the disease, or the symptoms, and the features for anyone are different from those of the next person.

### Why are there so many different individual patterns of the disease?

While puzzling, this is actually fairly common and not only in MSA, but also in other diseases as well. One way for people with MSA to better understand and benefit from each other is in self-help and support groups (small group meetings in individual homes or in community facilities). The multiple MSA societies (see Chapter 19) have helpful information for such support groups. However, whatever group is selected for participation, it must have direction and a positive focus, otherwise, it may turn into a negative experience. The experience must be a positive learning.

### When is information not helpful?

Misinformation (including from the Internet and from chat rooms) is not helpful and can cause much trouble and distress, and waste of time and money.

### How can I or my loved one help improve care for people with MSA?

Consider participating in a clinical trial so clinicians and scientists can learn more about MSA and related disorders. Clinical research uses human volunteers to help researchers learn more about a disorder and, perhaps, find better ways to safely detect, treat, or prevent disease.

All types of volunteers are needed—those who are healthy or may have an illness or disease—of all different ages, sexes, races, and ethnicities to ensure that study results apply to as many people as possible, and that treatments will be safe and effective for everyone who will use them.

For information about participating in clinical research visit NIH Clinical Research Trials and You. Learn about clinical trials currently looking for people with MSA at Clinicaltrials.gov.

## About seeking a healthcare provider

### When should I call my doctor?

Call your doctor right away if you have any sudden changes in your health, such as losing coordination or noticing severe muscle weakness. You should also see your doctor if you have:

- Vision problems or headaches.
- Slurred speech.
- Numbness, tingling, or loss of sensation in your arms or legs.
- Tremors or tics (random muscle movements).
- Changes in behavior or memory.
- Problems with coordination or moving your muscles.

### What should I discuss with my doctor?

Many of the earliest symptoms of MSA are ones that you should discuss with your healthcare provider. These include:

- Sexual dysfunction.
- Orthostatic hypotension (or any passing-out or dizziness that repeatedly happens without explanation).
- Sleep disturbances and sleep apnea (when you stop breathing while asleep).

If a healthcare provider diagnoses you with a movement condition like Parkinson's disease, it is important to talk to them if you notice changes in your symptoms. Your healthcare provider will schedule follow-up visits to monitor your condition, adjust medications, etc. Those visits are an opportunity for you to talk about any changes you have noticed in your symptoms. It is not uncommon for people with a Parkinson's disease diagnosis to later have that diagnosis modified to MSA because of new symptoms or when the medication Levodopa does not help symptoms as it should.

People with MSA often experience other symptoms, especially mental health issues. It is important to seek care for mental health concerns related to MSA, as well as care for your physical symptoms. Your healthcare provider can help you by recommending treatments or referring you to a provider specializing in mental healthcare.

## About normal living

### How does multiple system atrophy affect my body?

MSA causes deterioration in different brain areas. The symptoms depend on the areas affected. The parts of your brain most commonly affected include:

- **Basal ganglia:** These are structures near the center of your brain that link many different areas of your brain together. They create a critical network that allows different parts of your brain to work cooperatively.
- **Brainstem:** Your brainstem is responsible for managing many of your body's key autonomic processes. You need these elements to stay alive, but your body handles them automatically without you thinking about them. They include breathing, heart rate, blood pressure, etc.
- **Cerebellum:** This structure at the back of your head helps coordinate movements. It also works cooperatively with other brain areas. Researchers are still learning what it does, but some evidence suggests it even plays a role in other things like emotions and decision-making.

MSA symptoms can vary depending on which areas of your brain this condition affects. As the affected areas deteriorate, you will have more and more difficulty with the abilities those areas control. For example, deterioration of your brainstem causes problems with autonomic processes like blood pressure.

### How do I keep my nervous system healthy?

Your nervous system is the command center for your entire body. It needs care to keep working correctly. See your doctor regularly, eat a healthy diet, avoid drugs, and only drink alcohol in moderation. The best way to avoid nerve damage from disease is to manage conditions that can injure your nerves, such as diabetes.

### How do I take care of myself?

People who have MSA have symptoms that get progressively worse. That means people who have this condition cannot live independently once their symptoms reach a certain point. The condition also eventually causes problems with your ability to think, speak, and make choices for yourself. Because of all these factors, it is a good idea to talk with loved ones about your wishes for the future, and to make plans for what should happen with your medical care once you can no longer choose for yourself.

### How can I reduce my risk or prevent this condition?

Experts do not know what causes MSA or if there are factors that contribute to having it. Because of that, it is impossible to prevent it or reduce your risk of developing it.

### Can I live a normal life with MSA?

After an MSA diagnosis, patients and their healthcare teams typically will work together to come up with a suitable care plan. This plan often involves:

- Regular appointments with a neurologist to monitor disease progression.
- The use of available disease-modifying drugs/therapies (DMD/Ts) to prevent relapses and slow the disease progression.
- Other medications or therapies to help manage individual symptoms.

Certain changes in lifestyle also may help some MSA patients to better manage their disease. These can include:

- Quitting smoking.
- Exercising and losing weight.
- Finding strategies to reduce stress.

MSA is a lifelong disease, and disease manifestations vary substantially from person to person. For some people with MSA, the disease causes noteworthy disability shortly after it manifests, whereas others may go years without ever developing symptoms that substantially interfere with their daily life.

### Will I end in a wheelchair with MS?

MSA can make it difficult to walk and some patients will eventually rely on a wheelchair to help them get around and retain their independence. Though there is substantial variability from person to person, it is estimated that about one-quarter of patients receiving modern treatments will require a wheelchair within a few years of their diagnosis.

## About the disease course

### Do MSA symptoms become worse with age?

Sometimes. There are various forms of MSA, and the symptoms of each vary.

### How do I choose a health care provider?

Choosing a healthcare provider to support a lifelong condition is a personal decision. Finding a specialist that aligns with the patient's treatment and management goals is important.

## About symptoms management and treatments

### How to take care of myself/manage symptoms?

MSA is a condition that only a trained, qualified healthcare provider can diagnose. Because of that, you should not try to self-diagnose or manage the symptoms without first talking to a healthcare provider.

### What medications or treatments are used?

Many medications can help in treating the symptoms of MSA. The medications you receive depend partly on the symptoms you have as well as many other factors. Your healthcare provider is the best person to recommend medications to you, as the information they provide will be the most relevant to your situation. They can also explain the possible side effects of the treatments they recommend.

### How is MSA treated, and is there a cure?

MSA is a severe, ultimately fatal disease. Unfortunately, at this time, there is no way to cure or treat this condition directly. However, many of its symptoms are treatable, and there may be ways to minimize the effects and symptoms. Thus, treatments almost always focus on keeping symptoms from posing a problem for as long as possible. The possible treatments for MSA symptoms depend on many factors, especially the symptoms a person has and their severity. With treatment, many people can preserve their quality of life for years, giving them valuable time to spend with loved ones and making the most of their time.

## About prognosis and life expectancy

### How long does MSA last?

MSA is a permanent condition that lasts the rest of a person's life. The average survival time for this condition is six to 10 years. In less severe cases, people can survive up to 15 years. However, in very severe cases, survival time may be much lower. These cases usually involve the following features and characteristics:

- Autonomic symptoms that reach severe levels before motor symptoms begin.

- Older age at time of diagnosis.
- Movement symptoms that cause repeated falls.

### What is the outlook for this condition?

The outlook for MSA is poor. The symptoms of this condition get progressively worse and always disrupt body function, leading to deadly complications. The complications that may lead to death include:

- Pneumonia.
- Urinary tract infections (UTIs) that lead to sepsis.
- Sudden death (usually at night, because of disruptions in how your brain controls breathing while you sleep).

### Would knowing my prognosis be helpful?

Research suggests that people with MSA have mixed feelings about knowing their likely disease course. Some aim to live in the moment and try not to worry about what the future might hold, so they avoid finding out too much about later stage MSA. However, for others, knowing their prognosis could reduce their anxiety from not knowing what is likely to happen, and enable them to make plans.

Much research effort is currently aimed at understanding what factors like brain volume and optic nerve size in an attempt to find markers that might be linked to better or worse disease pathways. It is still early days, but the aim is to help people understand their likely prognosis and make it easier for them to choose the right treatment.

## About fatality and terminal illness

### Is MSA fatal?

MSA is usually lethal, Complications associated with it like infections, cardiovascular disease, and accidents can cause the lifespan of someone with MSA to be shorter than people who are not living with MSA. But, treating these complications can greatly reduce the risk of a shortened lifespan.

Living well despite MSA may require some lifestyle adjustments, such as exercising and cutting back smoking, as well as treatment and regular monitoring to improve long-term outcomes. As the disease progresses, it may impair patients' ability to function independently, reduce quality of life, and cause cognitive difficulties. These changes also may require patients to make adjustments and find accommodations in day-to-day life.

## About the Research Registry

### What is the World MSA Research Registry & Support hub?

The Registry is designed as a way for patients and caregivers to build supportive networks and to connect with vital research opportunities worldwide. It is open for sign-ups for patients with MSA or their caregivers, from all over the world.

### How do I join the Registry?

The Registry is free of charge to all registered individuals (patients with MSA and their caregivers all over the world). Registration can be done online by connecting with the Autonomic Disorders Consortium (ADC) organization (www.adc.org) and filling-out a simple registration form.

## Take-away points

- It is important for the MSA patient to have concerns addressed and questions answered.
- The frequently asked questions by people who are afflicted by MSA, and others, have been categorized as about: the disease; learning from others; seeking a health provider; normal living; the disease course; symptoms management; and treatments; prognosis and life expectancy; fatality and terminal illness; and the Research Registry.

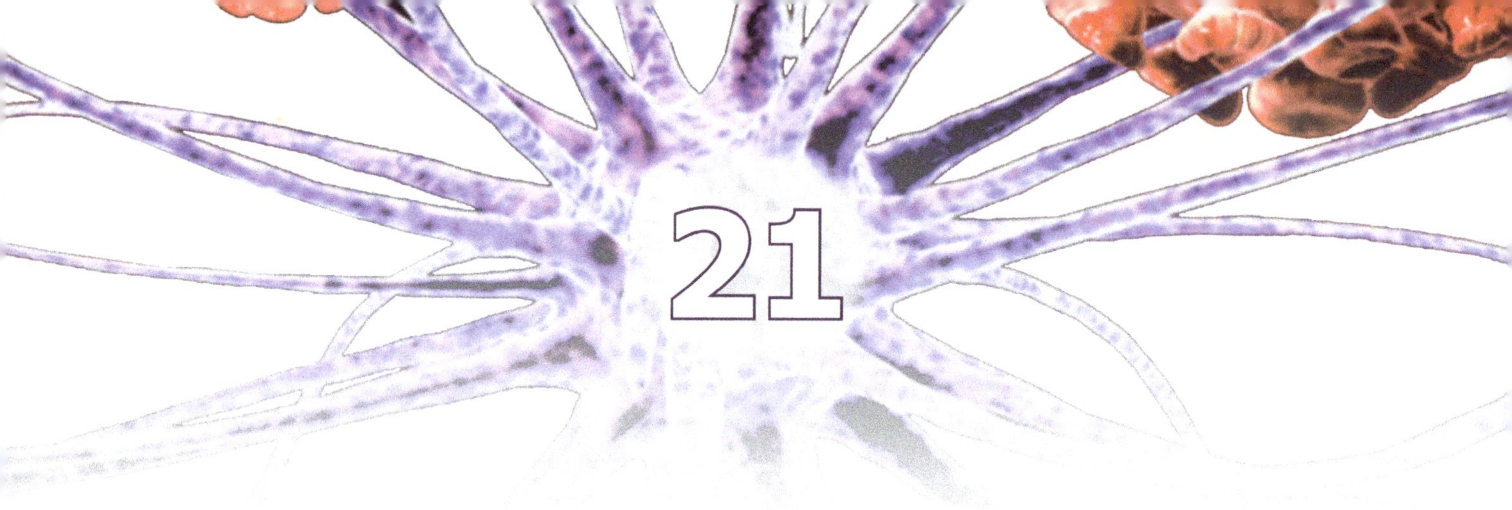

# 21 MSA and COVID-19

During COVID-19, the medical establishment has faced major hurdles. To confront such challenges, numerous measures were taken, including the following:

## From the European Commission

### COVID-19 Clinical Management Support System" (CMSS)

The aim of the CMSS is to support clinicians in hospitals that are currently facing the coronavirus emergency all over Europe. It helps to create rapid connections across Europe among the hospitals indicated as reference centers for COVID-19. Within CMSS, clinicians can set up web conferences and exchange with their peers in Europe on possible treatments, and on how to handle severe and complex cases. This synergy aims to speed up the adoption of specific treatment options and help reduce some of the uncertainties due to the unknown aspects of the virus. Ultimately, it is in the vital interest of the patients infected with COVID-19 that their doctors can discuss their cases, and get the best advice possible.

### Guidance to manage clinical trials during the COVID-19 pandemic

The impact of the pandemic on European health systems and more broadly on society, make it necessary for sponsors to adjust how they manage clinical trials and the people who participate in these trials. The guidance provides concrete information on changes and protocol deviations which may be needed in the conduct of clinical trials to deal with extraordinary situations, e.g. if trial participants need to be in self-isolation or quarantine, access to public places (including hospitals) is limited due to the risk of spreading infections, and healthcare professionals are being reallocated.

The guidance also includes a harmonized set of recommendations, to ensure the utmost safety of trial participants across the European Union while preserving the quality of the data generated by the trials. It also advises how these changes should be communicated to authorities.

There is specific advice on the initiation of a robust trial methodology in new clinical trials for COVID-19 treatments and vaccines, and in particular on the need for large, multinational trial protocols. It provides a harmonized approach in the conduct of trials, in order to mitigate the negative effects of the pandemic.

## From the Autonomic Disorders Consortium

### Survey to highlight the impact of COVID-19 on the rare disease community

A preliminary analysis of more than 3,400 responses to a recent survey of people living with rare diseases and their caregivers is shedding new light on their experiences during the COVID-19 pandemic (see Figure 20.1).

While only 71 responses indicated a positive COVID-19 diagnosis, a significant number of respondents were uncertain of their COVID-19 infection status due to difficulties accessing testing and medical advice. Most who reported COVID-19 infection experienced a mild infection, with serious interventions (e.g., mechanical ventilation) reported only by a few. Many reported some interaction between the infection and their rare disease, with one increasing the severity of the symptoms of the other.

The survey responses also indicated that the pandemic negatively affected rare disease patients in terms of access to regular health care, treatment for the rare disease, special diet, and special treatment and hospitalization, even among those who reported acquiring the infection.

### Preliminary data analyses

Results presented here reflect the 3,413 survey responses submitted through the closing date of December 15, 2020.

Individuals from the entire country participated in the survey, with 26 states contributing 50 or more surveys. Participants were predominantly women (64%) and white (89%). Minorities were under-represented in all subgroups of rare diseases. About 80% of the participants were adults.

More than 130 distinct rare disease diagnoses were reported by respondents. The five most common diagnoses were myasthenia gravis, amyotrophic lateral sclerosis, eosinophilic esophagitis, mitochondrial disease and primary ciliary dyskinesia.

While 71 respondents reported acquiring a confirmed COVID-19 infection, 566 respondents (17% of the total) were not sure if they acquired the infection.

**Figure 20.1 - Preliminary results of a survey of people living with rare diseases and their caregivers during the COVID-19 pandemic**

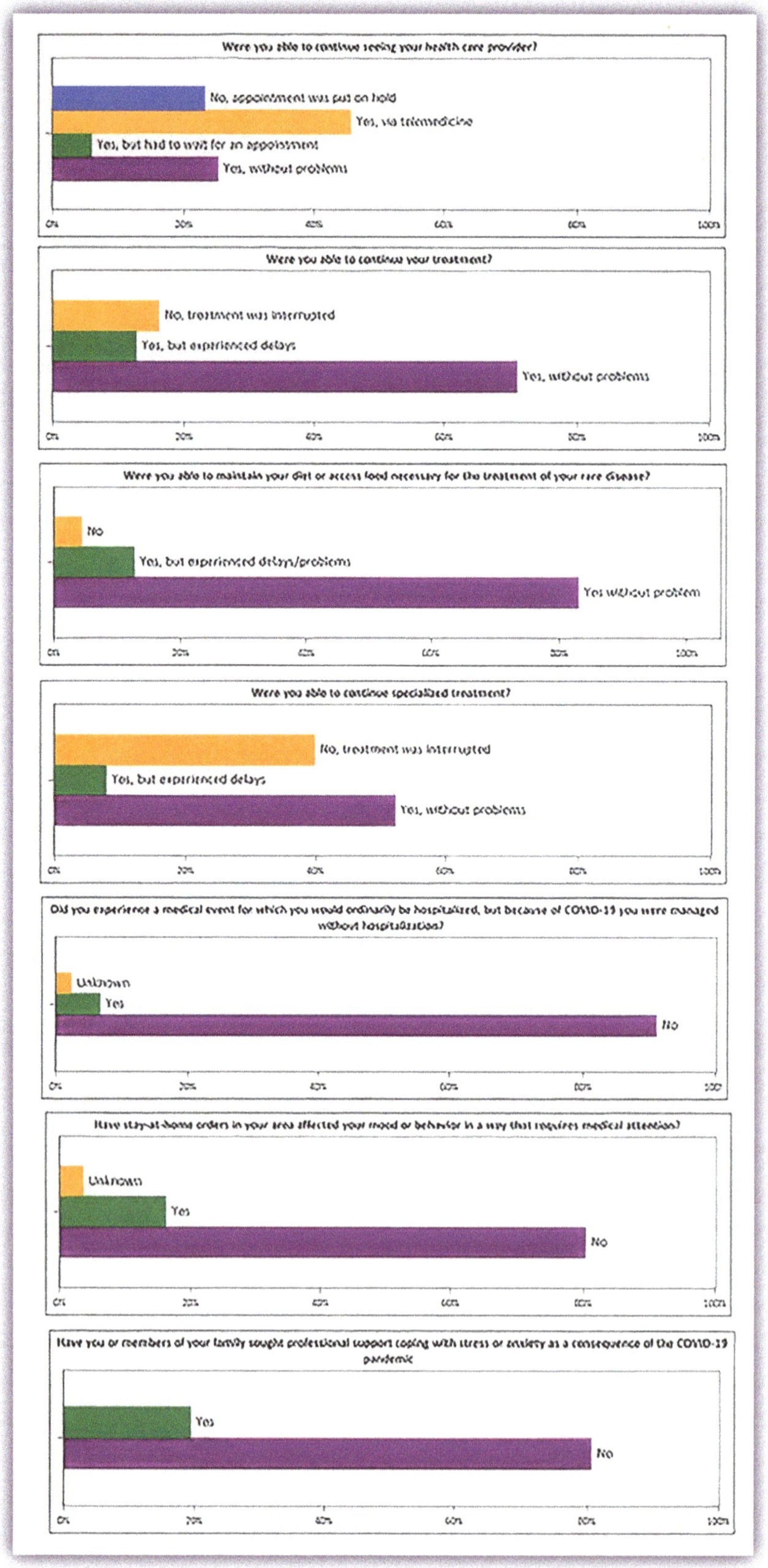

The charts of Figure 20.1 show reported COVID-19 infection status: Those who acquired COVID-19 are shown in blue color; those who did not acquire COVID-19 are shown in orange; and those unsure of a diagnosis are shown in grey.

Obtaining access to testing/advice on COVID-19 was more difficult among those who did not know if they acquired COVID. This finding raises concerns that the infection may have been under-diagnosed in that community.

Participants who reported that they had acquired COVID-19 had increased cough, fever greater than 100.5, new or increased shortness of breath, headache, loss of taste, and confusion much more often than participants who reported that they had not acquired COVID-19. Those with unsure infection status often reported symptoms consistent with COVID-19 infection, reinforcing suspicion that COVID-19 infection was under-diagnosed.

### Impact of the pandemic

The survey responses indicated that the pandemic negatively affected rare disease patients and their caregivers in terms of access to regular health care, treatment for the rare disease, special diet, and special treatment and hospitalization, even among those who reported acquiring the infection. Some respondents had difficulty receiving treatments, especially those requiring special diets, occupational therapies, and physical therapies. The pandemic also caused mood changes, anxiety, and stress in both the patients and their family members to an extent that required medical attention.

(Note: Due to the current global COVID-19 pandemic, some brain banks are not back to full capacity in their operations.)

## Take-away points

1. During COVID-19, the medical establishment has faced major hurdles that required extraordinary measures to confront its challenges.
2. The impact of the pandemic made it necessary to adjust how clinical trials are managed including changes and protocol deviations needed in their conduct such as, for example, self-isolation or quarantine of participants, access to public places (including hospitals), and reallocation of healthcare professionals.
3. The pandemic negatively affected rare disease patients in terms of access to regular health care, treatment, hospitalization, and special diet even among those who reported acquiring the infection.

# E. HOPE FOR THE FUTURE

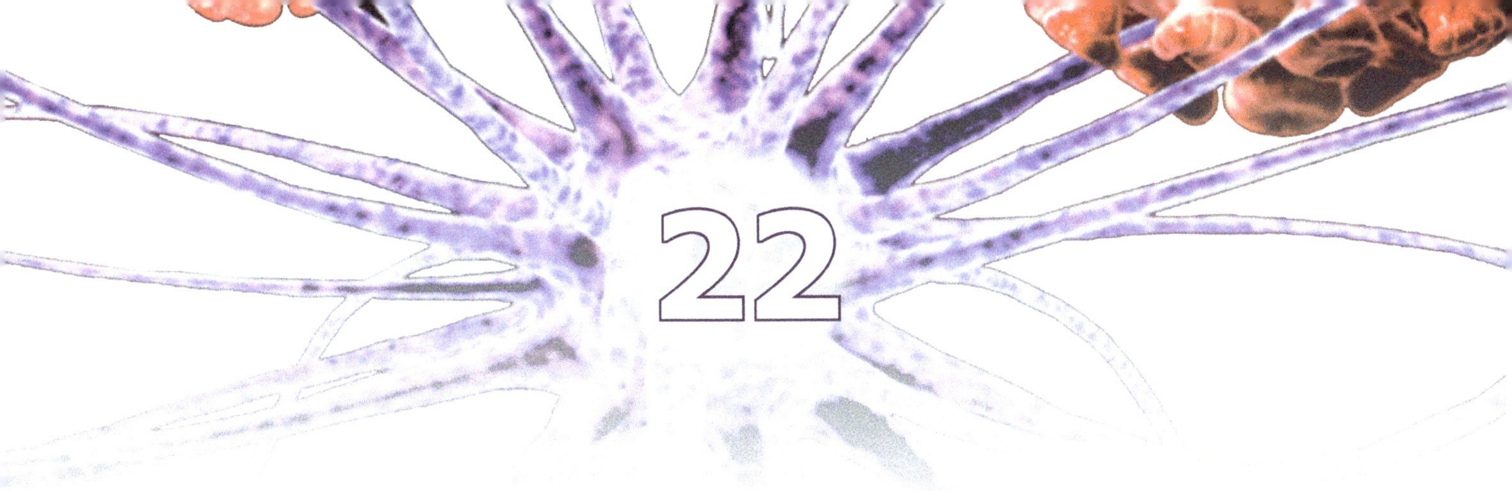

22

# Research and latest developments

People with MSA face significant challenges learning about current research, especially given the rarity of the disease. Moreover, patients often need extra help locating further support resources. For them, research is a priority as it leads to a better understanding of their disease, quicker and more accurate diagnosis, innovative treatments and cures, and better health care. It represents hope for the millions of people living with MSA or other rare disease and their families.

While improvements have been made in the past decades with dedicated public funding and coordinated actions, rare disease research faces political and practical obstacles such as inadequate funding, small patient populations for clinical trials, and a lack of coordinated resources for patient registries. This translates into insufficient knowledge of these diseases and delays in both diagnosis and the development of much-needed treatments.

Research on rare diseases covers a whole spectrum – from basic research (understanding of disease mechanisms in laboratories), to pre-clinical (development of disease models including animal and cell-based systems to test potential therapies), to translation (how to make research results translate into real benefits for patients), to clinical trials. Scientific advancements in rare disease research also contribute to progress for more common diseases and the health outcomes of individuals.

## Rare diseases research in Europe

In Europe, rare diseases are a priority area for research funding. Major investments have been allocated to rare disease research innovation programs and in recognition of the added value of cross-country and multidisciplinary cooperation in this field.

### Initiatives

Several initiatives have been supported to improve rare disease research including the:

- **International Rare Diseases Research Consortium (IRDiRC).**
- **European Joint Program on Rare Diseases (EJPRD):** Develop an ecosystem to allow a virtuous circle between research, care, and medical innovation.
- **Past projects:** Like EPIRARE, TREAT-NMD, RD-Connect and RARE Best Practices.
- **Ongoing initiatives:** Such as the:
    1. **European Rare Diseases Registries Infrastructure (ERDRI).**
    2. **European Reference Networks.**
    3. **European research infrastructures:** Such as BBMRI and ECRIN.
    4. **Solve-RD.**
    5. **Orphanet.**

But, there is still work to be done as most rare diseases lack effective and curative treatments and unmet medical needs of people living with rare diseases are still vast.

## Participation in research

People living with a rare disease can be directly implicated in each step of the rare disease research process. For example, they could: advocate for research when there is none by connecting with researchers working on similar diseases; help researchers design studies that reflect their needs; start or contribute to a registry so that researchers can find patients' data; and participate in research activities.

Often patient organizations can support researchers to recruit patients and encourage them to donate samples to boost research.

Patient representatives can participate in the EURORDIS Open Academy on Scientific Innovation and Translational Research to become valued partners in rare disease research by developing their knowledge and capacities in this area. All EURORDIS Open Academy training courses are free and provided through a blend of e-learning courses and webinars.

## Advocacy

Rare diseases are a prime example of a research area that can strongly benefit from coordination and collaboration on a national, European, and international scale.

The patient community in Europe, supported by EURORDIS, has effectively advocated for increased European cooperation in research on rare diseases. In turn, EURORDIS has also promoted the need for rare disease research and budget as a priority at the national level, in particular through rare disease national plans.

As a result, funding opportunities for research have increased in recent decades. Between 2007 and 2017 the European Commission (EC) invested over 874 M€ in research on rare diseases. The EU Orphan Drug Regulation has also provided incentives (such as market exclusivity) that encourage companies to invest in rare disease research. However, there remains a lack of research to cover every one of the 6,000+ rare diseases.

EURORDIS promoted rare diseases as a research priority in EU research framework programs such as 'Horizon 2020' and in the upcoming 'Horizon Europe 2021-2027', and played an instrumental role in the creation of the:

- **International Rare Diseases Research Consortium (IRDiRC).**
- **European Joint Program on Rare Diseases (EJPRD).**
- **European Reference Networks (ERN).**
- **EURORDIS Position Paper on Rare Disease Research:** It set out the ethical, social, economic, and scientific grounds of rare disease research and shaped research priorities.

## Rare diseases research in the U.S.

From the:

**National Center for Advancing Translational Sciences (NCATS):**

- **Rare Diseases Clinical Research Network (RDCN):** This program is designed to advance medical research on rare diseases by providing support for clinical studies and facilitating collaboration, study enrollment, and data sharing. Through the RDCRN consortia, physician-scientists and their multidisciplinary teams work together with patient advocacy groups to study more than 200 rare diseases at sites across the nation.
- **Gene Therapy and Gene Editing Programs - The Accelerating Medicines Partnership® Bespoke Gene Therapy Consortium (BGTC):** This program is part of the Accelerating Medicines Partnership® (AMP®) program, a public–private partnership among NIH, FDA, multiple pharmaceutical and life sciences companies, and non-profit and other organizations. The AMP program aims to improve current models for developing diagnostics and therapies. The BGTC is establishing platforms and standards to speed the development and delivery of customized or "bespoke" gene therapies that could treat millions of people affected by rare diseases, including diseases too rare to be of commercial interest. It is the first AMP initiative focused on rare diseases and the first to focus on a therapeutic platform.
- **Therapeutics for Rare and Neglected Diseases (TRND):** This program supports preclinical development of therapeutic candidates intended to treat rare or neglected disorders, with the goal of enabling an Investigational New Drug (IND) application.
- **The Genetic and Rare Diseases (GARD) Information Center:** Sources of information include the National Library of Medicine, Orphanet, Human Phenotype

Ontology, patient support groups and other NIH Institutes and Centers. It offers information on genetic and rare disorders clinical trials, It uses translational science to improve the research process to get more treatments to more people more quickly.

- **The Rare Diseases Registry Program (RaDaR)**: This living website provides the rare diseases community with easily accessible guidance on how to set up and maintain high-quality registries. A registry is a collection of information about individuals, usually focused around a specific diagnosis or condition. The goal is to enable rare diseases patient organizations to better promote and support patient-focused research. Its content includes additional instructions, best practices, testimonials and shared resources from the rare diseases community in a phased approach.
- **Rare diseases research and resources:** NCATS is committed to using research to address the public health crisis presented by rare diseases. Speeding development of treatments for patients requires innovation in science and technology and engaging patients and their support organizations as essential partners.

## (U.S.) National Institutes of Health (NIH)

- **NIH Blueprint for Neuroscience Research:** It aims "to accelerate transformative discoveries in brain function in health, aging, and disease" by pooling the resources and expertise of various NIH entities to confront challenges too large for any single Institute or Center. Topics have ranged from transforming our understanding of dynamic neuroimmune interactions to enhancing our fundamental knowledge of interception, supporting the development of innovative tools and technologies to monitor and manipulate biomolecular condensates, and more.
- **Grand Challenges:** Their aim is to catalyze research with the potential to transform our basic understanding of the brain and our approaches to treating brain disorders.
  1. **Human Connectome Project (HCP):** An ambitious effort to map all the connections within the human brain.
  2. **Chronic Neuropathic Pain:** Supports research to understand the changes in the nervous system that cause acute, temporary pain to become chronic.
  3. **The Blueprint Neurotherapeutics Network (BPN):** Helps small laboratories develop new drugs for nervous system disorders.

- **The BRAIN Initiative®:** A coordinated effort among public and private institutions and agencies aimed at revolutionizing our understanding of the human brain.

## American Academy of Neurology (AAN)

Has an active research funding program on neurology and neurosciences.

## Multiple System Atrophy Coalition (MSAC)

It has a dedicated MSA Research Fund to support scientific study into the cause, treatments and a cure for MSA. It is used to encourage and finance critically important MSA research leading to the identification of causes, improved diagnostic methods, and more effective symptomatic and disease modifying treatments:

## National Organization for Rare Disorders (NORD)

The NORD Patient Registry allows patients and advocacy organizations to share experiences, so researchers better understand how to diagnose and treat rare diseases. The platform is easy-to-use, allowing patients to own their data, benefit from knowledge gained, generate clinical-grade data, and have a voice in the design and scope of research.

## Cure PSP

CurePSP is devoted to accelerate the development of diagnostic tests and be a catalyst in treatments to prevent, slow, halt or even reverse disease progression. In particular, it partners with pharmaceutical and biotechnology companies interested in designing and implementing clinical trials aimed at new ways to diagnose and treat MSA.

## NYU Langone Health

NYU Langone's Dysautonomia Center is a founding member of the Autonomic Disorders Consortium (ADC). It offers the following research programs:

- **Multiple System Atrophy Research Program:** The Division of Autonomic Disorders, in conjunction with NYU Langone's Dysautonomia Center boasts a comprehensive translational clinical research program dedicated to MSA. They aim to provide direct access to clinical care and support to people living with MSA. They offer patients the opportunity to participate in research studies focused on understanding the causes and evolution of MSA, developing and approving new symptomatic treatments of MSA, and discovering treatments that can stop or slow the progression of neurodegeneration in MSA.
- **Global Multiple System Atrophy Patient Registry:** In collaboration with the Rare Diseases Clinical Research Network, a Global MSA Patient Registry (GloMSAR) - a shared project among leading academic medical centers around the world treating people with MSA has been established. It connects people who have MSA and their caregivers to physicians and researchers focused on the disease; provides updates on treatments, news, and clinical trial opportunities; and enables neurologists who specialize in treating MSA to contact eligible patients to participate in clinical trials and speed up the testing of potential new therapies.
- **Preparing for clinical trials:** NYU Langone Health is the main site of an international collaborative project to define and understand the natural history of

MSA, to map how and when the disease begins, and how it evolves over time. Data collected is key in planning clinical trials that test new therapies for MSA.

- **Testing and developing new drug treatments for MSA and its symptoms:** NYU Langone's Dysautonomia Center has a long history of developing and helping approve drugs for the symptomatic treatment of MSA: Midodrine, Droxidopa (Northera), and TD-9855 for the treatment of orthostatic hypotension). It is also currently the only clinical research center in the U.S. that is actively recruiting patients to test Sirolimus (a disease-modifying drug for MSA).
- **Institutional collaboration:** NYU Langone's Dysautonomia Center is the central site of the largest-ever natural history study of MSA, coordinating more than 20 recruiting sites around the world. It shares research data and biospecimens. It also collaborates on research studies to understand the genome, blood-borne biomarkers of disease, and neuroimaging changes.

## Latest updates on multiple system atrophy

Researchers hope to learn why the protein alpha-synuclein accumulates in glial cells in MSA and neuronal (nerve) cells in Parkinson's disease. Recent studies have demonstrated that the alpha-synuclein taken from brain tissue of people with MSA is a potent inducer of alpha-synuclein clumping when injected into the brain of experimental animals. One area of ongoing research is aimed at blocking the spread of the clumping problem throughout the brain.

Using cell models of MSA, scientists were able to show that damage to mitochondria (cellular "powerhouses") and the generation of abnormal alpha-synuclein aggregates may contribute to the development of MSA. Research in animal models may determine if drugs that reduce the abnormal alpha-synuclein accumulation might be promising treatments for MSA.

Scientists are developing non-invasive trait markers that can distinguish MSA from other movement disorders and also track disease-specific changes in neurodegeneration over time.

Other researchers are using diagnostic imaging of specific nerves in the brain and heart to measure the levels of several nerve cell types.

Additionally, MSA is one of the diseases being studied as part of the Parkinson's Disease Biomarkers Program (PDBP). This major NINDS initiative is discovering ways to identify individuals at-risk for developing Parkinson's disease and related disorders and to track the progression of the disease. Identifying biomarkers (signs that may indicate risk of a disease and improve diagnosis) may speed up the development of novel therapeutics.

Additional research on neurodegenerative diseases such as multiple system atrophy can be found using NIH RePORTER, a searchable database of current and past research projects supported by NIH and some other federal agencies. RePORTER also includes links to publications and patents citing support from these projects.

### Brain donations

Brain donations could help researchers find the cause(s), more treatments, and a cure for MSA. The examination of brain tissue is vital in this research process. A brain donation involves a simple procedure and it does not hinder the funeral or any burial plans. For many, a brain donation is the ultimate gift for generations to come - because MSA brain research could help bring about more treatments, more ways to help diagnose MSA and, eventually, a cure!

There are several institutions in the U.S.A., Canada, and other countries as well, that are currently doing MSA-related brain research and desperately need brain donations. Defeat MSA Alliance does not require a fee in order to help donate a brain to any brain bank.

## The Bespoke Gene Therapy Consortium (BGTC)

Launched in October 2021, the BGTC will generate gene therapy resources that the research community can use to streamline gene therapy development for rare disorders, making the process more efficient and less costly.

One of the BGTC's goals is to improve the understanding of the basic biology of the harmless adeno-associated virus (AAV), a common gene-delivery vehicle or vector, how they carry genes to the correct place in cells, how those genes get into cells, and how the newly transported genes are turned on in the target cells. This information will help improve the effectiveness of AAV gene therapies.

Another important BGTC goal is to improve the efficiency of both vector manufacturing and production quality control testing by developing a standard and broadly applicable set of analytic tests that can be used to manufacture viral vectors.

The BGTC clinical component aims to streamline the path from animal studies to human testing, will develop strategies for streamlining the regulatory processes for FDA approval of safe and effective gene therapies, and will also develop standardized approaches to preclinical testing (e.g., toxicology studies).

### Sidebar 22.1 – The Global MSA Registry

The **Global MSA Registry (GloMSAR)** is a joint project between the Autonomic Disorders Consortium (ADC), the (U.S.) National Institutes of Health (NIH), the MSA Coalition, and leading academic medical centers around the world treating people with MSA. It administers surveys to its participants to better understand specific features of MSA and capture each patient's perspective of the challenges of living with MSA.

The overall goals of the Registry are to:

- Connect people who have MSA and their caregivers to physicians and researchers focused on the disease and keep them up to date on clinical trial opportunities.
- Administer surveys to better understand the features of MSA.
- Contact eligible patients to participate in trials and speed up the testing of potential therapies.

The Registry is free of charge. Patients with MSA or their caregivers, from all over the world, can register themselves online and by filling-out standard information, they can help scientists understand disease traits.

More than 1,000 people with MSA are part of the Registry, which also provides them with updates on treatments, news, and clinical trial opportunities. The registry also enables neurologists who specialize in treating MSA to contact eligible patients to participate in clinical trials and speed up the testing of potential new therapies.

23

# Conclusions

Multiple system atrophy is a sporadic, progressive, and fatal neurodegenerative synucleinopathic disease. It affects both the autonomic nervous system and the motor system, and is characterized by autonomic failure. Its varied clinical presentation and symptoms reflect the death of different types of nerve cells in the brain and spinal cord and the progressive loss of associated functions. It is a member of a class of neurodegenerative diseases known as synucleinopathies that have in common an abnormal accumulation of the alpha-synuclein protein in various parts of the brain. It has itself sub-types (parkinsonism, cerebellar, mixed) and variants with combined features of dementia with Lewy bodies or frontotemporal lobar degeneration. The hallmark of the disease is the widespread glial cytoplasmic inclusions that are mainly constituted of misfolded, hyperphosphorylated, fibrillary alpha-synuclein protein– the same protein that is involved in Parkinson's disease.

While multiple system atrophy can be explained as cell loss and gliosis, its root cause(s) remain unknown although genetics, environmental processes (toxins), and lifestyle factors (trauma) may contribute to the underlying pathological processes. Tests can only help determine whether the diagnosis is 'probable MSA' or 'possible MSA' but no laboratory or imaging studies are able to definitively confirm the diagnosis. Reaching a diagnosis can be challenging and difficult, particularly in the early stages, in part because of many confounding diseases. Because of this difficulty, some people are actually never properly diagnosed or may not ever be diagnosed. From the wide panoply of available tests, none can provide a definitive diagnosis. The main differential diagnoses seek to rule-out any one or more of a long list of confounding factors so that a definitive diagnosis can only be attained pathologically *post mortem*.

Pharmacological therapy is required because the disorder is progressive and fatal, but there are currently no treatments available to delay or arrest the progressive neurodegeneration of the disease, and there is no cure. The condition varies in its gradual progression, does not go into remission, and eventually leads to death. There is no neuroprotective treatment available. However, potential drug candidates have been considered as well as growth hormone therapy, immunotherapy, gene therapy and mesenchymal stem cell therapy. Orphan, repurposed, off-label, compassionate use medicines, and experimental disease-modifying drugs/therapies are available. Numerous clinical trials are ongoing in attempts to develop 'better' drugs with the overriding goal to determine if a new test or treatment is safe and effective.

The majority of the developed therapeutic approaches have been focused on enhancing the degradation of the alpha-synuclein protein and preventing or disrupting its aggregation. Despite the existence of prominent therapeutic strategies, major obstacles and open questions remain. Unfortunately, these will not lead to a cure as the alpha-synuclein processes are only symptoms, not the root cause(s) of the disease.

Another major obstacle in the search for an early diagnosis is the absence of useful biomarkers (whether early in the disease or as the disease progresses). Other obstacles are the discrepancies in the design of preclinical and clinical studies, the failure of treatment outcome measurements in clinical trials, and the failure in defining the best therapeutic target(s) for disease modification.

Currently, the prognosis and future outlook for multiple system atrophy is poor. The disease progresses without remission at a variable rate and symptoms get progressively worse, always disrupt body function, and lead to deadly complications.

Living with a rare disease such as multiple system atrophy is accompanied by numerous issues including immense personal and economic burdens and the absence of a cure. Fortunately, however, valuable assistance is available with access care aid, caregiver aid, emergency relief, educational support, and end-of-life issues. In addition, numerous available patient advocacy and support organizations offer many valuable services and often drive the research and development of treatments.

The COVID-19 pandemic presented major hurdles that the medical establishment had to face, requiring extraordinary measures to confront its challenges. It also negatively affected patients in terms of access to regular health care, treatment, hospitalization, and special diet even among those who reported acquiring the infection. It is hoped that the lessons learned during that period of time will be helpful when other epidemics/ pandemics, will strike again.

But, thee still is hope for the future as research across the world is being conducted and there has been excellent progress especially in the development of new treatments to prevent exacerbations of the disease. New discoveries are constantly changing treatment options and helping to reduce disease-related disability. However, to this date, researchers have not yet been able to identify the root cause(s) of multiple system atrophy with any certainty. As with most other neurodegenerative disorders, the proximal trigger is unknown. Regardless, what is clear is that understanding the mechanisms of chronic progression is currently the major challenge because this is the phase that contributes most to irreversible disability. The lack of insight into mechanisms of progression is largely responsible for the extremely limited treatment options currently available.

A shift in thinking about the disease is needed with greater consideration given to a potential underlying degenerative etiology. This will spur new and original research directions that will eventually unravel the mystery, provide more effective therapeutics to mitigate the disabling progressive phase of the disease, and eventually a cure..

# References

## History


Adams R, van Bogaert L, and van der Eecken H (1961). "Dégénérescences nigro-striées et cerebello- nigro-striées". *Psychiat Neurol.* **142:**219–59. [in French]

Bannister R and Oppenheimer DR (1972). "Degenerative diseases of the nervous system associated with autonomic failure". *Brain* **95:**457–74.

Bradbury S and Eggleston C (1925). "Postural hypotension. A report of three cases". *Am Heart* J **1**:73– 86.

Dejerine J and Thomas AA (1900). "L'atrophie olivo-ponto-cérébelleuse". *Nouv Iconog de la Salpêtrière* **13:**330–70. [in French]

Gilman S, Low P, Quinn N *et al.* (1999). "Consensus statement on the diagnosis of multiple system atrophy". *J Neurol Sci* **163:**94–8.

Gilman S, Wenning GK, Low PA *et al.* (2008). "Second consensus statement on the diagnosis of multiple system atrophy". *Neurology* **71:**670–6.

Graham JG, Oppenheimer DR (1969). "Orthostatic hypotension and nicotine sensitivity in a case of multiple system atrophy". *J Neurol Neurosurg. Psychiatry* **32:**28–34.

Klockgether T (2010). "Sporadic ataxia with adult onset: classification and diagnostic criteria". *Lancet Neurol* **9:**94–104.

Kollensperger M, Geser F, Seppi K *et al.* (2008). "Red flags for multiple system atrophy". *Mov Disord* **23:**1093–9.

Lin DJ, Hermann KL, and Schmahmann JD (2014). "Multiple system atrophy of the cerebellar type: Clinical state of the art". *Mov Disord* **29:**294–304.

O'Sullivan SS, Massey LA, Williams DR *et al.* (2008). "Clinical outcomes of progressive supranuclear palsy and multiple system atrophy". *Brain* **131:**1362–72.

Ozawa T, Paviour D, Quinn NP *et al.* (2004). "The spectrum of pathological involvement of the striatonigral and olivopontocerebellar systems in multiple system atrophy: Clinicopathological correlations." *Brain* **127:**2657–71.

Papp M, Kahn JE, Lantos PL (1989)."Glial cytoplasmic inclusions in the CNS of patients with multiple system atrophy (striatonigral degeneration, olivopontocerebellar atrophy and Shy- Drager syndrome)". *J Neurol Sci* **94:**79–100.

Quinn N (1989) Multiple system atrophy: The nature of the beast". *J Neurol Neurosurg Psychiatry* **52**((suppl)):78–89.

Quinn N (2015). "A short clinical history of multiple system atrophy". *Clin Auton Res* **25**(1):3–7. doi: 10.1007/s10286-014-0265-7; https://doi.org/10.1007/s10286-014-0265-7

Shy GM and Drager GA (1960). "A neurologic syndrome associated with orthostatic hypotension: A clinical-pathologic study. *Arch Neurol.* **2:**511–27.

Schrag A, Ben-Shlomo Y, and Quinn NP (1999). "Prevalence of progressive supranuclear palsy and multiple system atrophy: A cross-sectional study". *Lancet* **354:**1771–5.

Schrag A, Selai C, Mathias C *et al.* (2007). "Measuring health-related quality of life in MSA: The MSA-QoL". *Mov Disord* **22:**2332–8.

Spillantini MG, Crowther RA, Jakes R, Cairns NJ, Lantos PL, and Goedert M (1998). "Filamentous alpha-synuclein inclusions link multiple system atrophy with Parkinson's disease and dementia with Lewy bodies". *Neurosci Lett.* **251:**205–208.

Watanabe H, Saito Y, Terao S *et al.* (2002). "Progression and prognosis in multiple system atrophy. An analysis of 230 Japanese patients". *Brain* **125:**1070–83.

Wenning GK, Shlomo YB, Magalhães M, Danie SE, and Quinn NP (1994). "Clinical features and natural history of multiple system atrophy.:An analysis of 100 cases". *Brain* **117:**835–45.

Wenning GK, Tison F, Ben Shlomo Y, Daniel SE, and Quinn NP (1997). "Multiple system atrophy: A review of 203 pathologically proven cases". *Mov Disord.* 12:133–47.

Wenning GK, Tison F, Seppi K *et al.* (2004). Multiple System Atrophy Study Group, "Development and validation of the Unified Multiple System Atrophy Rating Scale (UMSARS)". *Mov Disord* **19:**1391–402.

Wenning GK, Geser F, Krismer F *et al.* (2013). European Multiple System Atrophy Study Group, "The natural history of multiple system atrophy: A prospective European cohort study". *Lancet Neurol* **12:**264–74.

## Thomas Willis

Arráez-Aybar L-A (2015). "Thomas Willis, a pioneer in translational research in anatomy (on the 350th anniversary of Cerebri anatome)". *J. of Anatomy* **226**(3):289–300. doi:10.1111/joa.12273.

Dewhurst D (1964). "Thomas Willis as a Physician", Los Angeles: University of California Press.

Dewhurst D (1981). "Willis' Oxford casebook", Oxford: Sandford Publications, ISBN 0-9501528-5-4.

Encyclopedia Britannica: Thomas Willis.

Hughes JT (1991)."Thomas Willis (1621–1675): His Life and Work", *London: Royal Society of Medicine.*

Isler H (1965). "Thomas Willis: Ein Wegbereiter der modernen Medizin, 1621–1675", *Stuttgart: Wissenschaftliche Verlagsgesellschaft.*

Martenson RL (2007). "Willis, Thomas (1621–1675)]". Oxford Dictionary of National Biography (online ed.). Oxford University Press. doi:10.1093/ref:odnb/29587.

Molnár Z (2004). "Timeline: Thomas Willis (1621–1675), the founder of clinical neuroscience". *Nature Reviews Neuroscience* **5** (4):329–35. doi:10.1038/nrn1369.

Moore N (1900). "Willis, Thomas (1621-1675)" . In Lee, Sidney (ed.). Dictionary of National Biography. Vol. 62. London: Smith, Elder & Co. pp. 25–6.

Pyle A (editor) (2000), "The Dictionary of Seventeenth Century British Philosophers", Thoemmes Press (two volumes), article Willis Thomas, p. 896. ISBN 1855067048.

Rengachary, Setti S, Xavier A, Manjila S, Smerdon U, Parker B, Hadwan S, and Guthikonda M (2008). "The legendary contributions of Thomas Willis (1621–1675): The arterial circle and beyond". *J. Neurosurg.* **109** (4):765–75. doi:10.3171/JNS/2008/109/10/0765.

SciHi.org: "Thomas Willis and the anatomy of the nervous system". SciHiBlog

Simonazzi M (2004). "Thomas Willis e il sistema nervoso", in Id., *La malattia inglese. La melanconia nella tradizione filosofica e medica dell'Inghilterra moderna*, Bologna: Il Mulino, pp. 185–252.

Symonds C (1960). "Thomas Willis, F.R.S. (1621–1675)". *Notes and Records of the Royal Society of London*. **15:** 91–97. doi:10.1098/rsnr.1960.0008.

## General

Arslan O (2001). "Neuroanatomical basis of clinical neurology". CRC Press. p.368. ISBN 1439806136. Berne RM and Levy MN (2000). "Principles of physiology" (3rd edition), Chapter 9. Mosby, Inc. (2000) ISBN 0-323-00813-5.

Bullock TH, Bennett MV, Johnston D, Josephson R, Marder E, and Fields RD (2005). "Neuroscience. The neuron doctrine, redux". *Science* **310**(5749):791–3. doi:10.1126/science.1114394.

Costanzo LS (2010). *Physiology.* LWW. ISBN 978-0781798761.

DeMyer W (1998). "Neuroanatomy". Williams & Wilkins. ISBN 9780683300758.

Fanciulli A and Wenning GK (2005). "Multiple-system atrophy", *N Engl J Med,* **372**:249-63.

Finger S(1994). Origins of neuroscience : a history of explorations into brain function. Oxford University Press. p. 47. ISBN 9780195146943.

Geser F, Seppi K, and Stampfer-Kountchev M (2005). "The European Multiple System Atrophy-Study Group (EMSA-SG)", *Neural Transm,* **112:**1677-86.

Gilman S, Wenning GK, Low PA, *et al.* (2008). "Second consensus statement on the diagnosis of multiple system atrophy" **71:**670-6.

Hall AC and Guyton JE (2005). "Textbook of medical physiology" (11th ed.). Philadelphia: W.B. Saunders. pp. 687–90. ISBN 978-0-7216-0240-0.

Kandel ER, Schwartz JH, and Jessell TM (2000). "Principles of neural science" (4th ed.). New York: McGraw-Hill. ISBN 0-8385-7701-6.

Peters A, Palay SL, and Webster HS (1991). "The fine structure of the nervous system" (3rd ed.). New York: Oxford University Press. ISBN 0-19-506571-9.

Présentation synthèse de l'Atrophie Multisystématisée - Source Association Parkinson Canada Association ARAMISE.

Ramón y Cajal S (1933). "Histology" (10th ed.). Baltimore: Wood.

Roberts A and Bush BM (1981). "Neurones without Impulses". Cambridge: Cambridge University Press. ISBN 0-521-29935-7.

Snell RS (2010). "Clinical neuroanatomy". Lippincott Williams & Wilkins. ISBN 978-0-7817-9427-5.

Stefanova N, Bucke P, Duerr S, et al. (2009). "Multiple system atrophy: An update", *Lancet Neurol.* **8**(12):1172-8.

Vitrikas K, Dalton H; and Breish D (2020). "Cerebral palsy: An overview". *American Family Physician* **101**(4):213–20.

Wenning GK, Geser F, Krismer F, *et al.* (2013). "The natural history of multiple system atrophy: A prospective European cohort study" *Lancet Neurol,* **12:**264-74.

Wenning GK and Krismer F (2013). "Multiple system atrophy" *Handb Clin Neurol.* 117:229-41. doi: 10.1016/B978-0-444-53491-0.00019-5.

Young PA (2007). "Basic clinical neuroscience" (2nd ed.). Philadelphia, Pa.: Lippincott Williams & Wilkins pp. 69–70. ISBN 9780781753197.

Yuan R, Di X, Taylor PA, Gohel S, Tsai Y-H, and Biswal BB (2015). "Functional topography of the thalamocortical system in human". *Brain Structure and Function* **221**(4):1971–84. doi:10.1007/s00429-015-1018-7.

## Nervous system

MedlinePlus (2016). "Neurosciences". https://medlineplus.gov/ency/article/007456.htm.

National Institute of Neurological Disorders and Stroke (2018). "Brain basics: Know your brain". https://www.ninds.nih.gov/Disorders/Patient-Caregiver-Education/Know-Your-Brain.

Puves D (2012). "Neuroscience" 5th Ed. Sinauer Associates. pp. 560–80. ISBN 978-0878936465.

Society for Neuroscience (2012). "Brain facts". Washington, DC. http://www.brainfacts.org/The-Brain- Facts-Book.

## Autonomic nervous system

Costanzo LS (2007). "Physiology". Hagerstwon, MD: Lippincott Williams & Wilkins. p. 37. ISBN 978-0-7817-7311-9.

Furness J (2007). "Enteric nervous system". *Scholarpedia* **2**(10):4064. doi:10.4249/scholarpedia.4064.

Gibbins and Blessing W. "Autonomic nervous system", *Scholarpedia.*

Goldstein D (2016). Principles of autonomic medicine", National Institute of Neurological Disorders and Stroke, National Institutes of Health. Bethesda, Maryland: ISBN 9780824704087.

Jänig W (2008). "Integrative Action of the Autonomic Nervous System: Neurobiology of Homeostasis" Cambridge University Press. p. 13. ISBN 978052106754-6.

Johnson JO (2013), "Autonomic nervous system physiology", *Pharmacology and Physiology for Anesthesia*, Elsevier, pp. 208–17, doi:10.1016/b978-1-4377-1679-5.00012-0, ISBN 978-1- 4377-1679-5.

Langley JN (1921). "The autonomic nervous system - Part 1". Cambridge: W. Heffer.

Moore KL and Agur AMR (2002). "Essential Clinical Anatomy". Lippincott Williams & Wilkins. 2nd ed. Page 199. ISBN 978-0-7817-5940-3.

Neil A, Campbell JN, and Reece JB (2003). "Biologie. Spektrum"-Verlag Heidelberg-Berlin. ISBN 3- 8274-1352-4.
Pocock G (2006). "Human Physiology" (3rd ed.). Oxford University Press. pp.63–4. ISBN 978-0-19- 856878-0.
Pranav K (2013). "Life Sciences: Fundamentals and Practice". Mina, Usha. (3rd ed.). *New Delhi: Pathfinder Academy*. ISBN 9788190642774.
Schmidt, A and Thews G (1989). "Autonomic nervous system". In Janig, W (ed.). Human Physiology (2 ed.). New York, NY: Springer-Verlag. pp. 333–370.
Willis WD (2004). "The autonomic nervous system and its central control". In Berne, Robert M. (ed.). Physiology (5. ed.). St. Louis, Mo.: Mosby. ISBN 0323022251.

## Motor system

Purves D, Augustine GJ, Fitzpatrick D, Hall WC, Lamantia AS, Mooney RD, Platt ML, Michael L, and VandenBos GR, ed. (2015). "Motor System". APA Dictionary of Psychology (2nd ed.). Washington, DC: American Psychological Association. p. 672. doi:10.1037/14646-000. ISBN 978-1-4338- 1944-5.- "The motor system: Part 1 – Lower motoneurons and the pyramidal system". Human Neuroanatomy. San Diego, CA: Academic Press. 15.1. Regions involved in motor activity, p. 259. ISBN 978-0-12-068251-5.
Rizzolatti G and Luppino G (2001). "The cortical motor system". *Neuron* **31:**889-901.
White LE, eds. (2018). "Neuroscience "(6th ed.). Sinauer Associates. Glossary, motor system, p. G-18. ISBN 9781605353807.

## Neurons

Callaway E (2011). "How to make a human neuron". *Nature.* doi:10.1038/news.2011.328.
Davies M (2002). "The neuron: Size comparison". *Neuroscience: A journey through the brain.*
Giménez C (1998). "Composition and structure of the neuronal membrane: Molecular basis of its physiology and pathology". *Revista de Neurologia* **26**(150) 232–9..
Guillery RW (2005). "Observations of synaptic structures: Origins of the neuron doctrine and its current status". *Philosophical Transactions of the Royal Society of London*. Series B, Biological Sciences **360**(1458):1281–307. doi:10.1098/rstb.2003.1459.
Kempermann G, Gage FH, Aigner L, Song H, Curtis MA, Thuret S, Kuhn HG, Jessberger S, Frankland PW, Cameron HA, Gould E, Hen R, Abrous DN, Toni N, Schinder AF, Zhao X, Lucassen PJ, and Frisén J (2018). "Human adult neurogenesis: Evidence and remaining questions". *Stem Cell* **23**(1):25–30. doi:10.1016/j.stem.2018.04.004.
Levitan, Irwin B.; Kaczmarek, and Leonard K. (2015). "Electrical signaling in neurons". *The Neuron.* Oxford University Press. pp. 41–62. doi:10.1093/med/9780199773893.003.0003. ISBN 978-0- 19-977389-3.
Llinás RR (2014). "Intrinsic electrical properties of mammalian neurons and CNS function: A historical perspective". *Frontiers in Cellular Neuroscience* **8:**320. doi:10.3389/fncel.2014.00320.

López-Muñoz F, Boya J, and Alamo C (2006). "Neuron theory, the cornerstone of neuroscience, on the centenary of the Nobel Prize award to Santiago Ramón y Cajal". *Brain Research Bulletin* **70**(4– 6): 391–405. doi:10.1016/j.brainresbull.2006.07.010.

Patlak J and Gibbons R (2000). "Electrical activity of nerves". *Action Potentials in Nerve Cells.*

Sabbatini RM (2003). "Neurons and synapses: The history of its discovery". *Brain & Mind Magazine* 17.

von Bartheld CS, Bahney J, Herculano-Houzel S (December 2016). "The search for true numbers of neurons and glial cells in the human brain: A review of 150 years of cell counting". *The Journal of Comparative Neurology* **524**(18):3865–3895. doi:10.1002/cne.24040.

Williams RW and Herrup K (1988). "The control of neuron number". *Annual Review of Neuroscience* 11(1):423–53. doi:10.1146/annurev.ne.11.030188.002231.

## Glial cells

Aw BL (2015). "Five reasons why glial cells ere so critical to human intelligence". *Scientific Brains.* https://www.researchgate.net/profile/Jacopo-Meldolesi.

Barres BA (2008). "The mystery and magic of glia: A perspective on their roles in health and disease". *Neuron* **60**(3):430–40. doi:10.1016/j.neuron.2008.10.013.

Bassotti G, Villanacci V, Antonelli E, Morelli A, and Salerni B (2007). "Enteric glial cells: New players in gastrointestinal motility?". *Laboratory Investigation* **87**(7):628–32. doi:10.1038/labinvest.3700564.

Brodal, Per (2010). "Glia". The central nervous system: structure and function. Oxford University Press. p. 19. ISBN 978-0-19-538115-3.

Campbell K and Götz M (2002). "Radial glia: Multi-purpose cells for vertebrate brain development". *Trends in Neurosciences* **25**(5):235–8. doi:10.1016/s0166-2236(02)02156-2.

Cserép C, Pósfai B, Lénárt N, Fekete R, László ZI, and Lele Z (2020). "Microglia monitor and protect neuronal function through specialized somatic purinergic junctions". *Science* 367(6477):528– 37. doi:10.1126/science.aax6752.

Fan X and AgidY (2018). "At the origin of the history of glia". *Neuroscience* **385:**255–71. doi:10.1016/j.neuroscience.2018.05.050.

Halassa MM, Fellin T, and Haydon PG (2007). "The tripartite synapse: Toles for gliotransmission in health and disease". *Trends Mol Med.* **13**(2):54–63. doi:10.1016/j.molmed.2006.12.005.

Hanani M (2005). "Satellite glial cells in sensory ganglia: From form to function". *Brain Res. Rev.* **48:**457–476.

Jessen KR and Mirsky R (1980). "Glial cells in the enteric nervous system contain glial fibrillary acidic protein". *Nature* 286(5774):736–7. doi:10.1038/286736a0.

Jessen KR and Mirsky R (2005). "The origin and development of glial cells in peripheral nerves". *Nature Reviews. Neuroscience* **6**(9):671–82. doi:10.1038/nrn1746.

Kettenmann and Ransom "Neuroglia", Oxford University Press, 2012, ISBN 978-0-19-979459-1 | http://ukcatalogue.oup.com/product/9780199794591.do#.UVcswaD3Ay4%7C

Kettenmann H, Verkhratsky A (2008). "Neuroglia: The 150 years after". *Trends in Neurosciences* **31**(12):653–9. doi:10.1016/j.tins.2008.09.003.

Peters A (2004). "A fourth type of neuroglial cell in the adult central nervous system". *Journal of Neurocytology* **33**(3):345–57. doi:10.1023/B:NEUR.0000044195.64009.27.

Santello M, Calì C, and Bezzi P (2012). Gliotransmission and the tripartite synapse". *Advances in Experimental Medicine and Biology* **970:**307–31. doi:10.1007/978-3-7091-0932-8_14. ISBN 978-3-7091-0931-1.

Valori CF, Brambilla L, Martorana F, and Rossi D (2013). "The multifaceted role of glial cells in amyotrophic lateral sclerosis". *Cellular and Molecular Life Sciences* **71**(2):287–97. doi:10.1007/s00018-013-1429-7. ISSN 1420-682X.

Volterra A and Steinhäuser C (2004). "Glial modulation of synaptic transmission in the hippocampus". Glia **47**(3):249–57. doi:10.1002/glia.20080.

von Bartheld CS, Bahney J, and Herculano-Houzel S (2016). "The search for true numbers of neurons and glial cells in the human brain: A review of 150 years of cell counting". *The Journal of Comparative Neurology* **524**(18):3865–95. doi:10.1002/cne.24040. ISSN 1096-9861.

Yiu G and He Z (2006). "Glial inhibition of CNS axon regeneration". *Nature Reviews. Neuroscience* **7** (8):617–27. doi:10.1038/nrn1956.

## Signs & symptoms

Jecmenica-Lukic M, Poewe W, Tolosa E, and Wenning GK (2012). "Premotor signs and symptoms of multiple system atrophy", *Lancet Neurol,* **11:**361-8.

McKay JH and Cheshire WP (2018). "First symptoms in multiple system atrophy", *Clin Auton Res.* **28**(2):215-21. doi: 10.1007/s10286-017-0500-0.

## Incidence and prevalence - Epidemiology

Bjornsdottir A, Gudmundsson G, Blondal H, *et al.* (2013). "Incidence and prevalence of multiple system atrophy: A nationwide study in Iceland", *J Neurol Neurosurg Psychiatry.* 84(2):136-40. doi: 10.1136/jnnp-2012-302500.

## Types and nature

Jellinger KA (2018). "Multiple system atrophy: An oligodendroglioneural synucleinopathy1", *J Alzheimers Dis.* **62**(3):1141-179. doi: 10.3233/JAD-170397.

Papp MI, Kahn JE, and Lantos PL (1989). "Glial cytoplasmic inclusions in the CNS of patients with multiple system atrophy (striatonigral degeneration, olivopontocerebellar atrophy and Shy- Drager syndrome)", *J Neurol Sci,* **94:**79-100.

Sakakibara R, Hattori T, Uchiyama T, *et al.* (2000). "Urinary dysfunction and orthostatic hypotension in multiple system atrophy: which is the more common and earlier manifestation? *J Neurol Neurosurg Psychiatry* **68:**65-9.

Tu PH, Galvin JE, Baba M, *et al.*(199). "Glial cytoplasmic inclusions in white matter oligodendrocytes of multiple system atrophy brains contain insoluble alpha-synuclein", *Ann Neurol,* **44:**415-22.

## Alzheimer's disease

Fymat AL (2018a). "Alzheimer's disease: A review", *J Current Opinions in Neurological Science* **2**(2);415-436.

Fymat AL (2018b). "Alzheimer's disease: Prevention, delay, minimization, and reversal", *J Clinical Research in Neurology* **1**(1):1-16.

Fymat AL (2018c). "Is Alzheimer's an autoimmune disease gone rogue", *J Clinical Research in Neurology* **2**(1):1-4.

Fymat AL (2018d). "Is Alzheimer's a runaway autoimmune disease? And how to cure it?" *Proc European Union Academy of Sciences* 379-83.

Fymat AL (2019). "Alzhei ... Who? Demystifying the disease and what you can do about it", Tellwell Talent Publishers, pp 236, ISBN: 978-0-2288-2420-6; 978-0-2288-2419-0.

Fymat AL (2020a). "Is Alzheimer's an autoimmune disease gone rogue? The Role of Brain Immunotherapy", *J Clinical Research in Neurology* **3**(2):1-3.

Fymat AL (2020b). "Alzheimer's: What do we know about the disease and what can be done about it?" *EC J of Psychology & Psychiatry* **9**(11):69-74.

Fymat AL (2020c). "Alzheimer's: Will there ever be a cure? "*J Clinical Psychiatry and Neuroscience* **3**(4): 1-5.

Fymat AL (2022). "Alzheimer's disease: A path to a cure", *Current Opinions in Neurological Science* **3**(1):1-16.

Fymat AL (2023). "Alzheimer's disease: A path to a cure", *J Neurology and Psychology Research* 3(1):1-15.

## Dementias

Fymat AL (2018). "Dementia treatment: Where do we stand?, *J Current Opinions in Neurological Science* **3**(1):1-3. 599.603.

Fymat AL (2019a). "On dementia and other cognitive disorders", *J Clinical Research in Neurology* **2**(1):1-14.

Fymat AL (2019b). "Dementia: A review", *J Clinical Psychiatry and Neuroscience* **1**(3):27-34.

Fymat AL (2019). "Dementia with Lewy bodies: A review", *J Current Opinions in Neurological Science* **4**(1);15-32.

Fymat AL (2019c). "What do we know about Lewy body dementias?" *J Psychiatry and Psychotherapy* (Editorial) **2**(1)-013:1-4. doi:10.31579/JPP.2019/018

Fymat AL (2020a). "Dementia: Fending off the menacing disease... and what you can do about it", Tellwell Talent Publishers, pp 488, **ISBN: 978-0-2288-4145-3; 978-0-2288-4145-6.**

Fymat AL (2020b). "Dementia: Should we Reorient our Approach to Treatment?", *EC J Psychology & Psychiatry* **9**(12):1-3.

Fymat AL (2021a). "Dementia: What is its Causal Etiology?", *International J Neuropsychology and Behavioral Sciences* **1**(1):19-22.

Fymat AL (2021b). "On Potentially Reversible Forms of Dementia", *J Current Opinions in Neurological Science* **6(**1):101-8.

Fymat AL (2022). "Dementia: Eliminating its Potentially Reversible Forms", *Proc. European Union Academy of Sciences* pp 270-7**.**

## Multiple sclerosis

Fymat AL (2022). **Multiple Sclerosis: The progressive demyelinating autoimmune disease, Tellwell Talent Publishers pp 509, 2022 ISBN: 978-0-2288-9292-2 (Hardcover); 978-0-2288-3 (Paperback).** https://portal.tellwell.ca/Tellwell/Design/212669.

## Parkinson's disease and parkinsonism

Anderson D, Beecher G, and Ba F (2017). "; Deep brain stimulation in Parkinson's disease: New and emerging targets for refractory motor and nonmotor symptoms.", *Parkinsons Dis.* **2017:**5124328. doi: 10.1155/2017/5124328.

Barbosa AF, Chen J, Freitag F, *et al;* (2016). "Gait, posture and cognition in Parkinson's disease", *Dement Neuropsychol.* **10**(4):280-6. doi: 10.1590/s1980-5764-2016dn1004005.

Cabreira V and Massano J (2019). "Parkinson's disease: Clinical review and update", *Acta Med Port.* **132**(10):661-70. doi: 10.20344/amp.11978.

EFNS/MDS-ES (2013). "recommendations for the diagnosis of Parkinson's disease", *European Journal of Neurology* (Janury).

Freitas ME and Fox SH (2016). Nondopaminergic treatments for Parkinson's disease: Current and future prospects", *Neurodegener Dis Manag.* **6**(3):249-68. doi: 10.2217/nmt-2016-0005.

Fymat AL (2018a). "Parkinson's Disease and Other Movement Disorders: A review", *J Current Opinions in Neurological Science* **2**(1):316-43.

Fymat AL (2018b). "Neurological Disorders and the Blood Brain Barrier: 2. Parkinson's Disease and Other Movement Disorders", *J Current Opinions in Neurological Science* **2**(1)362-83.

Fymat AL (2019). "Viruses in the Brain...? Any Connections to Parkinson's and Other Neurodegenerative Diseases?", *Proc European Union Academy of Sciences* pp 249-52.

Fymat AL (2020a). "Parkinson's: What is known about the disease and what can be done about it?", *J Clinical Research in Neurology* **3**(2):1-12.

Fymat AL (2020b). "Recent research developments in Parkinson's disease", *Current Opinions in Neurological Science* **5**(1):12-30,

Fymat AL (2020c). "Parkin... ss..oo..nn: Elucidating the Disease... and What You Can Do About It," Tellwell Talent Publishers, pp 258, *ISBN: 978-0-2288-2874-7; 10-0-2228-2874-0.*

Lees AJ, Hardy J, and Revesz T (2009). "Parkinson's disease", *Lancet.* **13373**(9680):2055-66.
Lemke MR (2008). "Depressive symptoms in Parkinson's disease", *Eur J Neurol.* Apr15 Suppl **1:**21-5.
NICE U.K. (2022). "Parkinson's disease;", *NICE U.K.*
NICE U.K. (2017). "Parkinson's disease in adults", *NICE Guideline* (July).
NICE U.K. (2023). "Devices for remote monitoring of Parkinson's disease", *NICE Diagnostics guidance* (January 2023)
Parkinson's UK "Drug-Induced Parkinsonism".
Raccagni C, Nonnekes J, Bloem BR, *et al.* (2020). ";Gait and postural disorders in parkinsonism: A clinical approach", *J Neurol.* **267**(11):3169-76. doi: 10.1007/s00415-019-09382-1.
Riboldi GM, Frattini E, Monfrini E, *et al* (2022). "A practical approach to early-onset Parkinsonism. *J Parkinsons Dis.* **12**(1):1-26. doi: 10.3233/JPD-212815.
Rizek P, Kumar N, and Jog MS (2016). "An update on the diagnosis and treatment of Parkinson's disease", *CMAJ.* 1188(16):1157-65. doi: 10.1503/cmaj.151179.
Scottish Intercollegiate Guidelines Network (2010). "Diagnosis and pharmacological management of Parkinson's disease,", *Scottish Intercollegiate Guidelines Network* – SIGN.
Shagam JY (2008). "Unlocking the secrets of Parkinson disease", *Radiol Technol.* **79**(3):227-39.
Sveinbjornsdottir S (2016). "The clinical symptoms of Parkinson's disease", *J Neurochem.* **139 Suppl 1:**318-24. doi: 10.1111/jnc.13691.
Tolosa E, Garrido A, Scholz SW, et al; (2021). "Challenges in the diagnosis of Parkinson's disease", *Lancet Neurol.* **20**(5):385-97. doi: 10.1016/S1474-4422(21)00030-2.

## Neuropathology and pathophysiology

Ahmed Z, Asi YT, Sailer A, *et al.* (2012). "The neuropathology, pathophysiology and genetics of multiple system atrophy", *Neuropathol Appl Neurobiol,* **38:**4-24.
Ubhi K, Low P, and Masliah E (2011). "Multiple system atrophy: A clinical and neuropathological perspective". *Trends Neurosci.* 34(11):581-90. doi: 10.1016/j.tins.2011.08.003.

## Phenoconversion

Kaufmann H, Norcliffe-Kaufmann L, Palma JA, Biaggioni I, Low PA, Singer W, Goldstein DS, Peltier AC, Shibao CA, Gibbons CH, Freeman R, and Robertson D (2017). "Autonomic Disorders Consortium. Natural history of pure autonomic failure: A United States prospective cohort", *Annals of Neurology* 81(2):287-97. www.ncbi.nlm.nih.gov/pubmed/28093795

## Causes - Genetics

Ahmed Z, Asi YT, Sailer A, *et al.* (2012). "The neuropathology, pathophysiology and genetics of multiple system atrophy", *Neuropathol Appl Neurobiol,* **38:**4-24.

Ferguson MC, Garland EM, Hedges L *et al.* (2014). "SHC2 gene copy number in multiple system atrophy (MSA)", *Clin Auton Res,* **24:**25-30.

Hara K, Momose Y, Tokiguchi S, *et al.* (2007). "Multiplex families with multiple system atrophy, *Arch Neurol,* **64:**545-51.

The Multiple-System Atrophy Research Collaboration (2013). "Mutations in COQ2 in familial and sporadic multiple-system atrophy", *N Engl J Med,* 369:233-44.

## Diagnosis

Palma JA, Norcliffe-Kaufmann L, and Kaufmann H (2018). "Diagnosis of multiple system atrophy", *Auton Neurosci.* 211:15-25. doi: 10.1016/j.autneu.2017.10.007.

Treglia G, Stefanelli A, Cason E, *et al* (2011). "Diagnostic performance of iodine-123-metaiodobenzylguanidine scintigraphy in differential diagnosis between Parkinson's disease and multiple-system atrophy: A systematic review and a meta-analysis", *Clin Neurol Neurosurg.* 113(10):823-9. doi: 10.1016/j.clineuro.2011.09.004.

## Effects - Cognitive impairment

Brown RG, Lacomblez L, Landwehrmeyer BG, et al. (2010). "Cognitive impairment in patients with multiple system atrophy and progressive multiple system atrophy: An update", *Brain.*

Stankovic I, Krismer F, Jesic A, *et al.* (2014). "Cognitive impairment in multiple system atrophy: A position statement by the Neuropsychology Task Force of the MDS Multiple System Atrophy (MODIMSA) study group ", *Mov Disord,*;29:857-67.

## Progression and prognosis

Figueroa JJ, Singer W, Parsaik A, *et al* (2014). "Multiple system atrophy: Prognostic indicators of survival", *Mov Disord.* **29**(9):1151-7. doi: 10.1002/mds.25927.

Watanabe H, Saito Y, Terao S, *et al.* (2002). "Progression and prognosis in multiple system atrophy: An analysis of 230 Japanese patients", *Brain* **125:**1070-83.

## Management and treatment

Kuzdas-Wood D, Stefanova N, Jellinger KA, et al. (2014). "Towards translational therapies for multiple system atrophy". *Prog Neurobiol.* **118C**:19-35. doi: 10.1016/j.pneurobio.2014.02.007.

## Outcomes

May S, Gilman S, Sowell BB, *et al.* (2007). "Potential outcome measures and trial design issues for multiple system atrophy". *Mov Disord,* 22:2371-7.

## Survival

Ben-Shlomo Y, Wenning GK, Tison F, AND Quinn NP (1997). "Survival of patients with pathologically proven multiple system atrophy: A meta-analysis", *Neurology* 48:384-93.

## Drug delivery across the blood-brain barrier

Fymat AL (2017a). "Nanoneurology: Drug Delivery Across the Brain Protective Barriers," *J Nanomedicine Research* **5**(1):1-4, 00105. **doi: 10:15406/jnmr/2017.05.00105**

Fymat AL (2017b). "Therapeutics Delivery Behind, Through and Beyond the Blood Brain Barrier", *Open Access J Surgery* ***5***(1): 1-9; 555654. **doi: 10.19080/OAJS.2017.05.555654**

Fymat AL (2018). "Blood Brain Barrier Permeability and Neurological Diseases", *J Current Opinions in Neurological Science* (Editorial). **2**(2);411-4.

## Brain immunotherapy

Fymat AL (2017a). "Synthetic Immunotherapy with Chimeric Antigen Receptors", *J. Cancer Prevention & Current Research 7*(5):1-3. 00253: **doi: 10.15406/jcpcr.2017.07.00253**.

Fymat AL (2017b). "Immunotherapy of Brain Cancers and Neurological Disorders", *J Cancer Prevention & Current Research 8*(6):1-7; 00301. **doi: 10.15406/jcpcr2017.08.00301**

Fymat AL (2018a). "Regulating the Brain's Autoimmune System: The End of All Neurological Disorders?" *J Current Opinions in Neurological Science 2*(3):475-9.

Fymat AL (2018b). "Harnessing the Immune System to Treat Cancers and Neurodegenerative Diseases" *J Clinical Research in Neurology* **1**(1):1-14.

## Neurodegenerative diseases treatment

Fymat AL (2018). "Neutrophils-Mediated Treatment of Neurodegenerative and Other Inflammatory Diseases, *J Clinical Research in Neurology* **1**(1):1-5.

Fymat AL (2019a). "The Pathogenic Brain", J Current Opinions in Neurological Science 3(2);669-71.

Fymat AL (2019b). "On the Pathogenic Hypothesis of Neurodegenerative Diseases", J Clinical Research in Neurology 2(1):1-7.

Fymat, AL (2019c). "Our Two Interacting Brains – Etiologic Modulations of Neurodegenerative and Gastroenteric Diseases", J Current Opinions in Neurological Science 4(2):50-4.

Fymat AL (2019d). "Electromagnetic Therapy for Neurological and Neurodegenerative Diseases: I. Peripheral Brain Stimulations". Open Access J Neurology and Neurosurgery 12(2):30-47. doi:10.19080/OAJNN.2019.12.555833

Fymat AL (2020a). "Neuroradiology and its Role in Neurodegenerative Diseases", *J Radiology and Imaging Science* **1**(1):1-14. (Journal closed and transferred to: *J Neuroradiology and Nanomedicine* **5**(1):1-14.

Fymat AL (2020b). "Electromagnetic Therapy for Neurological and Neurodegenerative Diseases: II. Deep Brain Stimulation". *Open Access J Neurology and Neurosurgery* **13**(1):1-17. **doi: 19080/OAJNN.2020.13.555855**

Fymat AL (2020c). "Nanobiotechnology-based Drugs for the Treatment of Neurological Disorders", *J Pharmaceutical Bioprocessing* **8**(3):1-3.

Fymat AL (2020d). "On the Symbiosis Between our Two Interacting Brains"**,** *Proceedings of the European Union Academy of Sciences* 147-51, 2020.

## Additional references

Ahmed Z, Asi YT, Sailer A, Lees AJ, Houlden H, Revesz T *et al.* (2012). "The neuropathology, pathophysiology and genetics of multiple system atrophy". *Neuropathol Appl Neurobiol* **38**(1):4–24. https://doi.org/10.1111/j.1365-2990.2011.01234.x

Alarcón-Arís D, Recasens A, Galofré M, Carballo-Carbajal I, Zacchi N, Ruiz-Bronchal E et al. (2018). "Selective α-synuclein knockdown in monoamine neurons by intranasal oligonucleotide delivery: potential therapy for Parkinson's disease". *Mol Ther* **26**(2):550–67. https://doi.org/10.1016/j.ymthe.2017.11.015

Al-Chalabi A, Dürr A, Wood NW, Parkinson MH, Camuzat A, Hulot JS *et al.* (2009). "Genetic variants of the alpha-synuclein gene SNCA are associated with multiple system atrophy". *PLoS ONE* **4**(9):e7114. https://doi.org/10.1371/journal.pone.0007114

Anderson JP, Walker DE, Goldstein JM, de Laat R, Banducci K, Caccavello RJ *et al.* (2006). "Phosphorylation of Ser-129 is the dominant pathological modification of alpha-synuclein in familial and sporadic Lewy body disease". *J Biol Chem* **28**1(40):29739–52. https://doi.org/10.1074/jbc.M600933200

Attar A, Chan WT, Klärner FG, Schrader T, and Bitan G (2014). "Safety and pharmacological characterization of the molecular tweezer CLR01—a broad-spectrum inhibitor of amyloid proteins' toxicity". *BMC Pharmacol Toxicol* 15:23. https://doi.org/10.1186/2050-6511-15-23

Auluck PK, Caraveo G, and Lindquist S (2010). "α-Synuclein: membrane interactions and toxicity in Parkinson's disease". *Annu Rev Cell Dev Biol* **26:**211–33. https://doi.org/10.1146/annurev.cellbio.042308.113313

Bassil F, Fernagut PO, Bezard E, Pruvost A, Leste-Lasserre T, Hoang QQ *et al.* (2016). "Reducing C- terminal truncation mitigates synucleinopathy and neurodegeneration in a transgenic model of multiple system atrophy". *Proc Natl Acad Sci U S A* **113**(34):9593–8. https://doi.org/10.1073/pnas.1609291113

Bassil F, Canron MH, Vital A, Bezard E, Li Y, Greig NH *et al.* (2017). "Insulin resistance and exendin-4 treatment for multiple system atrophy". *Brain* **140**(5):1420–36. https://doi.org/10.1093/brain/awx044

Beck RO, Betts CD, and Fowler CJ (1994). "Genitourinary dysfunction in multiple system atrophy: clinical features and treatment in 62 cases". *J Urol* **151**(5):1336–41. https://doi.org/10.1016/s0022-5347(17)35246-1

Benarroch EE, Schmeichel AM, Sandroni P, Low PA, and Parisi JE (2006). Involvement of vagal autonomic nuclei in multiple system atrophy and Lewy body disease". *Neurology* **66**(3):378– 83. https://doi.org/10.1212/01.wnl.0000196638.98781.bb

Bensimon G, Ludolph A, Agid Y, Vidailhet M, Payan C, and Leigh PN (2009). "Riluzole treatment, s urvival and diagnostic criteria in Parkinson plus disorders: the NNIPPS study". *Brain* **132**(Pt 1):156–71. https://doi.org/10.1093/brain/awn291

Brettschneider J, Irwin DJ, Boluda S, Byrne MD, Fang L, Lee EB *et al.* (2017). "Progression of alpha- synuclein pathology in multiple system atrophy of the cerebellar type". *Neuropathol Appl Neurobiol* **43**(4):315–329. https://doi.org/10.1111/nan.12362

Brundin P, Dave KD, and Kordower JH (2017). "Therapeutic approaches to target alpha-synuclein pathology. *Exp Neurol* **298**(Pt B):225–35. https://doi.org/10.1016/j.expneurol.2017.10.003

Burré J, Sharma M, and Südhof TC (2018). "Cell Biology and pathophysiology of α-Synuclein". *Cold Spring Harb Perspect Med.* https://doi.org/10.1101/cshperspect.a024091

Castro Caldas A, Levin J, Djaldetti R, Rascol O, Wenning G, and Ferreira JJ (2017). "Critical appraisal of clinical trials in multiple system atrophy: toward better quality". **Mov Disord** 3**2**(10):1356- 64. https://doi.org/10.1002/mds.27080

Chen YP, Zhao B, Cao B, Song W, Guo X, Wei QQ *et al.* (2015). "Mutation scanning of the COQ2 gene in ethnic Chinese patients with multiple-system atrophy". *Neurobiol Aging* 36(2):1222.e7–1211. https://doi.org/10.1016/j.neurobiolaging.2014.09.010

Coon EA, Ahlskog JE (2021). "My treatment approach to multiple system atrophy". *Mayo Clinic Proc* **96**(3):708–19. https://doi.org/10.1016/j.mayocp.2020.10.005

Couch Y, Alvarez-Erviti L, Sibson NR, Wood MJ, and Anthony DC (2011). "The acute inflammatory response to intranigral α-synuclein differs significantly from intranigral lipopolysaccharide and is exacerbated by peripheral inflammation". *J Neuroinflammation* **8:**166. https://doi.org/10.1186/1742-2094-8-166

Cykowski MD, Coon EA, Powell SZ, Jenkins SM, Benarroch EE, Low PA *et al.* (2015). "Expanding the spectrum of neuronal pathology in multiple system atrophy". *Brain* **138**(Pt 8):2293–309. https://doi.org/10.1093/brain/awv114

Danzer KM, Haasen D, Karow AR, Moussaud S, Habeck M, Giese A *et al.* (2007). "Different species of alpha-synuclein oligomers induce calcium influx and seeding". *J Neurosci* **27**(34):9220–22. https://doi.org/10.1523/jneurosci.2617-07.2007

Diguet E, Fernagut PO, Scherfler C, Wenning G, and Tison F (2005). "Effects of riluzole on combined MPTP + 3-nitropropionic acid-induced mild to moderate striatonigral degeneration in mice. *J Neural Transm* (vienna) **112**(5):613–31. https://doi.org/10.1007/s00702-004-0206-z

Djajadikerta A, Keshri S, Pavel M, Prestil R, Ryan L, and Rubinsztein DC (2020). "Autophagy induction as a therapeutic strategy for neurodegenerative diseases". *J Mol Biol* **432**(8):2799– 821. https://doi.org/10.1016/j.jmb.2019.12.035

Dodel R, Spottke A, Gerhard A, Reuss A, Reinecker S, Schimke N *et al.* (2010). "Minocycline 1-year therapy in multiple-system-atrophy: effect on clinical symptoms and [(11)C](R)-PK11195 PET (MEMSA-trial)" *J. Mov Disord* **25**(1):97–107. https://doi.org/10.1002/mds.22732

El-Agnaf O, Overk C, Rockenstein E, Mante M, Florio J, Adame A *et al.* (2017). "Differential effects of immunotherapy with antibodies targeting α-synuclein oligomers and fibrils in a transgenic model of synucleinopathy". *J Neurobiol Dis* **104:**85–96. https://doi.org/10.1016/j.nbd.2017.05.002

Ettle B, Kerman BE, Valera E, Gillmann C, Schlachetzki JC, Reiprich S *et al.* (2016). "α-Synuclein- induced myelination deficit defines a novel interventional target for multiple system atrophy". *Acta Neuropathol* **132**(1):59–75. https://doi.org/10.1007/s00401-016-1572-y

Fanciulli A and Wenning GK (2015). "Multiple-system atrophy". *N Engl J Med* **372**(3):249–63. https://doi.org/10.1056/NEJMra1311488

Fellner L, Jellinger KA, Wenning GK, and Stefanova N (2011). "Glial dysfunction in the pathogenesis of α-synucleinopathies: emerging concepts". *Acta Neuropathol* **121**(6):675–93. https://doi.org/10.1007/s00401-011-0833-z

Fellner L, Irschick R, Schanda K, Reindl M, Klimaschewski L, Poewe W *et al.* (2013). "Toll-like receptor 4 is required for α-synuclein dependent activation of microglia and astroglia". *Glia* **61**(3):349–60. https://doi.org/10.1002/glia.22437

Ferreira N, Gram H, Sorrentino ZA, Gregersen E, Schmidt SI, Reimer L *et al.* (2021). "Multiple system atrophy-associated oligodendroglial protein p25α stimulates formation of novel α-synuclein strain with enhanced neurodegenerative potential". *Acta Neuropathol.* https://doi.org/10.1007/s00401-021-02316-0

Fujioka S, Ogaki K, Tacik PM, Uitti RJ, Ross OA, and Wszolek ZK (2014). "Update on novel familial forms of Parkinson's disease and multiple system atrophy". *Parkinsonism Relat Disord* **20** Suppl 1(0 1):S29–34. https://doi.org/10.1016/s1353-8020(13)70010-5

Fymat AL (2018). "Role of Nanomedicine in Clinical Neuroscience", *Global J Nanomedicine* **4**(1):1-3. **doi:10.19080/GJN.2018.04555629.**

Gai WP, Power JH, Blumbergs PC, and Blessing WW (1998). "Multiple-system atrophy: A new alpha- synuclein disease?" *Lancet* **352**(9127):547–8. https://doi.org/10.1016/s0140-6736(05)79256-4

Ganjam GK, Bolte K, Matschke LA, Neitemeier S, Dolga AM, Höllerhage M *et al.* (2019). "Mitochondrial damage by α-synuclein causes cell death in human dopaminergic neurons". *Cell Death Dis* **10**(11):865. https://doi.org/10.1038/s41419-019-2091-2.

Gerhard A, Banati RB, Goerres GB, Cagnin A, Myers R, Gunn RN *et al.* (2003). "[11C](R)-PK11195 PET imaging of microglial activation in multiple system atrophy". *Neurology* **61**(5):686–9. https://doi.org/10.1212/01.wnl.0000078192.95645.e6

Goedert M, Jakes R, and Spillantini MG (2017). "The synucleinopathies: twenty years on". *J Parkinson's Dis* **7**(s1):S51-69. https://doi.org/10.3233/jpd-179005

Graham JG and Oppenheimer DR (1969). "Orthostatic hypotension and nicotine sensitivity in a case of multiple system atrophy". *J Neurol Neurosurg Psychiatry* **32**(1):28–34. https://doi.org/10.1136/jnnp.32.1.28

Hebron ML, Lonskaya I, and Moussa CE (2013). "Nilotinib reverses loss of dopamine neurons and improves motor behavior via autophagic degradation of α-synuclein in Parkinson's disease models". *Hum Mol Genet* **22**(16):3315–28. https://doi.org/10.1093/hmg/ddt192

Heras-Garvin A, Weckbecker D, Ryazanov S, Leonov A, Griesinger C, Giese A *et al.* (2019). "Anle138b modulates α-synuclein oligomerization and prevents motor decline and neurodegeneration in a mouse model of multiple system atrophy". *Mov Disord* **34**(2):255–63. https://doi.org/10.1002/mds.27562

Heras-Garvin A, Refolo V, Schmidt C, Malfertheiner K, Wenning GK, Bradbury M *et al.* (2021). "ATH434 reduces α-synuclein-related neurodegeneration in a murine model of multiple system atrophy." *Mov Disord*. https://doi.org/10.1002/mds.28714

Herrera-Vaquero M, Bouquio D, Kallab M, Biggs K, Nair G, Ochoa J *et al.* (2019). "The molecular tweezer CLR01 reduces aggregated, pathologic, and seeding-competent α-synuclein in experimental multiple system atrophy". *Biochim Biophys Acta Mol Basis Dis* **1865**(11):165513. https://doi.org/10.1016/j.bbadis.2019.07.007

Holmberg B, Johansson JO, Poewe W, Wenning G, Quinn NP, Mathias C *et al.* (2007). "Safety and tolerability of growth hormone therapy in multiple system atrophy: A double-blind, placebo- controlled study". *Mov Disord* **22**(8):1138–44. https://doi.org/10.1002/mds.21501

Ishizawa K, Komori T, Sasaki S, Arai N, Mizutani T, and Hirose T (2004). "Microglial activation parallels system degeneration in multiple system atrophy". *J Neuropathol Exp Neurol* **63**(1):43– 52. https://doi.org/10.1093/jnen/63.1.43

Ishizawa K, Komori T, Arai N, Mizutani T, Hirose T (2008). "Glial cytoplasmic inclusions and tissue injury in multiple system atrophy: a quantitative study in white matter (olivopontocerebellar system) and gray matter (nigrostriatal system)". *Neuropathology* **28**(3):249–57. https://doi.org/10.1111/j.1440-1789.2007.00855.x

Iwai A, Masliah E, Yoshimoto M, Ge N, Flanagan L, de Silva HA *et al.* (1995). "The precursor protein of non-A beta component of Alzheimer's disease amyloid is a presynaptic protein of the central nervous system". *Neuron* **14**(2):467–75. https://doi.org/10.1016/0896-6273(95)90302-x

Jakes R, Spillantini MG, and Goedert M (1994), "Identification of two distinct synucleins from human brain. *FES Lett* **345**(1):27–32. https://doi.org/10.1016/0014-5793(94)00395-5

Jellinger KA (2014). "Neuropathology of multiple system atrophy: new thoughts about pathogenesis. *Mov Disord* **29**(14):1720–41. https://doi.org/10.1002/mds.26052

Jellinger KA (2017). "Potential clinical utility of multiple system atrophy biomarkers". *Expert Rev Neurother* **17**(12):1189–208. https://doi.org/10.1080/14737175.2017.1392239

Jellinger KA, Wenning GK (2016). "Multiple system atrophy: Pahogenic mechanisms and biomarkers". *J Neural Transm* (vienna) **123**(6):555–72. https://doi.org/10.1007/s00702-016-1545-2

Jellinger KA, Seppi K, and Wenning GK (2005), "Grading of neuropathology in multiple system atrophy: proposal for a novel scale". *Mov Disord* **20**(Suppl 12):S29-36. https://doi.org/10.1002/mds.20537

Kaindlstorfer C, Sommer P, Georgievska B, Mather RJ, Kugler AR, Poewe W *et al.* (2015). "Failure of neuroprotection despite microglial suppression by delayed-start myeloperoxidase inhibition in a model of advanced multiple system atrophy: Clinical implications". *Neurotox Res* **28**(3):185– 94. https://doi.org/10.1007/s12640-015-9547-7

Kallab M, Herrera-Vaquero M, Johannesson M, Eriksson F, Sigvardson J, Poewe W *et al.* (2018). "Region-specific effects of immunotherapy with antibodies targeting α-synuclein in a transgenic model of synucleinopathy". *Front Neurosci* **12:**452. https://doi.org/10.3389/fnins.2018.00452

Kiely AP, Murray CE, Foti SC, Benson BC, Courtney R, Strand C *et al.* (2018). "Immunohistochemical and molecular investigations show alteration in the inflammatory profile of multiple system atrophy brain". *J Neuropathol Exp Neurol* **77**(7):598–607. https://doi.org/10.1093/jnen/nly035

Kübler D, Wächter T, Cabanel N, Su Z, Turkheimer FE, Dodel R *et al.* (2019). "Widespread microglial activation in multiple system atrophy". *Mov Disord* **34**(4):564–8. https://doi.org/10.1002/mds.27620

Lee HJ, Suk JE, Patrick C, Bae EJ, Cho JH, Rho S *et al.* (2010). "Direct transfer of alpha-synuclein from neuron to astroglia causes inflammatory responses in synucleinopathies". *J Biol Chem* **285**(12):9262–72. https://doi.org/10.1074/jbc.M109.081125

Lee PH, Kim JW, Bang OY, Ahn YH, Joo IS, and Huh K (2008). "Autologous mesenchymal stem cell therapy delays the progression of neurological deficits in patients with multiple system atrophy". *Clin Pharmacol Ther* **83**(5):723–30. https://doi.org/10.1038/sj.clpt.6100386

Lee PH, Lee JE, Kim HS, Song SK, Lee HS, Nam HS *et al.* (2012). "A randomized trial of mesenchymal stem cells in multiple system atrophy". *Ann Neurol* **72**(1):32–40. https://doi.org/10.1002/ana.23612

Lema Tomé CM, Tyson T, Rey NL, Grathwohl S, Britschgi M, and Brundin P (2013). "Inflammation and α-synuclein's prion-like behavior in Parkinson's disease–is there a link?" *Mol Neurobiol* **47**(2):561–74. https://doi.org/10.1007/s12035-012-8267-8

Lemos M, Venezia S, Refolo V, Heras-Garvin A, Schmidhuber S, Giese A *et al.* (2020). "Targeting α- synuclein by PD03 AFFITOPE® and Anle138b rescues neurodegenerative pathology in a model of multiple system atrophy: Clinical relevance". *Transl Neurodegener* **9**(1):38. https://doi.org/10.1186/s40035-020-00217-y

Levin J, Maaß S, Schuberth M, Giese A, Oertel WH, Poewe W *et al.* (2019). "Safety and efficacy of epigallocatechin gallate in multiple system atrophy (PROMESA): A randomized, double-blind, placebo-controlled trial". *Lancet Neurol* 18(8):724–735. https://doi.org/10.1016/s1474- 4422(19)30141-3

Li F, Ayaki T, Maki T, Sawamoto N, and Takahashi R (2018). "NLRP3 inflammasome-related proteins are upregulated in the putamen of patients with multiple system atrophy". *J Neuropathol Exp Neurol* **77**(11):1055–65. https://doi.org/10.1093/jnen/nly090

Li W, West N, Colla E, Pletnikova O, Troncoso JC, Marsh L *et al.* (2005). "Aggregation promoting C- terminal truncation of alpha-synuclein is a normal cellular process and is enhanced by the familial Parkinson's disease-linked mutations". *Proc Natl Acad Sci U S A* **102**(6):2162–7. https://doi.org/10.1073/pnas.0406976102

Lim S, Chun Y, Lee JS, and Lee SJ (2016). "Neuroinflammation in synucleinopathies". *Brain Pathol* **26**(3):404–9. https://doi.org/10.1111/bpa.12371

Lopez-Cuina M, Guerin PA, Canron MH, Delamarre A, Dehay B, Bezard E *et al.* (2020). "Nilotinib fails to prevent synucleinopathy and cell loss in a mouse model of multiple system atrophy". *Mov Disord* **35**(7):1163–72. https://doi.org/10.1002/mds.28034

Lövestam S, Schweighauser M, Matsubara T, Murayama S, Tomita T, Ando T *et al.* (2021)."Seeded assembly in vitro does not replicate the structures of α-synuclein filaments from multiple system atrophy". *FEBS Open Bio* **11**(4):999–1013. https://doi.org/10.1002/2211-5463.13110

Low PA, Robertson D, Gilman S, Kaufmann H, Singer W, Biaggioni I *et al.* (2014). "Efficacy and safety of rifampicin for multiple system atrophy: a randomised, double-blind, placebo- controlled trial". *Lancet Neurol* **13**(3):268–75. https://doi.org/10.1016/s1474-4422(13)70301-6

Mahul-Mellier AL, Burtscher J, Maharjan N, Weerens L, Croisier M, Kuttler F *et al.* (2020). "The process of Lewy body formation, rather than simply α-synuclein fibrillization, is one of the major drivers of neurodegeneration". *Proc Natl Acad Sci U S A* **117**(9):4971–82. https://doi.org/10.1073/pnas.1913904117

Mandler M, Valera E, Rockenstein E, Weninger H, Patrick C, Adame A et al. (2014). "Next-generation active immunization approach for synucleinopathies: implications for Parkinson's disease clinical trials". *Acta Neuropathol* **127**(6):861–879. https://doi.org/10.1007/s00401-014-1256-4

Mandler M, Valera E, Rockenstein E, Mante M, Weninger H, Patrick C *et al.* (2015). "Active immunization against alpha-synuclein ameliorates the degenerative pathology and prevents demyelination in a model of multiple system atrophy". *Mol Neurodegener* **10:**10. https://doi.org/10.1186/s13024-015-0008-9

Maroteaux L, Campanelli JT, and Scheller RH (1988). "Synuclein: a neuron-specific protein localized to the nucleus and presynaptic nerve terminal". *J Neurosci* **8**(8):2804–15. https://doi.org/10.1523/jneurosci.08-and 08-02804.1988

Mazzulli JR, Zunke F, Isacson O, Studer L, Krainc D (2016). "α-Synuclein-induced lysosomal dysfunction occurs through disruptions in protein trafficking in human midbrain synucleinopathy models". *Proc Natl Acad Sci U S A* **113**(7):1931–6. https://doi.org/10.1073/pnas.1520335113

McKay JH and Cheshire WP (2018). "First symptoms in multiple system atrophy". *Clin Auton Res* **28**(2):215–21. https://doi.org/10.1007/s10286-017-0500-0

Meissner WG, Traon AP, Foubert-Samier A, Galabova G, Galitzky M, Kutzelnigg A *et al.* (2020). "A phase 1 randomized trial of specific active α-synuclein immunotherapies

PD01A and PD03A in multiple system atrophy". *Mov Disord* **35**(11):1957–65. https://doi.org/10.1002/mds.28218

Novak P, Williams A, Ravin P, Zurkiya O, Abduljalil A, and Novak V (2012). "Treatment of multiple system atrophy using intravenous immunoglobulin. *BMC Neurol* **12**:131. https://doi.org/10.1186/1471-2377-12-131

Numao A, Suzuki K, Miyamoto M, Miyamoto T, and Hirata K (2014). "Clinical correlates of serum insulin-like growth factor-1 in patients with Parkinson's disease, multiple system atrophy and progressive supranuclear palsy". Parkinsonism Relat Disord **20**(2):212–6. https://doi.org/10.1016/j.parkreldis.2013.11.005

Ogaki K, Fujioka S, Heckman MG, Rayaprolu S, Soto-Ortolaza AI, Labbé C *et al.* (2014). "Analysis of COQ2 gene in multiple system atrophy". *Mol Neurodegener* **9:**44. https://doi.org/10.1186/1750- 1326-9-44

Olanow CW, Savolainen M, Chu Y, Halliday GM, and Kordower JH (2019). "Temporal evolution of microglia and α-synuclein accumulation following foetal grafting in Parkinson's disease". *Brain* **142**(6):1690–700. https://doi.org/10.1093/brain/awz104

Ozawa T (2007). "Morphological substrate of autonomic failure and neurohormonal dysfunction in multiple system atrophy: impact on determining phenotype spectrum". *Acta Neuropathol* **114**(3):201–11. https://doi.org/10.1007/s00401-007-0254-1

Ozawa T, Paviour D, Quinn NP, Josephs KA, Sangha H, Kilford L *et al.* (2004). "The spectrum of pathological involvement of the striatonigral and olivopontocerebellar systems in multiple system atrophy: Clinicopathological correlations". *Brain* **127**(Pt 12):2657–71. https://doi.org/10.1093/brain/awh303

Palma JA, Fernandez-Cordon C, Coon EA, Low PA, Miglis MG, Jaradeh S *et al.* (2015). "Prevalence of REM sleep behavior disorder in multiple system atrophy: A multicenter study and meta- analysis". *Clin Auton Res* **25**(1):69–75. https://doi.org/10.1007/s10286-015-0279-9

Papp MI, Kahn JE, and Lantos PL (1989). "Glial cytoplasmic inclusions in the CNS of patients with multiple system atrophy (striatonigral degeneration, olivopontocerebellar atrophy and Shy- Drager syndrome)". *J Neurol Sci* **94**(1–3):79–100. https://doi.org/10.1016/0022- 510x(89)90219-0

Peng C, Gathagan RJ, Covell DJ, Medellin C, Stieber A, Robinson JL *et al.* (2018). "Cellular milieu imparts distinct pathological α-synuclein strains in α-synucleinopathies". *Nature* **557**(7706):558–63. https://doi.org/10.1038/s41586-018-0104-4

Poewe W, Seppi K, Fitzer-Attas CJ, Wenning GK, Gilman S, Low PA *et al.* (2015). "Efficacy of Rasagiline in patients with the parkinsonian variant of multiple system atrophy: A randomised, placebo-controlled trial". *Lancet Neurol* **14**(2):145–52. https://doi.org/10.1016/s1474- 4422(14)70288-1

Poewe W, Volc D, Seppi K, Medori R, Lührs P, Kutzelnigg A *et al.* (2021). "Safety and tolerability of active immunotherapy targeting α-synuclein with PD03A in patients with early Parkinson's disease: a randomized, placebo-controlled, phase 1 study". *J Parkinsons Dis.* https://doi.org/10.3233/jpd-212594

Radford R, Rcom-H'cheo-Gauthier A, Wong MB, Eaton ED, Quilty M, Blizzard C *et al.* (2015). "The degree of astrocyte activation in multiple system atrophy is inversely proportional to the distance to α-synuclein inclusions". *Mol Cell Neurosci* 65:68–81. https://doi.org/10.1016/j.mcn.2015.02.015

Refolo V and Stefanova N (2019). "Neuroinflammation and glial phenotypic changes in alpha- synucleinopathies". *Front Cell Neurosci* **13:**263. https://doi.org/10.3389/fncel.2019.00263

Saccà F, Marsili A, Quarantelli M, Brescia Morra V, Brunetti A, Carbone R *et al.* (2013). "A randomized clinical trial of lithium in multiple system atrophy". *J Neurol* **260**(2):458–61. https://doi.org/10.1007/s00415-012-6655-7

Sailer A, Scholz SW, Nalls MA, Schulte C, Federoff M, Price TR *et al.* (2016). "A genome-wide association study in multiple system atrophy". *Neurology* **87**(15):1591–8. https://doi.org/10.1212/wnl.0000000000003221

Sanchez-Guajardo V, Tentillier N, and Romero-Ramos M (2015). "The relation between α-synuclein and microglia in Parkinson's disease: recent developments". *Neuroscience* **302:**47–58. https://doi.org/10.1016/j.neuroscience.2015.02.008

Scherfler C, Sather T, Diguet E, Stefanova N, Puschban Z, Tison F *et al.* (2005). "Riluzole improves motor deficits and attenuates loss of striatal neurons in a sequential double lesion rat model of striatonigral degeneration (parkinson variant of multiple system atrophy). *J Neural Transm* (Vienna) **112**(8):1025–33. https://doi.org/10.1007/s00702-004-0245-5

Scholz SW, Houlden H, Schulte C, Sharma M, Li A, Berg D *et al.* (2009). "SNCA variants are associated with increased risk for multiple system atrophy". *Ann Neurol* **65**(5):610–4. https://doi.org/10.1002/ana.21685

Schweighauser M, Shi Y, Tarutani A, Kametani F, Murzin AG, Ghetti B *et al.* (2020). "Structures of α- synuclein filaments from multiple system atrophy". *Nature* **585**(7825):464–9. https://doi.org/10.1038/s41586-020-2317-6

Shahnawaz M, Mukherjee A, Pritzkow S, Mendez N, Rabadia P, Liu X *et al.* (2020). "Discriminating α-synuclein strains in Parkinson's disease and multiple system atrophy". *Nature* **578**(7794):273–7. https://doi.org/10.1038/s41586-020-1984-7

Singer W, Dietz AB, Zeller AD, Gehrking TL, Schmelzer JD, Schmeichel AM *et al.* (2019). "Intrathecal administration of autologous mesenchymal stem cells in multiple system atrophy". *Neurology* **93**(1):e77–e87. https://doi.org/10.1212/wnl.0000000000007720

Song YJ, Halliday GM, Holton JL, Lashley T, O'Sullivan SS, McCann H *et al.* (2009). "Degeneration in different parkinsonian syndromes relates to astrocyte type and astrocyte protein expression". *J Neuropathol Exp Neurol* **68**(10):1073–83. https://doi.org/10.1097/NEN.0b013e3181b66f1b

Sorrentino ZA and Giasson BI, Chakrabarty P (2019). "α-Synuclein and astrocytes: tracing the pathways from homeostasis to neurodegeneration in Lewy body disease". *Acta Neuropathol* **138**(1):1–21. https://doi.org/10.1007/s00401-019-01977-2

Spillantini MG, Crowther RA, Jakes R, Cairns NJ, Lantos PL, and Goedert M (1998). "Filamentous alpha-synuclein inclusions link multiple system atrophy with Parkinson's disease and dementia with Lewy bodies". *Neurosci Lett* **251**(3):205–8. https://doi.org/10.1016/s0304-3940(98)00504-7

Spillantini MG and Goedert M (2000.)" The alpha-synucleinopathies: Parkinson's disease, dementia with Lewy bodies, and multiple system atrophy". *Ann N Y Acad Sci* **920:**16–27. https://doi.org/10.1111/j.1749-6632.2000.tb06900.x

Stamler D, Bradbury M, Wong C, and Offman E (2019)."A First in human study of PBT434, a Novel small molecule inhibitor of α-synuclein aggregation (S4.001)". *Neurology* **92**(15 Supplement): S4.001

Stamler D, Bradbury M, Wong C, and Offman E (2020). "A phase 1 study of PBT434, a novel small molecule inhibitor of α-synuclein aggregation, in adult and older adult volunteers (4871)". *Neurology* **94**(15 Supplement):4871

Stefanis L, Larsen KE, Rideout HJ, Sulzer D, and Greene LA (2001). "Expression of A53T mutant but not wild-type alpha-synuclein in PC12 cells induces alterations of the ubiquitin-dependent degradation system, loss of dopamine release, and autophagic cell death". *J Neurosci* **21**(24):9549–60. https://doi.org/10.1523/jneurosci.21-24-09549.2001

Stefanova N (2018). "Translational therapies for multiple system atrophy: Bottlenecks and future directions". *Auton Neurosci* **211**:7–14. https://doi.org/10.1016/j.autneu.2017.09.016

Stefanova N, Tison F, Reindl M, Poewe W, and Wenning GK (2005). "Animal models of multiple system atrophy". *Trends Neurosci* **28**(9):501–6. https://doi.org/10.1016/j.tins.2005.07.002

Stefanova N, Reindl M, Neumann M, Kahle PJ, Poewe W, and Wenning GK (2007). "Microglial activation mediates neurodegeneration related to oligodendroglial alpha-synucleinopathy: Implications for multiple system atrophy". *Mov Disord* **22**(15):2196–203. https://doi.org/10.1002/mds.21671

Stefanova N, Poewe W, and Wenning GK (2008). "Rasagiline is neuroprotective in a transgenic model of multiple system atrophy". *Exp Neurol* **210**(2):421–7. https://doi.org/10.1016/j.expneurol.2007.11.022

Stefanova N, Fellner L, Reindl M, Masliah E, Poewe W, and Wenning GK (2011). "Toll-like receptor 4 promotes α-synuclein clearance and survival of nigral dopaminergic neurons". *Am J Pathol* **179**(2):954–63. https://doi.org/10.1016/j.ajpath.2011.04.013

Stefanova N, Georgievska B, Eriksson H, Poewe W, and Wenning GK (2012). "Myeloperoxidase inhibition ameliorates multiple system atrophy-like degeneration in a transgenic mouse model". *Neurotox Res* **21**(4):393–404. https://doi.org/10.1007/s12640-011-9294-3

Stemberger S, Jamnig A, Stefanova N, Lepperdinger G, Reindl M, and Wenning GK (2011). "Mesenchymal stem cells in a transgenic mouse model of multiple system atrophy: Immunomodulation and neuroprotection". *PLoS ONE* **6**(5):e19808. https://doi.org/10.1371/journal.pone.0019808

Sturm E and Stefanova N (2014). "Multiple system atrophy: Genetic or epigenetic?" *Exp Neurobiol* **23**(4):277–91. https://doi.org/10.5607/en.2014.23.4.277

Sturm E, Fellner L, Krismer F, Poewe W, Wenning GK, and Stefanova N (2016). "Neuroprotection by epigenetic modulation in a transgenic model of multiple system atrophy". *Neurotherapeutics* **13**(4):871–9. https://doi.org/10.1007/s13311-016-0447-1

Tada M, Onodera O, Tada M, Ozawa T, Piao YS, Kakita A *et al.* (2007). "Early development of autonomic dysfunction may predict poor prognosis in patients with multiple system atrophy". *Arch Neurol* **64**(2):256–60. https://doi.org/10.1001/archneur.64.2.256

Trojanowski JQ and Revesz T (2007). "Proposed neuropathological criteria for the post mortem diagnosis of multiple system atrophy". *Neuropathol Appl Neurobiol* **33**(6):615–20. https://doi.org/10.1111/j.1365-2990.2007.00907.x

Ubhi K, Rockenstein E, Mante M, Patrick C, Adame A, Thukral M *et al.* (2008). "Rifampicin reduces alpha-synuclein in a transgenic mouse model of multiple system atrophy". *NeuroReport* **19**(13):1271–6. https://doi.org/10.1097/WNR.0b013e32830b3661

Ubhi K, Rockenstein E, Mante M, Inglis C, Adame A, Patrick C *et al.* (2010). "NeurodegeneArticleration in a transgenic mouse model of multiple system atrophy is associated with altered expression of oligodendroglial-derived neurotrophic factors". *J Neurosci* **30**(18):6236–46. https://doi.org/10.1523/jneurosci.0567-10.2010

Ubhi K, Inglis C, Mante M, Patrick C, Adame A, Spencer B *et al.* (2012). "Fluoxetine ameliorates behavioral and neuropathological deficits in a transgenic model mouse of α-synucleinopathy". *Exp Neurol* **234**(2):405–16. https://doi.org/10.1016/j.expneurol.2012.01.008

Ueda M, Nakamura T, Suzuki M, Imai E, Harada Y, Hara K *et al.* (2020). "Association of orthostatic blood pressure with the symptoms of orthostatic hypotension and cognitive impairment in patients with multiple system atrophy". *J Clin Neurosci* **75:**40–4. https://doi.org/10.1016/j.jocn.2020.03.040

Ulusoy A, Febbraro F, Jensen PH, Kirik D, and Romero-Ramos M (2010). "Co-expression of C- terminal truncated alpha-synuclein enhances full-length alpha-synuclein-induced pathology". *Eur J Neurosci* **32**(3):409–22. https://doi.org/10.1111/j.1460-9568.2010.07284.x

Valera E, Ubhi K, Mante M, Rockenstein E, and Masliah E (2014). "Antidepressants reduce neuroinflammatory responses and astroglial alpha-synuclein accumulation in a transgenic mouse model of multiple system atrophy". *Glia* **62**(2):317–37. https://doi.org/10.1002/glia.22610

Venezia S, Refolo V, Polissidis A, Stefanis L, Wenning GK, and Stefanova N (2017). "Toll-like receptor 4 stimulation with monophosphoryl lipid A ameliorates motor deficits and nigral neurodegeneration triggered by extraneuronal α-synucleinopathy". *Mol Neurodegener* **12**(1):52. https://doi.org/10.1186/s13024-017-0195-7

Vieira BD, Radford RA, Chung RS, Guillemin GJ, and Pountney DL (2015). "Neuroinflammation in multiple system atrophy: response to and cause of α-synuclein aggregation". *Front Cell Neurosci* **9:**437. https://doi.org/10.3389/fncel.2015.00437

Volc D, Poewe W, Kutzelnigg A, Lührs P, Thun-Hohenstein C, Schneeberger A *et al.* (2020). "Safety and immunogenicity of the α-synuclein active immunotherapeutic PD01A in patients with Parkinson's disease: a randomized, single-blinded, phase 1 trial". *Lancet Neurol* **19**(7):591–600. https://doi.org/10.1016/s1474-4422(20)30136-8

Volpicelli-Daley LA, Luk KC, Patel TP, Tanik SA, Riddle DM, Stieber A *et al.* (2011). "Exogenous α- synuclein fibrils induce Lewy body pathology leading to synaptic dysfunction and neuron death". *Neuron* **72**(1):57–71. https://doi.org/10.1016/j.neuron.2011.08.033

Wakabayashi K, Yoshimoto M, Tsuji S, and Takahashi H (1998). "Alpha-synuclein immunoreactivity in glial cytoplasmic inclusions in multiple system atrophy". *Neurosci Lett* **249**(2–3):180–2. https://doi.org/10.1016/s0304-3940(98)00407-8

Wales P, Pinho R, Lázaro DF, and Outeiro TF (*2013*). "Limelight on alpha-synuclein: pathological and mechanistic implications in neurodegeneration". *J Parkinsons' Dis* **3**(4):415–59. https://doi.org/10.3233/jpd-130216

Watts JC, Giles K, Oehler A, Middleton L, Dexter DT, Gentleman SM *et al.* (2013). "Transmission of multiple system atrophy prions to transgenic mice". *Proc Natl Acad Sci U S A* **110**(48):19555– 60. https://doi.org/10.1073/pnas.1318268110

Wenning GK and Quinn NP (1997). "Parkinsonism. Multiple system atrophy". *Baillieres Clin Neurol* **6**(1):187–204

Wenning GK, Tison F, Elliott L, Quinn NP, and Daniel SE (1996). "Olivopontocerebellar pathology in multiple system atrophy". *Mov Disord* **11**(2):157–62. https://doi.org/10.1002/mds.870110207

Wilms H, Rosenstiel P, Romero-Ramos M, Arlt A, Schäfer H, Seegert D *et al.* (2009). "Suppression of MAP kinases inhibits microglial activation and attenuates neuronal cell death induced by alpha- synuclein protofibrils". *Int J Immunopathol Pharmacol* **22**(4):897–909. https://doi.org/10.1177/039463200902200405

Yoshida M (2007). "Multiple system atrophy: alpha-synuclein and neuronal degeneration". *Neuropathology* **27**(5):484–93. https://doi.org/10.1111/j.1440-1789.2007.00841.x

Zella SMA, Metzdorf J, Ciftci E, Ostendorf F, Muhlack S, Gold R *et al.* (2019). "Emerging immunotherapies for Parkinson disease". *Neurol Ther* 8(1):29–44. https://doi.org/10.1007/s40120-018-0122-z

Zhang W, Wang T, Pei Z, Miller DS, Wu X, Block ML *et al.* (2005). "Aggregated alpha-synuclein activates microglia: A process leading to disease progression in Parkinson's disease". *Faseb J* **19**(6):533–42. https://doi.org/10.1096/fj.04-2751com

# Illustrations

## Figures

Chapter Page



## Tables

## Sidebars

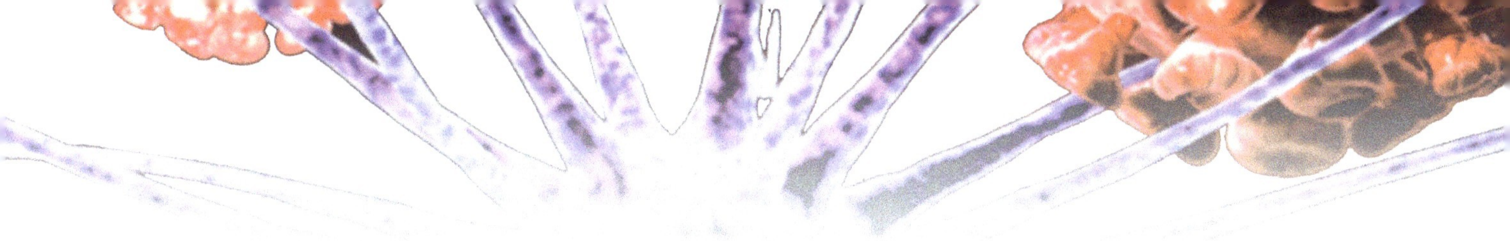

# Glossary

## A

**Abiotrophy:** Premature loss of vitality or degeneration of certain cells or tissues, usually of genetic etiology. Also, a genetic term applied to hereditary degenerative diseases.

**Acetylcholine: Neurotransmitter present in both central (brain and spinal cord) and peripheral nervous systems. In the brain, acetylcholine helps modulate attention, memory, and motivation. In the peripheral nervous system, acetylcholine is the primary neurotransmitter of the parasympathetic division (rest, repair, and regeneration) and is released at the neuromuscular junction of both smooth and skeletal muscles to stimulate contraction.**

**Advance directive: A legal document through which a person dictates the kind of medical care that should be provided in the event that he or she becomes incapable of making those decisions. A living will is a type of advance directive in which the patient details the types of care he or she wishes to receive or not receive. The patient can also name an individual and grant legal authority to that person to make healthcare decisions, known as durable power-of-attorney.**

Advanced Therapy Medicinal Product: **Medicines for human use that are based on genes, tissues or cells. They are highly relevant for the treatment of rare diseases.**

**Adverse Drug Reaction (ADR): A response to a medicinal product which is noxious and unintended. Response in this context means that a causal relationship between a medicinal product and an adverse event is at least a reasonable possibility. Adverse reactions may arise from use of the product within or outside the terms of the marketing authorization or from occupational exposure. Conditions of use outside the marketing authorization include overdose, misuse, abuse, and medication errors.**

**Adverse Event (AE) (or Adverse experience): Any untoward medical occurrence in a patient or clinical-trial subject administered a medicinal product and which does not necessarily have to have a causal relationship with this treatment. An adverse event can therefore be any unfavorable and unintended sign (e.g. an abnormal laboratory finding), symptom, or disease temporally associated with the use of a medicinal product, whether or not it is considered related to the medicinal product.**

**Age of onset: The most common ages for symptoms of a disease to begin.**

**Agonist: A chemical or drug that activates a neurotransmitter receptor, e.g. Dopamine agonists are drugs that imitate the actions of dopamine. Agonists closely mimic the actions of neurotransmitters but are generally less specific and less effective. Examples of dopamine agonists include Pramipexole, Ropinirole, Bromocriptine, and Apomorphine.**

**Aggregate: A clump or tangle of protein molecules, such as alpha-synuclein or tau proteins within neurons in Parkinson's related diseases.**

**Akinesia:** Inability to move ("freezing") or difficulty in beginning or maintaining voluntary movements (e.g., a body motion).

**Alpha-synuclein:** Protein found mainly at the ends of nerve processes in the brain and muscles and thought to control release and recycling of neurotransmitters. Alpha-synuclein accumulates in Multiple System Atrophy (MSA), Parkinson's disease, and Lewy Bodies Disease, and appears to play a key role in disease pathology.

**Alexander's technique:** This technique is a form of complementary therapy, pioneered at the turn of the century by FM Alexander. The principal aim is to teach people to stand and move more efficiently by improving movement awareness. Some MSA patients use it as a form of physical therapy.

**Amantadine:** An antiviral drug that also improves mild parkinsonian symptoms. Thought to stimulate the release of dopamine or inhibit acetylcholine. It is used as a single therapy or with L-DOPA and other medications. It has both an anti-Parkinson's effect and an anti-dyskinesia effect. It is usually not effective for MSA.

**Anhydrosis:** Decreased sweating.

**Anorgasmia:** A persistent, recurrent difficulty, delay in, or absence of attaining orgasm following sufficient sexual stimulation and arousal. Female orgasmic disorder.

**Anosmia:** Total loss of sense of smell. More common in Parkinson's disease than MSA. It occurs due to the accumulation of Lewy bodies.

**Antagonist:** A chemical or drug that blocks a neurotransmitter receptor. Dopamine antagonists can worsen parkinsonian symptoms and cause drug-induced Parkinsonism. Virtually all antipsychotic drugs have dopamine antagonist activity.

**Apathy:** Lack of interest, enthusiasm, or concern. In MSA, it can arise from damage to parts of the basal ganglia that relay with emotional centers in the brain.

**Apomorphine:** A type of dopamine agonist; highly powerful and effective but also causes a range of unpleasant effects, such as nausea, chest pain, dizziness, and fatigue.

**Artane (trihexyphenidyl HCL):** An anticholinergic drug that is often effective at reducing parkinsonian tremor. The most common side effects include anxiety, blurry vision, dry mouth, and nausea. It may also cause confusion.

**Antecollis:** A condition in which the neck bends forward and the head drops down.

**Anticholinergic:** A drug that blocks the action of acetylcholine, a neurotransmitter in the brain. Anticholinergic drugs are often effective in reducing the tremor of Parkinson's disease. In MSA patients, anticholinergics are typically used to treat muscle spasms and bladder control problems. Examples include Benzotropine, Biperidin, Procyclidine, and Scopolamine.

**Antiparkinsonian medication;** A medicine used **for treating symptoms of parkinsonism; mainly Levodopa, Dopamine agonists, and MAO-B inhibitors.**

**Artane (trihexyphenidyl HCL):** An anticholinergic drug that is often effective at reducing parkinsonian tremor. The most common side effects include anxiety, blurry vision, dry mouth, and nausea. It may also cause confusion.

**Astrocytes:** Support cells in the brain that assist neuron growth and repair, regulate communication between neurons, and detect and regulate glucose levels and blood flow in the brain. Also referred to as astroglia.

**Ataxia:** Inability to coordinate voluntary muscle movements, characterized by unsteady movements and staggering gait. A mobility-impairment condition marked by loss of balance and decreased coordination. Inability to coordinate the muscles in the execution of voluntary movement.

**Acute:** Progressive ataxia of cerebellar type developing after severe infections.

**Cerebellar ataxia;** The loss of muscular coordination as a result of disease in the cerebellum.

**Hereditary cerebellar:** A disease of later childhood and early adult life, marked by ataxic gait, hesitating and explosive speech, nystagmus, and sometimes optic neuritis.

**Ocular:** Nystagmus.

**Static:** Inability to preserve the equilibrium in standing through the loss of the deep sensibility.

**ATC: Anatomic, therapeutic, chemical. International system for classification of medicines.**

**Athetosis:** Slow, repetitive, involuntary movements, especially in the hands.

**Atrophy:** A wasting of tissues, organs, or the entire body, as from death and reabsorption of cells, diminished cellular proliferation, pressure, ischemia, malnutrition, decreased function, or hormonal changes.

**Cerebellar:** A degeneration of the cerebellum, particularly the Purkinje cells, as the result of abiototrophy or toxic factors such as alcoholism.

**Olivopontocerebellar:** Relating to the olivary nucleus, the basis pontis, and the cerebellum.

**Autonomic Nervous System (ANS):** Component of the peripheral nervous system that controls involuntary actions such as the heartbeat, the digestive and glandular systems, and smooth muscles of the bladder, bowel, and blood vessels. Consists of two divisions: sympathetic and parasympathetic.

**Autonomic dysfunction:** Any abnormal functioning of the autonomic nervous system resulting in problems with bodily functions such as bowel and bladder control, blood pressure control, sweating, drooling, and so forth.

**Autophagy**: Process whereby cells recycle or dispose of aged or damaged cellular components. Increases when cells are stressed or deprived of nutrients and/or growth factors as a way to regenerate needed substrates. Excessive autophagy can result in the production of dysfunctional organelles and misfolded protein molecules.

**Autosomes/autosomal:** All the chromosomes excluding the sex-related X and Y chromosomes.

**Autosomal recessive:** Passing on of a genetic trait or disease via transmission of two copies of a mutated gene to the offspring, one from each parent. Autosomal recessive inheritance guarantees that the offspring will manifest the trait or disease. MSA typically occurs in individuals with no family history and is not associated with inheritance patterns.

**Axon:** A nerve fiber that carries electrical impulses from the nerve cell body to other neurons or muscles.

## B

**Basal ganglia:** Large clusters of neurons deep within the brain that are responsible for voluntary movements such as walking and movement coordination. Include the caudate nucleus, globus pallidus, striatum, subthalamic nucleus, and the substantia nigra. **Cell death in the substantia nigra contributes to Parkinsonian signs.**

**Big data**: A system of data analysis that devises ways to accommodate data sets that are too large or complex for traditional methods.

**Bilateral surgery:** Surgery performed on both sides of the brain.

**Bilevel Positive Airway Pressure (BIPAP):** A machine that assists patients with sleep-related breathing disorders. Uses a mask-like device that is placed over the nose and mouth. A motor near the patient's bed sends pressurized air through a tube connected to the mask to keep the patient's airways open. The inhalation air pressure delivered by a BIPAP machine can be set to a different level from the exhalation pressure, which improves removal of carbon dioxide compared to that from a CPAP (continuous positive airway pressure) machine, which uses uniform pressure on both phases of respiration. See also CPAP.

**Biomarker:** A chemical substance or imaging finding that is used as an early indicator that a person may have a disease. **A sign that may indicate risk of a disease and improve diagnosis.** A biomarker, if present, could indicate that the person has a disease before symptoms of that disease appear. Currently, no biomarkers have been identified for MSA; however, some researchers have suggested that a characteristic thinning of the retinal nerve fiber layer in MSA patients may qualify as a biomarker.

**Biotechnology: It is** used in two ways: first it describes the traditional biological methods which living organisms use to produce or modify chemical compounds (e.g. antibiotics and vitamins); second, it includes gene technology, which is based on the ability to isolate, replicate, cut and recombine DNA and to transfer DNA from one cell to another. Organisms whose genetic material has been altered in a way that does not occur naturally are called genetically modified organisms (GMOs).

**Blood-brain barrier (BBB): A selective, semi-permeable thin membrane consisting of packed capillary cells and astrocyte nerve endings that separates the central nervous system from the body's blood stream. It filters the blood as**

**it enters the brain and protects the brain from being exposed to potentially harmful substances,** including certain drugs, from entering the brain.

**Braak staging:** A method to classify the degree of pathology in parkinsonian conditions on brain autopsy. Based on the idea that more brain regions contain alpha-synuclein pathology as diseases progresses over time. There is also a (different) Braak staging for Alzheimer's disease.

**Bradykinesia:** The slowing down of initiation of voluntary movement, progressive reduction in speed and amplitude or repetitive actions, and loss of spontaneous and voluntary movement. **It is commonly (but erroneously) used synonymously with akinesia and hypokinesia. Bradykinesia is a clinical hallmark of parkinsonism.**

**Bradyphrenia:** Slowness of thought or information processing common to many brain disorders.

**Brain stem:** The posterior portion of the brain between the cerebral hemispheres and the spinal cord, comprising three sections: medulla oblongata, pons, and midbrain. The brain stem contains centers that command vital functions such as heart and breathing rates, relays information between the brain and spinal cord, maintains consciousness, and regulates sleep and wakefulness cycles. The substantia nigra, which is damaged in MSA, is located in the midbrain of the brain stem.

**Bromocriptine: The generic name of a dopamine agonist drug that can alleviate Parkinson's symptoms. The most common brand name is Parlodel.**

**Bronchopneumonia:** An acute inflammation of the walls of the smaller tubes, with irregular areas of consolidation due to the spread of the inflammation into peribronchiolar alveoli and the alveolar ducts, It may become confluent or may be hemorrhagic. Complications include: necrosis and abscess formation.

## C

**C-Abl: A** gene involved in the processes of cell differentiation, cell division, cell adhesion, and stress response. It is over-active in parkinsonian diseases and implicated in the loss of dopamine- producing neurons.

**Cachexia (or wasting syndrome):** A general lack of nutrition and wasting occurring in the course of a chronic disease or emotional disturbance.

**Calcium:** An essential mineral. Calcium is important for neurological "signaling" and is involved in many chemical reactions within neurons and in mitochondria function. Calcium overload in the substantia nigra has been postulated as one mechanism that could contribute to the death of these neurons.

**Camptocormia:** An abnormal forward-flexed posture (e.g., forward flexion of the spine), which is noticeable when standing or walking but disappears when lying down. It is becoming an increasingly recognized feature of Parkinson's disease and dystonic disorders.

C**arbidopa:** A drug often used in conjunction with Levodopa—as in the drug Sinemet—to increase Levodopa's efficacy by allowing more to reach the brain. Carbidopa blocks the enzyme that converts Levodopa to dopamine in the peripheral tissues, thereby allowing more Levodopa to reach the brain. Carbidopa also reduces Levodopa's unpleasant side effects such as nausea.

**Carer/Care Partner: A name used to describe anyone who provides help or support of any kind to a relative or friend.**

Case manager: **A form of integrated service at an individual level.**

**Caudate nucleus:** A nucleus located in the basal ganglia. It is important in learning and memory as well as motor function. It is one component of the basal ganglia called the striatum. The other component is the putamen. Studies have shown that the caudate nucleus is spared relative to the putamen in MSA.

**Central Nervous System (CNS): Consists of the brain, brain stem, and spinal cord.**

**Centralized Procedure: Since 1995, medicinal products can be evaluated via the Centralized procedure. Medicinal products that have been approved via this procedure are issued a marketing authorization that is valid throughout the EU. This marketing authorization is granted by the European Commission. The use of this procedure is compulsory for medicinal products derived from a biotechnological process, for anticancer treatments, or for medicines to treat diabetes, AIDS/HIV infection, rare diseases, immune diseases, and neurological diseases. For other innovative products, such as products with a new active substance, a company can choose whether to follow this procedure or the Mutual recognition procedure. In the case of the Centralized procedure, a dossier must be submitted to the European Agency for the Evaluation of Medicinal Products (EMA) in London.**

**Cerebellum:** Part of the hindbrain. It coordinates movement. Damage to the cerebellum results in ataxia. In some MSA patients, cerebellar symptoms are more prevalent than parkinsonian symptoms and this type of MSA is designated MSA-C.

**CerebroSpinal Fluid (CSF):** A watery fluid generated within the brain's ventricles. CSF cushions the brain and spinal cord from physical impact and removes waste products as part of the brain's lymphatic system. Small amounts can be harvested in humans by lumbar puncture to measure chemicals coming from the brain.

**Chemokines**: Signaling proteins that are part of the cytokine family and an important component of the inflammatory response. Their activity has been found to be altered in MSA.

**Chorea: A general term for nervous disorders characterized by involuntary, random, jerking movements of muscles in the body, face, or extremities. A type of dystonia.**

**Chronic: (opposite: acute) Chronic diseases are of long-term duration, typically with subtle onset. The term does not imply anything about the severity of a disease.**

**Clinical Trials:** A clinical trial is a research study conducted in human participant volunteers to evaluate the safety and efficacy of a medicine to improve patient's health. Clinical trials conducted on new medicines and sponsored by pharmaceutical companies can only be started after a compound has survived rigorous pre-clinical development work, which involves laboratory testing (chemical/biological/pharmacological/toxicological). It is only when these tests show favorable and promising results that a company can proceed to assess the medicine in humans.

**Coenzyme Q10:** Antioxidant enzyme involved in cellular energy production. Protects nerve cells against oxidative stress and protects against loss of dopamine. Several clinical trials have been completed showing the effectiveness for Parkinson's disease. A phase 2 trial for MSA is currently underway.

**Cognition:** Mental processes including attention, memory, producing and understanding language, solving problems and making decisions.

**Cognitive:** Relating to cognition. Cognitive impairment occurs in some MSA patients, with recent statistics showing a greater prevalence than previously thought.

**Cogwheeling: Also referred to as cogwheel rigidity. Stiffness of the muscles characterized by ratchet- like movements when arms and legs are moved against a resistance. A jerky or ratchet-like sensation felt by a physician when a patient's limb is moved around a joint.**

Colostomy: **The establishment of an artificial cutaneous opening into the colon for fecal incontinence.**

**Compassionate use: The use of a medicinal product available for patients with a chronically, seriously debilitating, or life threatening disease who cannot be treated satisfactorily by an authorized medicinal product or prior to the drug's receiving regulatory approval.**

**Complementary therapies:** These are non-medical treatments, which many people use in addition to conventional medical treatments; examples include Alexander's technique, acupuncture, aromatherapy, music and art therapies, reflexology, and osteopathy.

**Computed Tomography (CT or CAT scan):** A technique that uses a series of X-rays to form image "slices" of the body from different orientations to create a two-dimensional imag. This presentation of images is known as tomography. The term CAT scan (computed axial tomography) refers to a specific orientation of images.

**COMT (catchol-O-methyltransferase) inhibitor**: **One of the enzymes that break down dopamine, adrenaline (also called epinephrine) and noradrenaline (also called norepinephrine).**

**COMT Inhibitor:** A drug that increases dopamine levels by blocking an enzyme that breaks down dopamine. COMT inhibitors include Entacapone (Comtan) and Tolcapone (Tasmar). It is used to treat Parkinson's symptoms.

**Consumer:** A person who is not a healthcare professional such as a patient, lawyer, friend or relative / parent / child of a patient.

**Continuous Dopaminergic Stimulation (CDS):** A therapeutic concept for the management of Parkinson's disease and MSA that proposes that continuous (as opposed to discontinuous or pulsatile) stimulation of striatal dopamine receptors will delay or prevent the onset of Levodopa-related motor complications. It may also be effective for some MSA patients.

**Continuous Positive Airway Pressure (CPAP):** A machine that assists patients with sleep apnea and other conditions in which breathing is impaired during sleep. Uses a mask-like device that is placed over the nose and mouth. A motor near the patient's bed sends pressurized air through a tube connected to the mask to keep the patient's airways open. See also BIPAP.

**Contractures:** The chronic shortening of muscles or tendons around joints in the hands or limbs, which prevents the joints from moving freely.

**Contralateral synkinesis:** An opposite limb action.

**Controlled release drugs**: Drug delivery system whereby the drug is released into the body slowly and steadily rather than all at once. Controlled release maintains a steadier level of the drug in the bloodstream than the 'ordinary' version of the same drug.

**CoQ10 (CoenzymeQ10):** Compound produced by the body and found in all cells. It is vital for energy production and also functions as an antioxidant.

**Cytokines:** A family of small proteins that are secreted by specific cells of the immune system and carry signals locally between cells. Some cytokines are "pro-inflammatory, which is beneficial against infections but may also cause death of the body's own cells whereas other cytokines are "anti-inflammatory". MSA patients tend to have higher levels of pro-inflammatory cytokines.

## D

**DaTscan: A type of neuroimaging that evaluates the brain's dopamine system using a radioactive tracer that attaches to the dopamine transporter molecule in the brain. It can be used to differentiate between parkinsonian syndromes,**

**Deep Brain Stimulation (DBS): A surgical treatment that involves the implantation of a medical device (electrical stimulator) that acts as a brain pacemaker sending electrical impulses to the specific area in which an electrode connected to a programmable power source inserted in the chest wall (similar to a cardiac pacemaker). was implanted. In Parkinson's patients, the device is typically inserted in either the subthalamic nucleus or the globus pallidus, depending upon the specific problem.**

**Dementia:** A decline in cognitive function due to damage or disease in the brain beyond what might be expected from normal aging. Areas particularly affected include memory, attention, judgment, language, planning and problem solving.

**Dendrites:** (from Greek meaning, "tree") Highly branched nerve fibers that project from the nerve cell body and receive incoming signals from other neurons and convert these chemical signals into electrical ones that travel to the nerve cell body.

**Deprenyl:** The generic name of the drug that inhibits the enzyme monoamine oxidase type B (MAO- B), thereby increasing the level of dopamine in the brain. The most common side effects include nausea, dizziness, insomnia, agitation, and confusion.

**Depression: Feelings of sadness and/or a loss of interest in activities once enjoyed. It can decrease one's ability to function in daily activities.**

**Depression can be a clinical symptom of MSA due to cognitive impairment and/or emotional stresses imposed by the disease.**

**Diagnosis: The i**dentification or naming of a disease by its signs and symptoms.

**Disease: An illness; sickness; an interruption, cessation, or disorder of body functions, systems, or organs. A disease entity characterized usually by at least two of these criteria: a recognizable etiologic agent (or agents) and an identifiable group of signs and symptoms, or consistent anatomical alterations. (see also disorder, syndrome).**

**Disease modification**: Treatments or interventions that affect the underlying pathological processes of a disease and have a beneficial outcome on the course of the disease.

**Disequilibrium:** Unsteadiness or balance problems.

**Disorder: A disturbance of function, structure, or both resulting from a genetic or embryologic failure in development, or from exogenous factors such a poison, injury, or disease. (See also disease; syndrome.)**

**DJ-1:** A protein that inhibits alpha-synuclein aggregation and reduces oxidative stress. Mutations in the gene that codes for DJ-1 cause an autosomal recessive form of Parkinson's disease.

**Dopamine:** One of the brain's neurotransmitters that is involved in motivation, learning, and motor function (movement, balance, and walking). It is produced by cells within the substantia nigra. These cells project to the striatum in the basal ganglia. Deficiency of dopamine in the striatum due to the death of cells in the substantia nigra causes symptoms of parkinsonism.

**Dopamine agonist:** A compound other than dopamine that activates dopamine receptors. Examples include drugs such as Bromocriptine mesylate (Parlodel), Pergolide (Permax), Pramipexole (Mirapex), Ropinirole hydrochloride (Requip), Piribedil, Cabergoline, Apomorphine (Apokyn), Rotigotine (Neupro patch) and Lisuride. Dopamine agonists are the second most powerful type of anti-Parkinson medication after Levodopa. They can cause side effects such as sleepiness, sleep attacks, ankle swelling, hallucinations and impulse control problems, more commonly than Levodopa does.

**Dopaminergic pathways**: Neural pathways in the brain which utilize dopamine as their neuro- transmitter. There are four major groups:

- Nigrostriatal: Connects the substantia nigra to the striatum. Involved heavily in Parkinson's.
- Mesocortical: Connects the ventral tegmental area (adjacent to the substantia nigra) to the cerebral cortex. Closely associated with the mesolimbic pathway. Can cause hallucinations and schizophrenia if not functioning properly.
- Mesolimbic: Connects ventral tegmental area to areas involved in memory, motivation, emotional response, reward and addiction.
- **Tuberoinfundibular: from hypothalamus to pituitary gland involved in hormonal regulation, maternal behavior (nurturing), pregnancy and sensory processes.**

**Drug Repurposing**: Application of drugs for potential use with conditions other than those they were originally approved to treat.

**dx (dx'd):** Diagnosed (e.g. d5 is diagnosed 5 years ago).

**Dysarthria:** Impaired speech function. **A** general description referring to a neurological speech disorder characterized by poor articulation. Slurred or otherwise impaired speech. Depending on the involved neurological structures, dysarthria may be further classified as spastic, flaccid, ataxic, hyper/hypokinetic, or mixed.

**Dysautonomia (autonomic disorder):** A Functional abnormality of the autonomic nervous system. A disorder affecting the function of the autonomic division of the nervous system, which controls automatic functions necessary for life, such as heart and respiratory rate, blood pressure, and bowel and bladder function. Symptoms include dizziness, difficulty swallowing, blurred vision, orthostatic hypotension, constipation, and urinary Incontinence. Dysautonomia is a defining characteristic of MSA and is present to varying degrees in Parkinson's disease and numerous other conditions.

**Dyschezia: Constipation.**

**Dysequilibrium:** Unsteadiness or balance problems.

**Dyskinesia:** An involuntary movement disorder, also sometimes called hyperkinesia. Characterized by lurching, dance-like or jerky movements that are distinct from the rhythmic tremor commonly associated with Parkinson's disease. Often occurs as a side effect of long-term Levodopa therapy and can affect a single body part or the entire body. In MSA, dyskinesias often occur in the face, neck, or limbs.

**Dysphagia:** Difficulty in swallowing.

**Dystonia**: Abnormal and awkward posture or sustained movements of a hand, foot, or other part of the body. May be accompanied by rigidity and twisting. Persistent or sudden intermittent muscle contractions causing abnormal posture and/or rigid or twisting movements. Dystonias associated with MSA include antecollis – a forward flexion of the neck, diurnal laryngeal stridor, which affects the vocal cords, and dystonias of the mouth and face.

**Axial (or Truncal):** A type of dystonia that affects the midline muscles, i.e., the chest, abdominal cavity, and back muscles.

## E

**Eldepryl:**. The brand name for the version of Deprenyl, also known as Selegiline, an MAO-B inhibitor used to treat Parkinson's disease and MSA. Manufactured by Somerset Pharmaceuticals.

**Embryonic stem (ES) cell:** See stem cell.

**Encephalitis**: Inflammation of the brain. See neuroinflammation.

**Enzyme: A protein that catalyzes or speeds up chemical reactions.**

**Epitope (also known as antigenic determinant): The part of an antigen that is recognized by the immune system, specifically by antibodies, B-cells, or T-cells. Although epitopes are usually non-self proteins, sequences**

**derived from the host that can be recognized (as in the case of autoimmune diseases) are also epitopes. (See also paratope.)**

**Essential tremor:** A rapid tremor (about eight cycles per second) that is most pronounced when performing an action such as writing or bringing a hand to a target.

**Executive Dysfunction:** A deficit in executive functioning that may occur in Parkinson's dementia. Executive functioning allows the completion of tasks using higher level mental skills such as planning, organization, memory, flexible thinking, and self-regulation.

**Exosome:** Small spherical structures consisting of proteins, lipids, DNA, enclosed in cellular membrane. Exosomes are released by cells into surrounding tissues and bodily fluids such as blood, urine, and CSF. They may serve as a means of intercellular communication and molecular transport.

**Extraordinary means: Ways of continuing human life that go beyond simple nutrition and hydration (even if that nutrition or hydration is provided via a feeding tube and the like. See ordinary means.**

## F

**Festination:** An involuntary quickening of the gait and shuffling after starting to walk. It is characterized by short, accelerated steps combined with forward flexion of the torso; literally means "chasing the center of gravity".

**Free radicals:** Reactive molecules that form from the oxidation, or breakdown, of other molecules.

**Freezing:** A inability of Parkinson's patients to move that frequently occurs at a boundary such as a door or when exiting a car.

**Freezing of Gait (FOG)**: The sudden brief, abrupt and temporary inability of Parkinson's patients to walk or to continue walking; frequently occurs at a boundary such as a door or when exiting a car.

**Functional Magnetic Resonance Imaging (fMRi): An imaging technique designed specifically for the brain. It measures the rate at which oxygen is removed from the blood to the cells, therefore suggesting the activity of a particular area of the brain.**

## G

**Gait: The manner of walking.**

Antalgic: **Resulting from pain on weight bearing in which the stance phase of gait is shortened on the affected side.**

Ataxic: **An unsteady, staggering, or irregular gait.**

Calcaneal: **A gait disturbance due to paralysis of the calf muscles, seen following poliomyelitis and other neurologic diseases.**

Cerebellar: **A staggering gait, often with a tendency to fall to one or other side, forward or backward.**

Charcot's: **The gait of hereditary ataxia.**

Festinating: **See festination.**

**GABA (gamma amino butyric acid):** The principal inhibitory neurotransmitter in human brain. GABA-producing neurons are concentrated in the basal ganglia, substantia nigra, and cerebellum.

**GBA (Glucocerebrosidase):** An enzyme involved in maintaining cell membrane stability, cellular immune response, and intercellular bonds. Mutations in the GBA gene are associated with Parkinson's disease and MSA.

**GDNF:** Glial Cell line derived nerve growth factor. See growth factors.

**Gene therapy:** The insertion of genes into an individual's cells and tissues to treat hereditary diseases where deleterious mutant alleles can be replaced with functional ones. The genes are usually placed within a non-pathogenic virus, which serves as the vector to penetrate the cells. Gene therapy can also be used to correct non-genetic deficiencies such as the loss of dopamine in MSA, to modify the function of a group of cells (e.g. convert an excitatory structure to one that is inhibitory) or to provide a source of growth factors.

**Genetic:** Referring to genes, the inherited code ("DNA") for human structure and function.

**Genetic predisposition:** The inherited genetic pattern that may make some individuals more prone to certain conditions than others with a different genetic makeup.

**Genotype:** The collection of genetic material in an organism that gives rise to its characteristics.

**Glia:** Non-neural cells, commonly called neuroglia or simply glia (Greek for "glue"), that maintain homeostasis, form myelin, and provide support and protection for the brain's neurons. Astrocytes are one kind of glial cells.

**Gliosis: The proliferation of astrocytes in damaged areas of the central nervous system, forming a scar termed a glial scar.**

**Globus pallidus:** A component of the basal ganglia involved in movement control. It is split into two main parts: the internal globus pallidus (GPi), which, seems to be more affected, as evidenced by lower neuronal firing rates, in MSA than in Parkinson's disease and the external globus pallidus (GPe), which is equally affected in the two conditions.

**Glucose**: A simple sugar that is an important energy source in living organisms and is a component of many carbohydrates.

**Glutamate:** An amino acid and the main excitatory neurotransmitter in the human brain. The major input to the striatum is from the cerebral cortex and uses glutamate as a neurotransmitter. Excess glutamate is toxic to neurons and if the neurotransmitter is not well regulated can result in neuronal cell death.

**Glycation**: The bonding of a sugar molecule to a protein or lipid molecule without enzymatic regulation causing the bonded molecules to be non-functional. Glycation products accumulate in cells and cause damage.

**Glycosylceramide:** A type of cerebroside. Cerebrosides are important components of muscle and nerve cell membranes.

**Growth factors:** Naturally occurring substances (usually proteins) that help maintain the health of neurons and encourage cell growth, proliferation and differentiation. Some growth factors are being looked at to try to promote the survival of the neural cells that are affected in MSA and Parkinson's.

**Gut microbiome: The complex community of microorganisms that live in the digestive tracts of humans and other animals. Alterations in the gut microbiome have been noted in MSA patients and may be associated with increased inflammation and intestinal permeability, leading to absorption of neurotoxins.**

## H

**Healthcare professional: For the purposes of reporting suspected adverse reactions, healthcare professionals are defined as medically qualified persons, such as physicians, dentists, pharmacists, nurses, and coroners.**

**Health technology assessment: The assessment of whether a medicine is effective and cost effective in comparison to existing medicines available with the ultimate goal to have authorized medicines available, affordable, and accessible for rare disease patients.**

**Heterogeneity: The variable appearance of a condition.** Lacking uniformity in composition or character (as opposed to homogeneity, which is uniformity in composition or character).

**Hippocampus:** A complex neural structure (shaped like a sea horse) located in the temporal lobes of the brain. It is involved in memory storage, motivation and emotion as part of the limbic system.

**HMP:** Within the European Medicines Agency (EMA), the Committee for Human Medicinal Products is the scientific committee responsible for preparing the Agency's opinions on questions relating to the evaluation of medicinal products for human use.

**Hospice:** A type of non-curative, palliative approach to care given to terminally-ill patients for whom t here are no further viable options for long-term disease management. Hospice care is meant to reduce suffering as well as address a patient's emotional and spiritual needs.

**Hyperkinesia:** An abnormal increase in movement and/or muscle activity; sometimes used synonymously with dyskinesia.

**Hypokinesia:** Literally means reduced amplitude or/and number of movements. It is commonly used synonymously (but erroneously) with akinesia and bradykinesia.

**Hypomimia: Immobile, expressionless face with reduced blinking.**

**Hyposmia:** Diminished sense of smell.

**Hypothalamic Pituitary Adrenal (HPA) axis:** A network of feedback loops within three components of the endocrine system: the hypothalamus, pituitary gland, and the adrenal cortex. The HPA axis has a wide range of functions from stimulating the stress response to controlling digestion, the immune system, mood, sexuality and energy storage and consumption.

**Hypothalamus: A component of the brain that acts as a relay between the nervous system and the endocrine system. Important in maintaining hormone balance, body temperature, sleep cycles, and other aspects of homeostasis.**

## I

**Idiopathic:** Arising from an unknown cause.

**Immunotherapy** (or **biological therapy**)**:** The treatment of disease by activating or suppressing the immune system. Immunotherapies designed to elicit or amplify an immune response are classified as activation immunotherapies, while immunotherapies that reduce or suppress are classified as suppression immunotherapies.

**Impotence:** Inability to achieve or maintain an erection.

**Impulse control disorder (ICD):** A set of psychiatric disorders characterized by an inability to control one's actions, in particular those that might bring harm to oneself or others. Common ICDs in patients receiving dopamine agonists are pathologic gambling, compulsive eating, compulsive shopping, and hypersexuality.

**Informed consent:** The concept of informed consent (required to participate in clinical trials and sometimes for compassionate use) is based on the principle that a physician/doctor has the duty to disclose information to the patient (e.g. potential risks, benefits, and alternatives) that allows the patient to make reasonable decision regarding his or her treatment on a compassionate basis.

**Inherited form:** Can be passed down through families.

**Interdisciplinary care**: Multiple healthcare professionals collaborating to provide care with a common perspective, often involving joint consultations.

**iPS Cells:** Stem cells that can be generated directly from adult cells. See stem cells.

## L

**Learned voluntary movements: Movements that we learn to do, like walking and talking.**

**Lesion:** An area of cell damage or cell death.

**Levodopa (L-Dopa): (brand name is Sinemet in the U.S.) A precursor to dopamine (a chemical messenger in the brain responsible for smooth, coordinated movement, and other motor and cognitive functions. It can pass through the blood-brain barrier (whereas dopamine cannot). It helps restore dopamine levels in the brain. It is the most commonly administered drug for treating Parkinson's symptoms.**

**Lewy bodies:** Abnormal structures seen in dead or dying dopamine-producing cells of the substantia nigra in Parkinson's disease. They are frequently the most precise way to diagnose Parkinson's. They form aggregates of alpha-synuclein proteins in several brain regions, including the substantia nigra and locus ceruleus. It is a pathologic hallmark and distinguishing feature among parkinsonian conditions. In Parkinson's disease and dementia with Lewy bodies, the deposits accumulate within dopamine-producing nerve cells, while, in MSA, the deposits occur in glial cells.

**Linked clinical trials (LCT):** An international initiative to find potential drugs for treating a given disease from among existing drugs that are approved for other diseases. A designated scientific committee meets annually to choose which drugs to recommend for fast-tracking into clinical trials.

## M

**Magnetic Resonance Imaging (MRI):** A noninvasive medical imaging technique to visualize detailed internal structure and function of the body. MRI provides much greater contrast between the different soft tissues of the body than computed tomography (CT), making it especially useful in neurological (brain), musculoskeletal, cardiovascular, and oncological (cancer-related) imaging.

**Masking:** Also known as facial masking. A symptom in Parkinsonian conditions caused by loss of control of the facial muscles leading to a mask-like expression.

**MAO (MonoAmine Oxidase):** A family of enzymes that catalyze the breakdown of amine molecules, including some neurotransmitters. There are two MAO subtypes, with groups of drugs that target each:

**MAO-A inhibitors:** Drugs that inhibit the MAO-A enzyme, which is responsible for the metabolism of dietary tyramine. MAO-A inhibitors can cause tyramine-induced hypertension, the so-called "cheese effect" because tyramine can be found in high concentrations in some soft cultured cheeses.

**MAO-B inhibitors:** These drugs (e.g. Selegiline, Rasagiline) inhibit the breakdown of dopamine via MAO-B enzyme and do not cause the "cheese effect" of hypertension.

**Medication Error:** Any unintentional error in the prescribing, dispensing, or administration of a medicinal product while in the control of the healthcare professional, patient or consumer.

Mesenchyme: A type of loosely organized animal embryonic connective tissue of undifferentiated cells that give rise to most tissues, such as skin, blood or bone. The interactions between mesenchyme and epithelium help to form nearly every organ in the developing embryo.

**Microbiome:** The collection of microbes (bacteria, viruses, fungi) and their genetic material that live in or on the human body. See gut microbiome.

**Microelectrodes:** Thin metallic tubes inserted into the brain and guided stereotactically (surgically) to the target location. They are connected to the operating room computer and used to measure the electrical signal from brain cells during surgical procedures, such as pallidotomy.

**Microglia**: A type of glial cell. It provides the first immune defense mechanism in the brain and central nervous system. Widespread activation of microglia is associated with neuroinflammatory changes in the early stages of MSA.

**Micrographia:** The tendency to have very small, cramped handwriting due to difficulty with fine motor movements in Parkinson's disease.

**Mild Cognitive Impairment (MCI):** A decline in memory or intellectual functioning that is not as severe as that found in dementia.

**Mirapex:** The brand name of a dopamine agonist, Pramipexole, made by Pharmacia. It has been used in MSA patients who do not respond well to Levodopa.

**Mitochondria:** A specialized cell structure that contains genetic material and many enzymes important for metabolism, including those responsible for the conversion of food to usable energy.

**Mitophagy**: The selective degradation of mitochondria by autophagy. (See Mitochondria and Autophagy.)

**Monoamine oxidase inhibitors:** Drugs that enhance the effect of dopamine by inhibiting the enzymes that break them down. (See MAO.)

**Motor skills:** The degree of control or coordination provided by brain control of the skeletal muscles.

**Motor symptoms:** Symptoms that involve movement, coordination, physical tasks or mobility. These include, among others: resting tremor, bradykinesia, rigidity, postural instability, freezing, micrographia, mask-like expression, unwanted accelerations, stooped posture, dystonia, impaired motor dexterity and coordination, speech problems, difficulty swallowing, muscle cramping, and drooling of saliva. (See also non-motor symptoms.)

**Movement disorders:** Refers to several conditions, many of them neurodegenerative, that prevent normal movement. Some are characterized by either lack of movement (bradykinesia, hypokinesia, etc) or excessive movement (chorea, athetosis, dystonia, tremor). Besides Parkinson's, other conditions often defined as movement disorders include essential tremor, multiple system atrophy, progressive supranuclear palsy, Huntington's disease, Tourette's syndrome and cerebral palsy.

**Movement Disorder Specialist (MDS):** A neurologist who has special training and experience with movement disorders such as MSA.

**MPTP (N-methyl-4-phenyl-1,2,3,6-tetrahydropyridine): A precursor of the neurotoxin known as MPP+ that is taken up in dopamine nerve terminals and damages dopamine-producing cells. MPTP is catalyzed to MPP+ by MAO-B. MPTP is widely used to create an animal model of Parkinsonism by depleting substantia nigra dopamine neurons.**

**Multidisciplinary care**: Care given by multiple healthcare professionals each approaching the patient from their professional perspective, often involving separate, individual consultations.

**Multiple organ dysfunction:** The repetition of organ difficult or abnormal function several times, occurring in several parts at the same time.

**Multiple System Atrophy (MSA):** Formerly known as Shy-Drager syndrome, a progressive neurodegenerative disorder of dopamine-producing cells that affects autonomic (involuntary) and motor functions. Considered a form of parkinsonism, symptoms of MSA typically manifest between the ages of 50-60 years. Common autonomic symptoms include postural hypotension, irregular heartbeat, bowel and bladder incontinence, inability to control body temperature, sleep disorders, sexual dysfunction, and loss of emotional control. Two forms are recognized depending on the symptom pattern:

**MSA-P (Parkinsonian type):** Symptoms are predominantly similar to those of Parkinson's disease and include muscle rigidity, slowness of movement (bradykinesia), postural changes, and balance problems.

**MSA-C (Cerebellar type):** Symptoms are mostly related to problems with muscle coordination and balance and include ataxia (unsteady gait), slurred speech, blurred vision, and problems with swallowing.

**Multiple System Proteinopathy (MSP):** The absence of proteins in numerous systems. It is a more common muscle-wasting syndrome than multiple system atrophy..

**Myeloneuritis:** Neuritis combined with spinal cord inflammation.

## N

**Name of the medicinal product:** The name which may be either an invented name not liable to confusion with the common name, or a common or scientific name accompanied by a trade mark or the name of the marketing authorization holder. The common name is the international non-proprietary name (INN) recommended by the World Health Organization (WHO) or, if one does not exist, the usual common name. **The complete name of the medicinal product is the name of the medicinal product followed by the strength and pharmaceutical form.**

Neuritis: **Inflammation of a nerve marked by neuralgia, hyperesthesia, anesthesia, or paresthesia, paralysis, muscular atrophy in the region supplied by the affected nerve, and by abolition of the reflexes.**

Optic: **Inflammation of the nerves supplying the eyes.**

**Neurodegeneration:** Refers to conditions such as MSA that are characterized by the progressive loss of neurons, particularly those in the brain.

**Neurodegenerative disease:** Disease causing the progressive loss of nerve cells in the brain. Refers to conditions such as Parkinson's disease that are characterized by the loss of cells in the central nervous system.

**Neuroinflammation**: Swelling of the tissue of the nervous system. May be initiated in response to a number of triggers including infection, traumatic brain injury, toxic metabolites, or autoimmunity. Microglia are the immune cells of the nervous system that are activated in response to these cues.

**Neurological conditions**: Disorders caused by damage to or malfunctioning of the brain or nervous system.

**Neurologist: A physician specializing in diseases and disorders of the brain, spinal cord, nerves, and muscles, including stroke, Parkinson's disease, epilepsy, and Alzheimer's disease, and muscular dystrophy.**

**Neurology:** A branch of medicine dealing with the diagnosis and treatment of disorders of the nervous system.

**Neuromodulator:** A chemical substance other than a neurotransmitter, released by a neuron at a synapse (juncture) with another neuron and either enhances or dampens the activity of the target neuron.

**Neuromyelitis:** Inflammation of the bone marrow.

**Optica (Devic's disease):** Inflammation of the optic nerve. A demyelinating disorder associated with transverse myelopathy and optic neuritis.

**Neuron: The fundamental unit of the brain and nervous system. body.** A nerve cell that transmit information within the central nervous system through electrochemical signals to other cells or to muscles. It consists of a cell body, dendrites that convey information from other nerves toward the cell body, and an axon that conveys information away from the cell.

**Neuroplasticity:** The ability of the brain to change and form new connections even with aging. Involves neurons regenerating anatomically or functionally after partial injury, or changing (such as by making more numerous or more effective connections) in response to training and experience.

**Neuroprotection:** Mechanisms within the nervous system that would protect neurons from dying due to a degenerative disease or from other types of injury.

**Neuroprotective**: Serving to protect neurons from injury or degeneration or an effect that may result in salvage, recovery or regeneration of the nervous system, its cells, structure, and function.

**Neuropsychology:** The study of how the structure and function of the brain influence behavior and cognition.

**Neuroscience:** The scientific study of the nervous system that deals with the anatomy, biochemistry, molecular biology, and physiology of neurons and neural circuits.

**Neurosurgeon:** A doctor who specializes in surgical treatment of the brain and central nervous system.

**Neurotransmitter:** A chemical messenger in the nervous system that carries impulses permitting communication between two neuronal cells, often but not always across a synapse. The neurotransmitter is usually released from the nerve terminals on the axons. Examples of neurotransmitters include dopamine, acetylcholine, adrenaline, noradrenaline, serotonin, glutamate, and GABA.

**Neurotrophic factors**: A family of biomolecules that support the growth, survival, and differentiation of both developing and mature neurons.

**Non-motor symptoms:** Symptoms that do not involve movement, coordination, physical tasks or mobility. May include impaired sense of smell, constipation, sleep disturbances, mood disorders, orthostatic hypotension, bladder problems, sexual problems, excessive saliva, weight loss or gain, vision and dental problems, fatigue, depression, fear and anxiety, skin problems, and cognitive issues.

**Nystagmus:** Rhythmical oscillation of the eyeballs, either pendular or jerky.

## O

**Objective measurements:** The repetition of a unit amount that maintains its size, within an allowable range of error, no matter which instrument, intended to measure the variable of interest, is used and no matter who or what relevant person or thing is measured.

**Occupational Therapist (OT)**: An allied health professional trained to assess a person's home or work environment and devise ways to make them more manageable and less hazardous. An OT also works with patients to improve fine motor skills, as needed, as they apply to everyday activities such as dressing, writing, computer use, etc.

Off-label use: **The use of a medicine prescribed for a use different from what is authorized on the label.**

**Olfactory dysfunction:** An impaired ability to detect odors, impaired sense of smell. Thought to be an early sign of MSA but can occur in many situations not related to MSA.

**On-Off phenomenon:** A sudden loss of activity of Levodopa lasting minutes to hours after a brief period of effectiveness. The term also sometimes refers to a cyclical response to medication where the patient can function adequately at times but is too stiff and immobile to function at other times.

**Ordinary means:** Methods of preserving life that are commonly accessible, subject to widely accepted social norms for moral and obligatory measures, and in which there is reasonable expectation of successful outcome. Nutrition and hydration, are considered by some to be ordinary means. (For Catholics, the church requires members to provide nutrition and hydration, even by way of a feeding tube as along as the patient can *assimilate* such nutrition or hydration.)

**Orphan medicines:** Medicines not developed or marketed by the pharmaceutical industry because the high cost of bringing them to market may not be recovered by their. They are intended for the diagnosis, prevention or treatment of rare diseases.

**Orthostatic hypotension:** A sudden drop in blood pressure (>20 mm Hg systolic) when a person goes from lying down to sitting or from sitting to standing and accompanied by symptoms such as dizziness, fatigue, and syncope. Can occur as a complication of certain medications, but can sometimes be due to MSA itself.

**Oxidative stress:** Accumulation of free radicals within a cell, leading to cell damage.

## P

**Palliative care:** A collaborative approach to care involving healthcare professionals from multiple specialty areas to minimize pain and suffering and maximize quality of life for patients with life-threatening illnesses.

P**allidotomy:** A surgical procedure in which lesions are produced in the globus pallidus region of the brain in an effort to lessen Parkinson's symptoms such as tremors, rigidity, and bradykinesia.

**Generally associated with poor clinical outcomes in MSA patients.**

**Palsy:** Antiquated term referring to paralysis or an uncontrollable shaking of the body. Often used to connote partial paralysis or paresis. Parkinson's disease was originally called the "shaking palsy".

**Cerebral:** Defect of motor power and coordination related to damage of the brain.

**Paradoxical kinesia:** A characteristic of parkinsonian conditions in which an individual who experiences difficulty performing a simple movement may be able to perform a more complex movement.

**Paralysis agitans:** Antiquated name for Parkinson's disease.

**Paratope: The part of an antibody that binds to the epitope. (See also epitope.)**

**Parkinsonian gait: A slow, short paced gait with a tendency to shuffle, associated with decreased arm swing.**

**Parkinsonism:** A group of neurological diseases whose features include slowness and paucity of spontaneous movement (bradykinesia), resting tremors, rigidity of the muscles, loss of postural reflexes, flexed posture and freezing of gait. Several conditions cause these signs and symptoms, including Parkinson's disease, dementia with Lewy bodies, progressive supranuclear palsy, and multiple system atrophy. Also associated with Parkinson-like side effects. A number of medications produce this appearance.

**Parkinson-plus syndromes: A group of neurodegenerative diseases featuring the classical features of Parkinsonism (rigidity, akinesia/ bradykinesia, postural instability and less commonly tremor) with additional features that distinguish them from typical Parkinson's disease. Parkinson-plus syndromes include MSA, progressive supranuclear palsy (PSP), and corticobasal degeneration (CBD).**

**Parlodel: The brand name for the dopamine agonist Bromocriptine that is made by Novartis.**

**Pathogenesis: The underlying biologic mechanism responsible for a disease.**

**Peduncutolomy: The partial resection of the pyramidal tract either at the primary motor cortex or at the cerebral crus.**

**PEG (Percutaneous Endoscopic Gastrostomy):** A procedure in which a feeding tube is passed into the stomach through the abdominal wall.

**PEG-tube: Feeding tube used in a percutaneous endoscopic gastrostomy.**

**Pergolide:** The generic name of a Dopamine agonist used to treat Parkinson's disease. The brand name is Permax.

**Peripheral Nervous System:** The nervous system outside the brain and spinal cord, comprising two divisions:

- **Somatic nervous system** – includes sensory nerves and motor nerves involved with voluntary movement.
- **Autonomic nervous system – includes nerves involved with automatic functions such as the heartbeat, the digestive and glandular systems, and smooth muscles of the bladder, bowel, and blood vessels. Consists of two divisions: sympathetic and parasympathetic.**

**Permax:** The brand name for the dopamine agonist Pergolide that is made by Eli Lilly.

**PET scan: An acronym for "positron emission tomography", an imaging technique used to monitor and produce pictures of metabolic or biochemical activity in the brain.**

**Pharmacovigilance: The science and activities related to the detection, assessment, understanding, prevention of adverse effects or any other medicine-related problem, and reporting of side effects of a medicine, together with measures to minimize these risks. In line with this general definition, underlying objectives of the applicable EU legislation for pharmacovigilance are:**

- **Preventing harm from adverse reactions in humans arising from the use of authorized medicinal products within or outside the terms of marketing authorization or from occupational exposure; and**
- **Promoting the safe and effective use of medicinal products, in particular through providing timely information about the safety of medicinal products to patients, healthcare professionals and the public.**

**Pharmacovigilance is, therefore, an activity contributing to the protection of patients' and public health..**

**Pharmacovigilance glossary: A glossary of terms covering topics including adverse reactions and pharmacovigilance.**

**Phenotype:** The observable characteristics of an organism or person, such as appearance, development and behavior. Determined by the interaction between the genotype and the environment.

**Phosphorylation:** A process that modifies proteins by adding one or more phosphate groups. For proteins that function as enzymes, this results in activating or deactivating their function.

**PhysioTherapist (PT)**: An allied health professional trained to use physical means such as exercise and manipulation to help prevent or reduce stiffness in joints and restore muscle strength. PT's can also advise on aids and equipment to help with movement problems.

**Pill-rolling tremor: A characteristic tremor in Parkinson's, uncommon in MSA patients, in which the thumb and forefinger involuntarily move in a way that resembles rolling a small object such as a pill.**

**Pisa syndrome:** An abnormal posture in which the body appears to be leaning to one side like the Leaning Tower of Pisa.

**Placebo:** A simulated or inert form of treatment used in clinical trials along with the active drug being tested. Health professionals and/or participants involved in the trial do not know who receives the placebo or the drug. The difference in responses between the placebo and the drug is considered the true effect of the active drug. It is thought that benefits experienced from placebos, termed the 'placebo effect' may, in part, be associated with release of dopamine in the brains of patients who believe that they have received an active drug.

**Positron Emission Tomography (PET): A medical imaging technique in which radioactive isotopes are incorporated into a chemically active compound utilized by an organ in the body. The isotopes emit gamma rays that are detected by a special camera/scanner. A computer then generates an image to illustrate the location of the active compound in the organ being**

**studied. It produces pictures of metabolic or biochemical activity in the brain.**

PET scan: **In a PET scan of the brain, the compound fluorodeoxyglucose (FDG), is used to measure regional glucose metabolism. F-DOPA, a radioactive form of L-DOPA is another compound used in PET scans of the brain. F-DOPA is taken up in dopamine nerve terminals. The amount of uptake serves as a measure of the integrity of these nerve terminals.**

**Postural instability: A tendency to fall or the inability to keep oneself from falling; imbalance. The** retropulsion test is widely regarded as the gold standard to evaluate postural instability.

Difficulty with balance and inability to maintain stability while standing. One of the major motor symptoms of Parkinson's disease and MSA.

Priapism: **A painful or prolonged erection lasting 4 or more hours.**

**Prodromal: Referring to early signs or symptoms of a disease that manifest before the development of** definitive diagnostic signs and symptoms. In MSA, prodromal non-motor symptoms, such as sleep problems, respiratory problems, and other signs of autonomic failure may appear months to years before the onset of motor symptoms.

**Prognosis:** The expected future course of an illness.

**Progressive Supranuclear Palsy (PSP):** A rare degenerative brain disorder of unknown cause that causes progressive problems with control of gait and balance, along with complex eye movement and cognitive problems. A classic manifestation of the disease is the inability to move the eyes properly, particularly when looking up and down. PSP is one of the Parkinson- plus syndromes and is not helped consistently by Levodopa.

**Proteostatis:** The concept that there are biological pathways within cells that compete for control of the creation, folding, transporting, and degradation of proteins present within and outside the cell. A combination of the words protein and homeostasis. Loss of proteostasis can lead to misfolding and degradation of proteins.

**Proteasomes:** Protein complexes which degrade unneeded or damaged proteins. Proteasome dysfunction is implicated as one of the contributing factors in the disease process of MSA.

Protein:

- A class of food necessary for the growth and repair of the body tissues—sources of proteins include fish, meat, eggs and milk.
- Large biomolecules or macromolecules consisting of long chains of amino acid residues. Within organisms, proteins catalyze metabolic reactions (enzymes), replicate DNA, and transport molecules.

**Pulmonary embolus:** A blood clot in the lungs.

## R

**Raynaud's phenomenon (or disease): Spasm of the digital arteries with blanching and numbness of the fingers.**

**Receptor:** A protein structure typically embedded in the cell membrane with which neurotransmitters and drugs interact.

**Registry: A collection of information about individuals, usually focused around a specific diagnosis or condition. The goal is to enable patient organizations to better promote and support patient- focused research.**

**REM (Rapid Eye Movement)/ REM Behavior Disorder (RBD):** A sleep disorder that involves abnormal behavior during the sleep phase characterized by rapid eye movements – the stage of sleep in which dreaming occurs. In normal sleep, muscles are paralyzed during dreaming, except for the eye movements. In RBD, muscles are not paralyzed so that the dreamer acts out his or her dreams. RBD is common in people with Parkinson's disease or Multiple System Atrophy.

**Restless Leg Syndrome (RLS):** A neurological disorder characterized by unpleasant sensations in the legs, often described as the feeling of ants crawling underneath the skin with the urge to move the legs to alleviate the sensations, hence the term "restless legs." RLS usually occurs in the late evening and during sleep. The condition interferes with sleep and is common in people with MSA and PD. Medications, such as dopamine agonists, Levodopa and opioids, can be effective treatments.

**Rigidity: Abnormal stiffness in a limb or other body part. A type of muscle stiffness in which the muscles tend to pull against each other instead of working smoothly together. It is most apparent when an examiner moves a patient's limb — as in a form known as cogwheeling. A type of rigidity in MSA patients affects the cervical spine muscles causing a forward or backward head posture known as torticollis.**

## S

**Schwab & England Activities of Daily Living (ADL) Scale:** An estimation of the abilities of a person's degree of independence. The person (or a family member) can self-assess it on a scale of 0% to 100%.

**Second opinion:** The process of consulting with a second medical specialist in order to confirm a diagnosis, receive a new or more precise diagnosis, or discuss alternative options for treating a health condition. When a potential diagnosis includes a rare condition or where symptoms overlap considerably with other conditions, for example with MSA, a second opinion is important in order to avoid a possible misdiagnosis. A second opinion is also useful if symptoms persist following a course of treatment, or when a recommended treatment is especially risky.

**Senescence:** A natural aging process in cells that stops them from dividing. Can become activated when certain types of damage occur.

**Sepsis:** A systemic inflammatory response to an infection. The presence of various pus-forming and other organisms, or their toxins, in the blood or tissues. Sepsis is life threatening and can lead to organ damage and septic shock.

**Septic shock:** A condition in which impaired blood flow due to sepsis results in low blood pressure that does not respond to fluid replacement. Occurs most often in the very young, the elderly, and in people with compromised immune systems.

**Serious adverse reaction: A**n adverse reaction which results in death, is life-threatening, requires in- patient hospitalization or prolongation of existing hospitalization, results in persistent or significant disability or incapacity, or is a congenital anomaly/birth defect.

Life-threatening in this context refers to a reaction in which the patient was at risk of death at the time of the reaction; it does not refer to a reaction that hypothetically might have caused death if more severe. Medical and scientific judgement should be exercised in deciding whether other situations should be considered serious reactions, such as important medical events that might not be immediately life threatening or result in death or hospitalization but might jeopardize the patient or might require intervention to prevent one of the other outcomes listed above. Examples of such events are intensive treatment in an emergency room or at home for allergic bronchospasm, blood dyscrasias or convulsions that do not result in hospitalization, or the development of dependency or abuse. Any suspected transmission via a medicinal product of an infectious agent is also considered a serious adverse reaction.

**Serotonin:** A neurotransmitter that regulates mood, appetite, and sleep. It also has some cognitive functions, including memory and learning. The serotonin-producing neurons are located in the brain stem. Serotonin has a relaxing effect on smooth (non-voluntary) muscles and serotonin- enhancing drugs have been used to manage cerebellar ataxia and to alleviate chronic constipation and sleep apnea in MSA patients.

**Shaking palsy:** Prior term for Parkinson's disease.

**Shuffling gait:** A degenerative condition characterized by low blood pressure when standing. It may lead to parkinsonism, rigidity, ataxia, fainting, or incontinence. and MSA-P. Refers to short, slow steps, with feet close to the ground or dragging along the ground. This gait is often seen in people with advanced Parkinson's disease.

**Shy-Drager Syndrome:** An antiquated name for multiple system atrophy.

**Side effects**: A secondary reaction to a drug, usually adverse, that is additional to the intended therapeutic actions. Side effects vary in severity from person to person and can range from mild and/or tolerable to life-threatening.

**Sinemet:** The brand name of the most commonly prescribed version of the drug Levodopa, made by DuPont Pharmaceuticals

**Single Photon Emission Computed Tomography (SPECT):** A nuclear medicine imaging technique using gamma rays and able to provide 3D information via tomography, or imaging in sections. Commonly used to detect areas of reduced blood flow in the brain.

**Sleep apnea:** A sleep disorder characterized by abnormal pauses in breathing or instances of abnormally low breathing during sleep.

**Sporadic form: Without a known family history.**

**Sodium channel:** Voltage gated channels in nerve cell membranes that allow the generation of nerve impulses via the flow of positively charged sodium ions into a cell. After sodium enters the cell, it needs to be pumped back out. This process happens through the sodium-pump mechanism, which requires the expenditure of cellular energy. Sodium channel blocking drugs are used to control pain and treat epilepsy and may be a target for new drugs in Parkinson's and MSA.

**Spontaneous report (or notification):** An unsolicited communication by a healthcare professional or consumer to a company, regulatory authority or other organzation (e.g. the World Health Organization, a regional centre, a poison control centre) that describes one or more adverse reactions in a patient who was given one or more medicinal products and that does not derive from a study or any organized data collection scheme. Stimulated reporting can occur in certain situations, such as direct healthcare professional communication (DHPC), a publication in the press or questioning of healthcare professionals by company representatives, and adverse reaction reports arising from them.

Stem cells: Biological cells found in all multicellular organisms. They can divide and differentiate into diverse specialized cell types and self-renew to produce more stem cells. Stem cells are a potential line of treatment in MSA and Parkinson's, either by directly replacing the old nigrostriatal neuronal cells or by creating growth factor releasing cells. Problems have arisen due to the inability to stop growth, which may cause tumor development.

There are four types of stem cells:

- **Embryonic –** Cells formed prior to implantation in the uterus, 4-5 days after fertilization. They are obtained from human embryos and capable of giving rise to any type of cell (pluripotent). Ethical concerns over the use of embryonic stem cells is ongoing, with laws varying from country to country and, in the U.S., from state to state.
- **Fetal:** There are two types:
  - P*roper fetal* which come from fetal tissue and are generally obtained after an abortion. o Extra-embryonic from extra-embryonic membranes.
- **Induced Pluripotent (iPSC) –** Laboratory engineered cells made by converting tissue cells into embryonic-like stem cells. Research is ongoing into the development of iPSC's that will mature into dopamine-producing neurons that can be used for treating MSA.
- **Mesenchymal (MSC) –** Relating to the mesenchyma. Also known as **stromal** stem cells. Obtained from the connective tissues that surround organs in such places as bone marrow, fat, and umbilical cord blood. There is some controversy over what types of cells MSC's can generate. Autologous MSC's (derived from the patient's own tissues) have been used with some success in MSA. **They are**

**considered an efficient source of cells for therapy, because they can be safely harvested and transplanted to donors or patients, have low immunogenicity, and have broad therapeutic potential.**

- **Tissue-specific –** Also known as **somatic** or **adult** stem cells. Found within some tissues and organs, they give rise to one specific type of tissue. For example, bone marrow stem cells can produce red and white blood cells and platelets. They maintain and repair the tissue in which they are found.

**Stem cell potency:**

Oligopotency: ***Can* differentiate only into a few cell types.**

P**luripotent:** Can develop into each of the more than 200 cell types of the adult body. Can differentiate into a number of cell types, but only those of a closely related family of cells.

**Totipotent:** Formed by the fusion of an egg and a sperm, the cells can subsequently differentiate into embryonic and extra-embryonic cell types, and can construct a complete and viable organism.

**Stereotactic:** A minimally invasive brain surgery technique, guided by images from CAT or MRI scans, usually involving a metallic frame bolted to a patient's head to prevent any movement.

**Striatonigral degeneration:** Degeneration referring to the efferent connection of the striatum with the substantia nigra.

**Striatum:** Also known as the corpus striatum, it is the largest component of the basal ganglia in the brain and controls movement, balance, and walking. Collective name for the caudate nucleus and the putamen which together with the globus pallidus or pallidum form the corpus striatum. A large cluster of nerve cells that are part of the basal ganglia. The striatum controls movement, balance, and walking. It consists of two sectors: the caudate nucleus and the putamen. The striatum receives nerve inputs from many parts of the brain including dopamine neurons from the substantia nigra and glutamate neurons from the cerebral cortex. Acetylcholine and GABA neurons are located within the striatum. The striatum contains the largest concentrations of dopamine and acetylcholine in the brain.

**Stridor: Abnormal breathing at night or harsh breathing sound. A high pitched sound resulting from turbulent air flow in the upper airway.**

**Substantia nigra:** (Latin for black substance). Literally means "black substance" from the black pigment neuromelanin (hence, its name). A part of the basal ganglia, located in the midbrain along with the striatum (caudate nucleus, putamen), globus pallidus, and subthalamic nucleus. It is rich in dopamine-producing nerve cells and plays an important role in movement. Parts of the substantia nigra appear darker than neighboring areas due to high levels of neuromelanin in dopamine-producing neurons. The substantia nigra is the site of the brain's major collection of dopamine neurons, which project their axons to the striatum, the so-called nigrostriatal pathway. In Parkinson's, the loss of nerve cells from this region leads to a dopamine deficit and subsequently to Parkinson's symptoms. These neurons slowly die in PD and MSA.

**Subthalamic Nucleus (STN):** A nerve center near the substantia nigra and part of the basal ganglia. The STN may be targeted for deep brain stimulation (DBS) to reduce Parkinson's symptoms. Is relatively unaffected in MSA. It may be targeted for deep brain stimulation to reduce Parkinson's symptoms.

**Supine hypertension:** Dangerously high blood pressure levels while lying down.

**Suprapubic catheter:** A permanent catheter inserted into the bladder above the pubic bone.

**Synapse:** The narrow space between two neurons (axon to dendrite) or between a neuron and a muscle. Axons release neurotransmitters at the nerve terminal. The neurotransmitter crosses the synapse to activate or inhibit another nerve cell by acting on a receptor on the dendrite of the receiving cell.

**Synaptic plasticity:** The ability of synaptic activity to modify and adapt to changes in activity levels. Particularly important for learning and memory.

**Syndrome:** A group of symptoms that tend to occur together and which reflect the presence of a specific disorder or disease. Parkinson's syndrome, also called parkinsonism, comprises a group of disorders with symptoms and signs in common, such as bradykinesia, rigidity, tremor, loss of postural reflexes, flexed posture, and freezing of gait. A person with parkinsonism does not need to have all of these but must have bradykinesia according to one diagnostic criterion. Disorders that fall within Parkinson's syndrome include Parkinson's disease, atypical parkinsonism, Parkinson-plus syndromes, drug-induced parkinsonism, and normal pressure hydrocephalus.

**Synuclein:** A protein in the brain that helps nerve cells communicate, but whose function is not yet fully understood.

**Synucleinopathy:** A class of neurodegenerative diseases resulting from pathological accumulation of alpha-synuclein in neurons (Parkinson's, Lewy Body Dementia) or in a kind of glial cell called oligodendrocytes (Multiple System Atrophy).

## T

**Tasmar:** The brand name of the COMT inhibitor Tolcapone, that is made by Roche Laboratories.

**Tau proteins:** Proteins that stabilize microtubules, which are structural entities in axons. They are abundant in neurons in the central nervous system and are less common elsewhere. When tau proteins are defective and no longer stabilize microtubules properly, they can result in dementia (including Alzheimer's disease).

**Tauopathies: A class of neurodegenerative diseases resulting from the pathological aggregation of tau protein in so-called neurofibrillary tangles (NFT) in the human brain. Besides Alzheimer's, this is commonly seen in Pick's disease, progressive supranuclear palsy (PSP) and corticobasal degeneration (CBD). Tau pathology is relatively rare in MSA.**

**Thalamotomy:** A surgical procedure in which cells in the thalamus are destroyed in an effort to eradicate debilitating tremors. **A now uncommon surgical procedure used to treat Parkinson's tremor in which a small portion of the brain**

**area called the thalamus is destroyed. Thalamotomy is associated with significant secondary complications. The procedure has been replaced by medical therapies, such as L-Dopa and deep brain stimulation surgery.**

**Thalamus:** A mass of gray matter (nerve cells) located deep in the brain that is responsible for motor control and serves as a relay center for sensory signals. **A midline paired symmetrical structure situated between the cerebral cortex and brain stem. The thalamus acts as a relay and processing center for sensory information to reach higher brain centers for interpretation and for coordination of regulatory commands among areas of the cerebral cortex. Its functions also include regulating sleep, wakefulness, and consciousness.**

**Tolcapone:** A drug in the COMT inhibitor class that is sometimes prescribed in tandem with Levodopa. The drug has been known to cause serious liver problems and has been withdrawn from the Canadian and European markets.

**Toxicity:** The degree to which a chemical substance or a particular mixture of substances can damage an organism.

**Transcranial Magnetic Stimulation (TMS):** A method in which a changing magnetic field is used to cause electric current to flow to a small region of the brain. Some initial clinical trials have reported improvements in motor control in MSA patients with the use of TMS.

**Transcription factors:** Proteins that regulate the transcription (i.e. the expression) of genes.

**Translation: Also known as gene expression. The process by which protein molecules are assembled in accordance with a specific, corresponding genetic code. The process is preceded by transcription of the DNA into messenger RNA (mRNA).**

**Tremor: Involuntary** rhythmic movements (may be fast or slow) that may affect the hands, head, voice or other body parts.

**Postural:** Tremor triggered by holding a limb in a fixed position.

**Resting: Occurs when muscles are at rest. Becomes less noticeable or disappears when the affected muscles are moved. Often slow and coarse.**

**Tracheotomy: A surgical operation of opening into the trachea to preserve breathing ability.**

**Trigger event:** An external or environmental factor such as head trauma, exposure to a toxin, or stress that contributes to the development of a condition or disease.

**Tyramine-induced hypertension:** High blood pressure caused by an increase in tyramine, an amine compound that promotes blood pressure elevation, which forces noradrenaline/norepinephrine into circulation. This is the so-called "cheese effect" because some fermented cheeses (and other foods) contain high concentrations of tyramine. Normally, tyramine is broken down in the gut by MAO-A. When this enzyme is inhibited, as with a category of drugs called MAO inhibitors, the tyramine in food is able to enter the blood stream, resulting in a hypertensive crisis. MAO inhibitors are used in parkinsonian conditions because, in addition to preventing the breakdown of tyramine they also prevent the breakdown of dopamine.

Tyrosine: An amino acid used by cells to synthesize proteins. It is also the precursor of dopamine.

## U

**Ubiquitin:** A small regulatory protein found ubiquitously in most tissues, hence its name. Ubiquitin is involved in the degradation of damaged proteins. Mutated forms have been found in MSA patients.

**Ultra-compassionate use:** There are cases when a patient is at the end stage of the disease, suffering, or worsening. Aware that a new product is available, he or she is willing to take the risk, even if very little is known about the product, or even if the toxicity profile is not yet determined. This type of patient may prefer to rake the risk of dying from an adverse drug reaction if the product is finally not safe, because he or she will die soon anyway. And, if there is the faintest chance that the treatment benefits him or her, at least he or she will have tried. In such dramatic situations, some regulators take the stand that it is not their role to intervene: it is up to the doctor and the patient to decide. Any regulatory intervention, even in an emergency context, would take time and from their position, regulators do not feel at ease to decide. It is a debate close to the debate on end-of-life and euthanasia: when legal, the decision belongs to the patient and his/her doctor, there is no need to ask prior authorization from any authority.

**UMSARS (Unified MSA Rating Scale)** – A four-part rating scale for MSA comprising:

- Part I: Patient's history.
- Part II: Motor examination.
- Part III: Autonomic examination.
- Part IV: Global disability scale.

**Urostomy:** The establishment of an artificial cutaneous opening into the urethra for urinary incontinence.

## V

**Ventral Tegmental Area (VTA):** A group neurons located in the midbrain next to the substantia nigra and involved in cognition and motivation, including reward and addiction. Contains the cell bodies of dopamine-producing cells and one of the major dopamine producing centers in the brain.

**Vesicle:** An organelle in a cell that separates some molecules from the rest of the cell. In nerve cells, neurotransmitters are stored in vesicles at the terminal ends of axons, called synaptic vesicles, and are released by the vesicles into the synapse when the nerve fires.

## W

**Wasting syndrome (see Cachexia).**

**Wearable devices: Devices worn on the body, incorporating computers, electronics, software and/or sensors, often used to measure some aspect of function or physical manifestation, for example: activity trackers, accelerometers, gyroscopes, etc.**

**Wearing Off:** Loss of effectiveness of Parkinson's medications between doses, resulting in the return of symptoms. If the effectiveness of a medication does not last until the next dose is due, it "wears off".

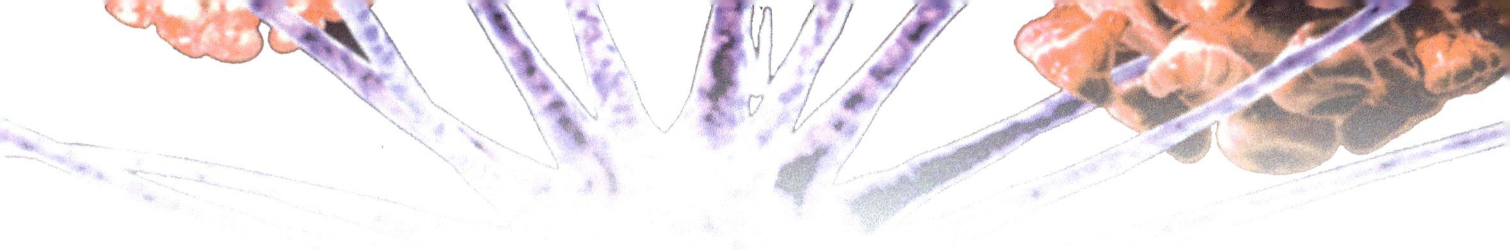

# Abbreviations, Acronyms & Mnemonics

## A

AADC: Amino Acid DeCarboxylase (a radiolabeled substrate)
AAN: American Academy of Neurology
AAV: Adeno-Associated Virus
AD: Alzheimer's Disease
ADC: Autonomic Disorders Consortium
ADL: **Activities of Daily Living**
**ADR: Adverse Drug Reaction**
**AE: Adverse Event**
ALS: Amyotrophic Lateral Sclerosis
AMP: (U.S.) Accelerating Medicines Partnership
AMS; Atrophie MultiSystématisée (in French)
ANS: Autonomic Nervous System
ASO: AntiSense Oligonucleotides
ATC: **Anatomic, Therapeutic, Chemical.**
ATMP: Advanced Therapy Medicinal Product
ATP: Adenosine TriPhosphate

## B

BBB: Blood-Brain Barrier
BG: Basal Ganglia
BGTC: (U.S.) Bespoke Gene Therapy Consortium
BN: Basal Nuclei
BP: Blood Pressure
BPAP: **Bilevel Positive Airway Pressure**
BPH: Benign Prostatic Hyperplasia
BPN: (U.S. NIH) Blueprint Neurotherapeutics Network
BRAIN: (NIH) Brain Research through Advancing Innovative Neurotechnologies®

## C

CAPS: Central – Astrocytes; Peripheral - Satellite
CAT: Computed Axial Tomography
CBD: Corticobasal degeneration
CDER: (FDA) Center for Drug Evaluation and Research
CDS: **Continuous Dopaminergic Stimulation**
CHMP: (Europe EMA) Committee for Medicinal Products for Human Use
CJD: Creutzfeldt-Jakob disease
CMSS: (Europe) Clinical Management Support System
CNS: Central Nervous System
**COMP: (Europe EMA) Committee for Orphan Medicinal Products**
**COMT: Catchol-O-MethylTransferase)**
COPS: Central - Oligodendrocytes; Peripheral – Schwann
CP: Cerebral Palsy
CPAP: Continuous Positive Airway Pressure
CRO: Contract Research Organization
CT: Clinical Trial
CT: Computed Tomography
CTP: Clinical Trial Protocol
CUP: Compassionate Use Program

## D

DBS: Deep Brain Stimulation
DHPC: Direct Healthcare Professional Communication
DMT: Disease-Modifying Therapy

## E

EC: European Commission
ED: Erectile Dysfunction
EJPRD: European Joint Program on Rare Diseases
EMA: European Medicines Agency
EMST: Expiratory Muscle Strength Training
ENS: Enteric Nervous System
ePMS: extraPMS
ERDRI: European Rare Diseases Registries Infrastructure
ERN: European Reference Networks
EU: European Union
EURORDIS: European Organization of Rare Disorders

## F

FDA: (U.S.) Food & Drug Administration
FDG: **FluoroDeoxyGlucose**
**FRS: Fellow of the Royal Society (England)**
FTLD: FrontoTemporal Lobar Degeneration

## G

GABA: Gamma-AminoButyric Acid
GARD: Genetic and Rare Diseases
GCI: Glial Cytoplasmic Inclusions
GD: Guam Disease (GD) (or LBS)
GFD: Gluten-Free Diet
GHT: Growth Hormone Therapy
GI: GastroIntestinal
GloMSAR: (U.S.) Global MSA Patient Registry
GMO: Genetically-Modified Organism
GWAS: Genome-Wide Association Studies

## H

HCP: Human Connectome Project
HD: Huntington's Disease
HMP: Human Medicinal Products
HTA: Health Technology Assessment

## I

ICD: **(WHO) International Classification of Diseases**
**IGF: Insulin Growth Factor**
**IND: Investigational New Drug**
INI: IntraNasal Insulin
INN: International Non-proprietary Name
IOC: Inferior Olivary Complex
ION: Inferior Olivary Nucleus
IP&MDS: International Parkinson & Movement Disorder Society
IRDIRC: International Rare Diseases Research Consortium
ISAN; International Society for Autonomic Neuroscience
IT: IntraThecal
IVIg: IntraVenous Immunoglobulins

## L

LBD: Lewy Bodies Dementias
LBS: Lytico-Bodig Syndrome
LCD: **Linked clinical trials**
LMN: Lower Motor Neuron

## M

MAO: **MonoAmine Oxidase**
**MCI: Mild Cognitive Impairment**
**MD: Muscular Dystrophy**
**MID: Multi-Infarct Dementia**
**MIM: Mendelian Inheritance in Man**
MOD: Multiple Organ Dysfunction
MOS: Multiple Organ System
MPLA: MonoPhosphoryl Lipid A
**MPTP (N-Methyl-4-Phenyl-1,2,3,6-TetrahydroPyridine)**

MRI: Magnetic Resonance Imaging
MS: Motor System
MSA: Multiple system atrophy
MSAC: Multiple System Atrophy Coalition
MSC: Mesenchymal Stem Cells
MSP: Multiple System Proteinopathy

## N

NA: Nucleus Accumbens
NCATS: (U.S.) National Center for Advancing Translational Sciences
NCTR: (U.S.) National Center for Translational Research
NDD: NeuroDegenerative Diseases/Disorders
NICHHD: (NIH's Eunice Kennedy-Shriver) National Institute of Child Health and Human Development
NIGMS: (U.S.) National Institute of General Medical Sciences
NIH: (U.S.) National Institutes of Health
NIMH): (U.S.) National Institute of Mental Health
NINDS: (U.S.) National Institute of Neurological Diseases and Stroke
NLM: (U.S.) National Library of Medicine
NMS: Neuroleptic Malignant Syndrome
NORD: National Organization for Rare Disorders
NS: Nervous system
NSAID: Non-Steroidal Anti-Inflammatory Drug
NYUCI: New York University Caregiver Counseling and Support Intervention

## O

OCD: Obsessive–Compulsive Disorder
OHT: Orthostatic HypoTension
ON: Olivary Nucleus
OPCA: OlivoPontoCerebellar Atrophy
OT: **Occupational Therapist**
**OTC: Over-The-Counter**

## P

PAF: Pure Autonomic Failure
PAG: Patient Advocacy Group
PD: Parkinson's Disease
PD: Peyronie's Disease
PD: PharmacoDynamic
PD: Pick's Disease
PDBP: Parkinson's Disease Biomarkers Program
PET: Positron Emission Tomography
PK: PharmacoKinetic
PKU: PhenylKetonUria
PLMS: Periodic Limb Movements in Sleep
PMS: Pyramidal Motor System
PNS: Parasympathetic Nervous System
PNS: Peripheral Nervous System
PSP: Progressive Supranuclear Palsy (or SROD)
PT: **PhysioTherapist**

## R

RaDaR: Rare Diseases Registry Program
RBD: REM sleep Behavior Disorder
RDCN: (U.S. NCATS) Rare Diseases Clinical Research Network
REM: Rapid Eye Movement
ROS: Reactive Oxygen Species
rTMS: Repetitive TMS

## S

S**AE: Srious Adverse Event**
SALT: Speech And Language Therapy
SANS: Sympathetic Nervous System
SCS: Spinal Cord Stimulation
SDS: Shy-Drager Syndrome
SND: StriatoNigral Degeneration
SNS: Somatic Nervous System
SOC: Superior Olivary Complex
SON: Superior Olivary Nucleus
sOPCA: sporadic OlivoPontoCerebellar Atrophy

SPECT: Single Photon Emission Computed Tomography
SROD: Steele-Richardson-Olszewski Disease
SSRI: Selective Serotonin Reuptake Inhibitors
STN: SubThalamic Nucelus

## T

TLR: Toll-Like Receptor
TMS: (Repetitive) Transcranial Magnetic Stimulation
TRBG: Tremor, Rigidity, Bradykinesia, Gait
TS: Tourette's Syndrome

## U

UMN: Upper Motor Neuron
UMSARS: Unified MSA Rating Scale
UTI: Urinary tract Infection

## V

VP: Ventral Pallidum
VSNS: Visceral Sensory Nervous System
VTA: Ventral Tegmental Area

## W

WD: Wilson's Disease

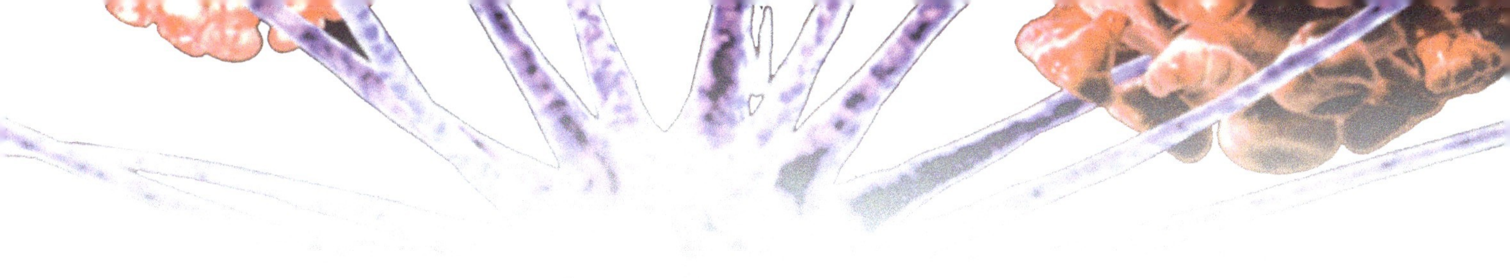

# Drugs

## A

Affitopac (R) PD01A (an alpha-synuclein therapy)
Aldesleukin
Alendronate
Amantadine
Amiodarone (a drug that affects heart rhythm QT prolongation)
Amphetamines
Ampreloxetine/TD-9855 (for symptomatic treatment)
Anticholinergic agents
Antidepressants (also for sleep problems)
Antiemetics
Antihistamines
Anti-Parkinson's drugs
Antispasmodic drugs
Antipsychotics
Apomorphine (Apokyn) (a dopamine agonist)
Artane (trihexyphenidyl HCl)
Aspirin (an NSAID)
Atomoxetine (for symptomatic treatment of orthostatic hypotension)
Atropine (an anticholinergic)
Avanafil

## B

Belladonna alkaloids
Belmacasan (VX-766) (an alpha-synuclein therapy)
Benotropine (n anti-cholinergic drug)
Beta-adrenergic blockers
BNN-20 (neuroprotective)
Boceprevir (a hepatitis C virus protease inhibitor)
Botilunum A toxin (for dystonia and for symptomatic treatment)
Bromocriptine mesylate (Parlodel) (a dopamine agonist)

## C

Cabergoline (a dopamine agonist)
Caffeine
Carbidopa
Celecoxib (an NSAID)
Chlorpromazine (a neuroleptic)
Clarithromycin (a macrolide antibiotic)
Clonazepam (for sleep problems)
Clopidogrel (an anti-platelet drug),
Cobicistat
Cyclosporine (an immunosuppressant)

## D

Dabigatran (a blood thinner)
DaTscanTM Iofluopane (12)
Dicyclomine (an antispasmodic)
Digoxin
Dihydroxyphenylserine (for orthostaict hypotension)
Dofetilide (a drug that affects heart rhythm QT

prolongation)
Dopa imaging (18-F)F
Dopamine
Dopaminergic agonists
Doxazosin (an alpha blocker)
Droxidopa (for orthostatic
hypotension)

### E

Entacapone (Comtan): a
COMT inhibitor
Erythromycin (a macrolide antibiotic)
Erythropoietin
Etidronate
Exonatide (neuroprotective)
Extendin-4 (Exenatide) (an
anti-diabetic drug)

### F

Fingolimod (FTY220) (an alpha-
synuclein therapy)
Fipamezole (JP-1730) (for
symptomatic treatment)
Flecainide
Fludrocortisone (for orthostatic
hypotension)
Fluorodopa
Fosamprenavir (an HIV-
protease inhibitor)

### G

Gene therapy (AAV 2-GDNF)
(neuroprotective)

### H

Haloperidol (a neuroleptic)
Hydrocortisone

### I

Ibuprofen
Indinavir (an HIV protease inhibitor)
Inosine 5 – Monophosphate
(neuroprotective)
Insulin (intranasal) (neuroprotective)
Isocarboxazid (an MAO inhibitor)
Isosorbide (a nitrate; an anti
chest pain/angina)
Itraconazole (an azole antifungal)

### K

Kalliterein-6 (an alpha-
synuclein therapy)
Ketoconazole (an azole antifungal)

### L

Larithromycin (a macrolide antibiotic)
Lenalidomide (an anti-inflammatory)
Levodopa or L-dopa (Sinemt)
(for motor issues and
Parkinson's disease)
Linezolid (an MAO inhibitor)
Lisuride ((a dopamine agonist)
Lithium (an anti-aggregate
of alpha-synuclein)
Lopinavir (an HIV protease inhibitor)
Lu AF82422 (an alpha-
synuclein therapy)

### M

Macrolide antibiotics
Melatonin (for sleep problems)
Metaxalone (an MAO inhibitor)
Methyldopa (an anti-high-
blood pressure drug)
Methylene blue (an MAO inhibitor)
Metoclopramide (an anti-
nausea drug)
Midodrine (for orthostatic
hypotension)
Mifepristone

Minocycline (a neuroprotective tetracycline)
Mirabegron
Mirapex (Pramipexole), a dopamine agonist
Moclobemide (an MAO inhibitor)
Monoamine oxidase inhibitors
Morphomer TM (a PET tracer specific for alpha- synuclein)
MPLA (an alpha-synuclein therapy)

## N

NBMI (an alpha-synuclein therapy)
NDMA modulator (for symptomatic treatment)
Nebivolol (for symptomatic treatment)
Nefazodone (a hepatitis C virus protease inhibitor)
Neuroleptics
Nilotinib (an anti-aggregate of alpha-synuclein)
Nitroglycerin (a nitrate; an anti chest pain/angina)
Non-steroidal anti-inflammatory drugs

## O

Oxybutynin (for bladder control)

## P

Parlodel (a dopamine agonist)
Pergolide (Permax) (a dopamine agonist)
Phenelzine (an MAO inhibitor)
Phenytoin (a barbiturate)
Pimozide (a drug that affects hearrtrhythm QT prolongation)
Piribedil (a dopamine agonist)
Potassium
Pramipexole (Mirapex) (a dopamine agonist)
Pramlintide
Prazosin (an alpha blocker)
Procainamide (a drug that affects heart rhythm QT prolongation)
Procarbazine (an MAO inhibitor)
Prochlorperazine (an anti-emetic)
Propafenone
Propantheline (an antispasmodic)

## Q

Quetiapine (an anti-psychotic)
Quinidine (a drug that affects heart rhythm QT prolongation)

## R

Ramsulosin (an alpha blocker)
Rapamycin (an anti-aggregate of alpha-synuclein)
Rasagiline (an MAO inhibitor)
Relaprevir (a hepatitis C virus protease inhibitor)
Ribociclib (a hepatitis C virus protease inhibitor)
Rifabutin (removes Fludorcortisone from the body)
Rifampicin (an anti- α-synuclein aggregation)
Rifampin (a hepatitis C virus protease inhibitor)
Rifamycin (removes Fludorcotisone from the body)
Riluzole (for symptomatic treatment)
Riociguat
Ritonavir (an HIV protease inhibitor)
Rituximab (an anti-inflammatory)
Ropinirole hydrochloride (Requip) (a dopamine agonist)
Rotigotine (Neupro patch) (a dopamine agonist)

## S

**Safinamide (an MAO inhibitor) (for symptomatic treatment)**
**Saquinavir (an HIV protease inhibitor)**
**Scopolamine (an anticholinergic)**
**Selective Serotonin Reuptake Inhibitors**
**Selegiline (an MAO inhibitor)**
**Sildenafil**
**Sirolinus (Rapamycin) (an alpha-synuclein therapy)**
**Sodium phenylbutyrate (an unspecific histone deacetylase inhibitor)**
**Somatostatin analogues**
**Sotalol (a drug that affects heart rhythm QT prolongation)**
**Stearoyl-coA (a desaterase inhibitor) (neuroprotective)**
Syncle**a**n-D

## T

**Tadalafil**
**TAK-34 (an alpha-synuclein therapy)**
**Tamsulosin (an alpha blocker)**
**Telaprevir (hepatitis C virus protease inhibitor)**
**Terazosin (an alpha blocker)**
**Tetrabenazine (an anti-high-blood pressure drug)**
**Thioridazine (a neuroleptic)**
**Tibociclib**
**Tiluzole**
**Titonavir (an HIV protease inhibitor)**
**Tolcapone (Tasmar) (COMT inhibitor)**
**Tolterodine (for bladder control)**
**Tranylcypromine (an MAO inhibitor)**
**Tricyclics**
**Trihexyphenidyl (an anti-Parlkinson's drug)**

## U

Ubiquinol (neuroprotective)

## V

V**ardenafil**
**Verdiperstat (BHV-3241) (neuroprotective)**
**Vericiguat**

## W

Warfarin (a blood thinner)

## Y

Yohimbine

## Z

Zoledronic acid (for symptomatic treatment)

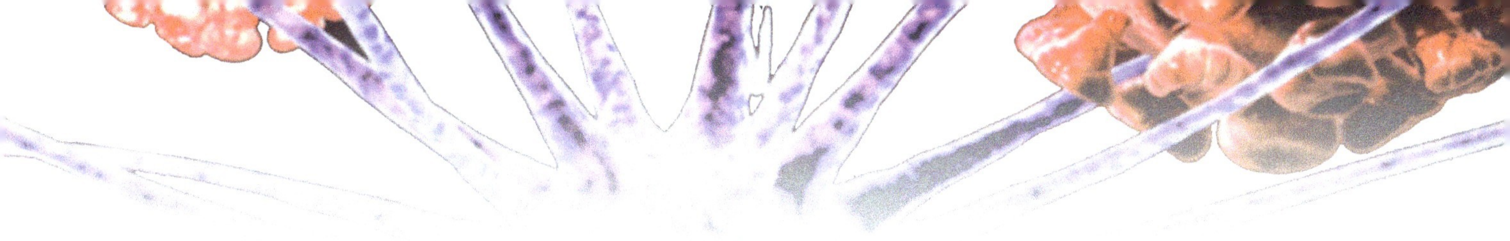

# Diseases & Disorders

**A**

Addiction
Addison's disease
Adrenocortical insufficiency
Adrenogenital syndrome
Alzheimer's disease
Amyotrophic lateral sclerosis (aka
    Lou Gehring's disease)
Anhydrosis
Antecollis
Anxiety
Ataxia
  Acute
  Cerebellar
  Gait
  Hereditary
  Limb
  Ocular
  Nystagmus
  Static

**B**

Bradykinesia

**C**

Camptocormia
Candidiasis
Cerebral palsy
Chorea
Cirrhosis
Congestive obstructive pulmonary disease
Corticobasal degeneration
Creutzfeldt-Jakob disease

**D**

Dementias
  Lewy bodies
  Multi-infarct
Depression
Devic's disease (or Neuromyelitis optica)
Diabetes mellitus (anciently
    known as Willis' disease)
Dysautonomia
Dyschezia
Dyskinesia
Dysphagia
Dysphonia
Dystonia

**E**

Encephalitis

**F**

Frontotemporal lobar degeneration

**G**

Gonorrhea
Guam disease (see Lytico-
    Bodig syndrome)

**H**

Hemiballismus
Hepatitis

Herpes
HIV
Huntington's disease
Hypokinsia

**K**

Kayser-Fleischer rings

**L**

Lytico-Bodig syndrome (see
  Guam disease)

**M**

Meningitis
Multiple sclerosis
Multiple System Atrophy (formerly
  known as Shy- Drager syndrome,
  Olivopontocerebellar atrophy)
Muscle contracture
Myeloneuritis

**N**

Neuritis
Neuroacanthocytosis
Neurodegenerative diseases/disorders
Neuroleptic Malignant Syndrome
Neuromyelitis optica (or Devic's disease)
Neurosarcoidosis
Neurosyphilis.
Nystagmus

**O**

Obsessive–compulsive disorder
Occulomotor dysfunction
Olivopontocerebellar atrophy (other
  name for multiple system atrophy)
Osteoporosis

**P**

Palsy
  Progressive supranuclear
  Pseudobulbar
Parkinson's disease
Parkinsonism
Periodic limb movements in sleep
Peyronie's disease
Phenylketonuria
Pick's disease
Pisa syndrome
Pneumonia
Progressive supranucleear palsy
  (see Steele- Richardson-
  Olszewski disease)
Psychosis

**R**

Rapid eye movement
Raynaud's syndrome

**S**

Schizophrenia
Septic shock
Shy-Drager syndrome (no longer used
  for multiple system atrophy)
Sleep apnea
Sleep behavior disorder
Steele- Richardson-Olszewski disease
  (see progressive supranuclear palsy)
Striatonigral degeneration
Stridor
Syphilis

**T**

Tourette's syndrome
Tremors
  Benign essential

Cerebellar
Drug- or toxin-induced
Psychogenic
Tuberculosis
Tumor

## V

Valley fever

## W

Willis' disease (or diabetes mellitus)
Wilson's disease

# Subject Index

## O



## N

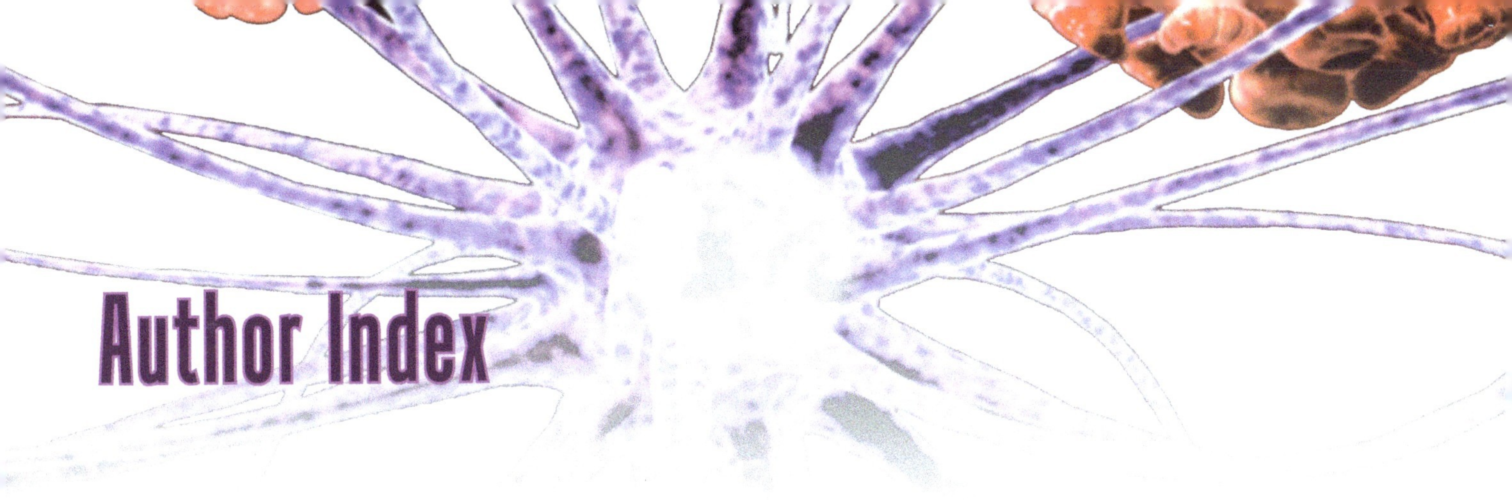

# Author Index

(**X.**y: **C**hapter or **R**eference number. **P**age number)

## C



## D

## E



## F



## G

## H



## I



## J

## K



## L

## M



## N

## O



## P



## Q



## R

## S

## W



## X



## Y



## Z

# About the Author

DR. ALAIN L. FYMAT is a medical-physical scientist and an educator. He is the current President/ CEO and Institute Professor at the International Institute of Medicine & Science with a previous appointment as Executive Vice President/Chief Operating Officer and Professor at the Weil Institute of Critical Care Medicine, California, U.S.A. He was formerly Professor of Radiology, Radiological Sciences, Radiation Oncology, Critical Care Medicine, and Physics at several U.S. and European Universities. Earlier, he was Deputy Director (Western Region) of the U.S. Department of Veterans Affairs (Office of Research Oversight). At the Loma Linda Veterans Affairs Medical Center, he was Scientific Director of Radiology, Director of the Magnetic Resonance Imaging Center and, for a time, Acting Chair of Radiology. Previously, he was Director of the Division of Biomedical and Biobehavioral Research at the University of California at Los Angeles/Drew University of Medicine and Science. He was also Scientific Advisor to the U.S. National Academy of Sciences, National Research Council, for its postdoctoral programs tenable at the California Institute of Technology and Member of the Advisory Group for Research & Development, North Atlantic Treaty Organization (NATO). He is Health Advisor to the American Heart & Stroke Association, Coachella Valley Division, California. He is a frequent Keynote Speaker and Organizing Committee member at several international scientific/medical conferences. He has lectured extensively in the U.S.A, Canada, Europe, Asia, and Africa. He has published in excess of 545 scholarly scientific publications and books. He is also Editor-in-Chief, Honorable Editor or Editor of numerous medical/scientific Journals to which he regularly contributes. He is a member of the New York Academy of Sciences and the European Union Academy of Sciences, a Board member of several institutions, and a reviewer for the prestigious UNESCO Newton Prize, United Kingdom National Commission for UNESCO.

Dr. Fymat's current research interests are focused on infectious and neurodegenerative diseases, cancer & glioblastoma, epigenetics & ecogenetics, neuroscience, and nanomedicine & nanobiotechnology. These are represented in part in his latest books: "**The Odyssey of Humanity's Diseases:** Epigenetic and ecogenetic modulations from ancestry through inheritance, environment, culture, and behavior" Volumes 1, 2, and 3; "**From the Heart to the Brain**: My collected works in medical science research (2016-2018)"; "**The Human Brain:** Wonders and Disorders"; **Cancer:** The pernicious, clonally-evolving disease braided in our genome"; "**Glioblastoma:** Management and treatment"; "**Nanomedicine:** My collected works in nanomedicine research"; "**Lyme disease:** The great invader, evader, and imitator"; "**Pandemics:** Prescription for prediction and prevention"; "**COVID-19:** Perspectives across Africa"; "**Alzhei... Who?** Demystifying the disease and what you can do about it"; "**Parkin..ss..oo..nn**: Elucidating the disease and what you can do about it"; "**Dementia:** Fending-off the menacing disease... and what you can do about it"; "**Epilepsy:** The electrical storm in the brain"; and "**Multiple sclerosis**: The progressive demyelinating autoimmune disease".